Pharmacology

D1147869

First and second edition authors:

Magali N F Taylor
Peter J W Reide
James S Dawson

CRASH COURSE

Third Edition

Pharmacology

Series editor
**Daniel
Horton-Szar**
BSc (Hons), MBBS
(Hons), MRCGP

Northgate Medical
Practice
Canterbury

Faculty advisor
Clive Page
BSc, PhD

Sackler Institute of
Pulmonary
Pharmacology
King's College
London, UK

Gada Yassin

BSc (Hons)
Fourth Year Medical Student,
Guy's, King's and St Thomas',
King's College London,
London, UK

MOSBY

ELSEVIER

Edinburgh • London • New York • Oxford • Philadelphia • St Louis • Sydney • Toronto 2007

MOSBY
ELSEVIER

An imprint of Elsevier Limited

Commissioning Editor	**Alison Taylor**
Development Editor	**Lulu Stader**
Project Manager	**Emma Riley**
Text Design	**Sarah Russell**
Cover Design	**Stewart Larking**
Icon Illustrations	**Geo Parkin**
Illustrations	**Marion Tasker**
Illustration Manager	**Merlyn Harvey**

First edition 2002
Second edition 2004
Third edition 2007

ISBN: 978 0 7234 3416 0

British Library Cataloguing in Publication Data
A catalogue record for this book is available from the British Library

Library of Congress Cataloging in Publication Data
A catalog record for this book is available from the Library of Congress

Note
Knowledge and best practice in this field are constantly changing. As new research and experience broaden our knowledge, changes in practice, treatment and drug therapy may become necessary or appropriate. Readers are advised to check the most current information provided (i) on procedures featured or (ii) by the manufacturer of each product to be administered, to verify the recommended dose or formula, the method and duration of administration, and contraindications. It is the responsibility of the practitioner, relying on their own experience and knowledge of the patient, to make diagnoses, to determine dosages and the best treatment for each individual patient, and to take all appropriate safety precautions. To the fullest extent of the law, neither the Publisher nor the Editors and Authors assumes any liability for any injury and/or damage to persons or property arising out or related to any use of the material contained in this book.

ELSEVIER your source for books,
journals and multimedia
in the health sciences

www.elsevierhealth.com

Working together to grow
libraries in developing countries

www.elsevier.com | www.bookaid.org | www.sabre.org

ELSEVIER BOOK AID International Sabre Foundation

The publisher's policy is to use **paper manufactured from sustainable forests**

Printed in China

Preface

The aim of this book is to explain pharmacology to medical students in a way that integrates the theory with practical clinical application. However, it will also be beneficial to other healthcare professionals, biomedical scientists and students interested in pharmacology.

A comprehensive, easy-to-understand introductory chapter explains the basic concepts of pharmacology, which are then drawn on and further elaborated in the following chapters. This new edition boasts clinical vignettes, designed to supplement the text and illustrations with modern teaching methods. New material has been added to include recent pharmacological advances. Information has been reorganized to make it even clearer than before and a new chapter on 'Pain and Anaesthesia' has been added. Updated multiple-choice questions and the new extended-matching questions can be used to test knowledge, as a learning tool or just for pre-exam practice! This book is very versatile and can be used alone or in conjunction with lecture notes.

Finally, I would like to wish you all the best in learning pharmacology and into what should prove an enlightening journey to understanding the body and drugs which act on it.

Gada Yassin

This volume of *Crash Course: Pharmacology* has been thoroughly revised from the previous two editions. Even more than ever it provides a comprehensive and approachable text on pharmacology for medical students and others interested in the study of pharmacology. As part of the *Crash Course* series, the overall style is user friendly, consisting of concise bulleted text with informative illustrations, many of which are new, along with a useful glossary of commonly used terms. The content provides a comprehensive overview of the core material needed to pass the pharmacology component of the undergraduate medical curriculum. At the end of the book, there is a self-assessment section consisting of multiple-choice questions, short-answer questions and extended-matching questions which test the reader's understanding of the topic.

In line with the new style of curriculum recommended by the General Medical Council, the pharmacology is organized logically into body systems and the clinical relevance of the pharmacology is stressed throughout.

I have no doubt that this volume will be a useful study and revision aid for students. It provides a refreshing means of bringing the medical student up to speed in pharmacology and many congratulations go to Gada Yassin for the professional way she has updated this volume, significantly increasing its usefulness as a revision aid for students.

Clive Page
Faculty Advisor

More than a decade has now passed since work began on the first editions of the *Crash Course* series, and over four years since the publication of the second editions. Medicine never stands still, and the work of keeping this series relevant for today's students is an ongoing process. These third editions build upon the success of the preceding books and incorporate a great deal of new and revised material, keeping the series up to date with the latest medical research and developments in pharmacology and current best practice.

As always, we listen to feedback from the thousands of students who use *Crash Course* and have made further improvements to the layout and structure of the books. Each chapter now starts with a set of learning objectives, and the self-assessment sections have been enhanced and brought up to date with modern exam formats. We have also worked to integrate points of clinical relevance into the basic medical science material, which will not only add to the interest of the text but will reinforce the principles being described.

Despite fully revising the books, we hold fast to the principles on which we first developed the series: *Crash Course* will always bring you all the information you need to revise in compact, manageable volumes that integrate basic medical science and clinical practice. The books still maintain the balance between clarity and conciseness, and providing sufficient depth for those aiming at distinction. The authors are medical students and junior doctors who have recent experience of the exams you are now facing, and the accuracy of the material is checked by senior faculty members from across the UK.

I wish you all the best for your future careers!

Dr Dan Horton-Szar
Series Editor

Acknowledgements

Firstly, I would like to thank Professor Clive Page for his invaluable suggestions and encouragement throughout. Secondly, I would like to thank everybody at Elsevier involved in bringing this book to print, in particular Lulu Stader, for her patience and understanding. A depth of gratitude to all my friends and family, who showed me great support during this time. In particular, thanks to my friends Asma Abdul Sattar, Tayyaba Akhtar, Karen Cheung-Hing, Kerwant Gill, Jaysal Patel and Zaid Shalchi, who took time to read through a few clinical scenarios each and discuss them with me. I would also like to thank everybody at Guy's, King's and St. Thomas' Medical School for helping to shape my learning of medicine and pharmacology. Finally, a very special thanks to my mother, father and brother ... for everything.

Figure credits

Figures 1.3–1.5, 1.15, 2.1–2.4, 5.3, 5.5, 5.12, 5.21–5.23, 6.1–6.5, 6.7, 6.11, 6.18, 7.2, 7.4–7.6, 8.2, 10.8–10.10 and 10.13 redrawn with kind permission from *Integrated Pharmacology*, 2nd edn, edited by Professor C Page, Dr M Curtis, Professor M Sutter, Professor M Walker and Professor B Hoffman, Mosby, 2002

Key to Icons

Dedication

I would like to dedicate this book to my beloved brother, Ali Yassin (may he rest in peace), who tragically died prematurely, aged 20, during the course of preparing this book. He was the inspiration, light and hero for me and many people who were fortunate enough to have him touch their lives. It is because of his encouragement and support that I have been able to complete my most noteworthy achievements, which includes the making of this book. I am sure he would have been proud to see this book published and benefiting students around the world.

Contents

Preface   v
Acknowledgements   vii
Glossary   xi

Part I: Principles of Pharmacology 1

1. **Introduction to pharmacology** 3
   Molecular basis of pharmacology 3
   Drug–receptor interactions 8
   Pharmacokinetics 11
   Drug interactions and adverse effects 18
   Drug history and drug development 20

Part II: Clinical Pharmacology . . 23

2. **Cardiovascular system** 25
   The heart 25
   The circulation 37
   Haemostasis and thrombosis 47
   The blood and fluid replacement 53

3. **Respiratory system** 55
   Basic concepts 55
   Obstructive airways diseases 56
   Respiratory stimulants and pulmonary
   surfactants 62
   Antitussives and mucolytics 62

4. **Peripheral nervous system** 65
   Nerve conduction 65
   Somatic nervous system 67
   Autonomic nervous system 71
   Nitrergic nervous system 80

5. **Central nervous system** 81
   Basic concepts 81
   Parkinson's disease and parkinsonism 82
   Dementia 86
   Anxiety and sleep disorders 86
   Affective disorders 90
   Psychotic disorders 95
   Nausea and vertigo 100
   Epilepsy 100
   Drug misuse 105
   The eye 113

6. **Endocrine and reproductive systems** 119
   The thyroid gland 119
   The endocrine pancreas and diabetes
   mellitus 123
   Adrenal corticosteroids 128
   The reproductive system 134
   Bone and calcium 140

7. **Kidney and urinary system** 143
   Basic concepts 143
   The kidney 143
   Diuretics 146
   The urinary system 149

8. **Gastrointestinal system** 153
   The stomach 153
   Nausea and vomiting 157
   The intestines 159
   The pancreas and gall bladder 164

9. **Pain and anaesthesia** 167
   Basic concepts 167
   Opioid analgesic drugs 170
   Headache and neuralgic pain 172
   Local anaesthesia 173
   General anaesthesia 176

10. **Inflammation, allergic diseases and
    immunosuppression** 183
    Inflammation 183
    Allergic disorders and drug therapy 194
    Immunosuppressants 196

11. **Infectious diseases** 201
    Antibacterial drugs 201
    Antiviral drugs 211
    Antifungal drugs 217
    Antiprotozoal drugs 219
    Anthelmintic drugs 224

12. **Cancer** 227
    Concepts of cancer chemotherapy 227
    Cytotoxic chemotherapy 228
    Endocrine therapy 233
    Immunotherapy 234
    The future 234

ix

Contents

Part III: Self-assessment 237

Multiple-choice questions (MCQs) 239
Short-answer questions (SAQs) 249
Extended-matching questions (EMQs) 251
MCQ answers 255

SAQ answers 267
EMQ answers 273

Index 277

Glossary

Aetiology The science of causation or origin of disease.

ACh (Acetylcholine) A neurotransmitter mainly used in parasympathetic neurotransmission.

Agonist A ligand that binds to receptors, thus activating the receptor and causing a response.

Agranulocytosis A serious condition in which white blood cells decrease to dangerously low numbers. Drugs which can cause this include antiepileptics, antithyroid drugs and some antipsychotics (such as clozapine).

Anaphylaxis An immediate and severe allergic reaction to a substance (e.g. certain foods or drugs). Symptoms of anaphylaxis include breathing difficulty, loss of consciousness and a drop in blood pressure, or it could even be fatal.

Antagonist A ligand that binds to receptors and reduces the chance of an agonist binding, but which itself is unable to activate the receptor.

Ascites An abnormal collection of fluid in the abdominal cavity.

β-Blockers Drugs which antagonize β-adrenergic receptors.

BMI (Body mass index) is the weight (kg) of a person divided by the square of the height (m). Generally, normal is 20–25; below this is underweight and above is overweight.

cAMP (Cyclic adenosine monophosphate) A second messenger produced by conversion of adenosine triphosphate (ATP) by the enzyme adenyl cyclase.

Central nervous system Comprises the brain and the spinal cord

Congestive cardiac failure (CCF) Impaired ability of the heart to fill with or pump sufficient blood around the body, affecting both left and right sides of the heart.

CT (Computerized tomography) is a form of X-ray examination in which the X-ray source and detector rotate around the object to be scanned, to produce cross-sectional images.

Dementia A neurological condition characterized by a gradual, progressive decline in intellectual functioning as a result of damage or disease of the brain.

Dyskinesia Impaired ability to control movement with involuntary muscular activity.

Dyspnoea Shortness of breath.

ECG (Electrocardiogram) Record of the electric current produced by the contraction of the heart muscle.

Endogenous Produced within the body.

Exogenous Produced outside the body.

First-pass metabolism The phenomenon of a drug which taken orally is absorbed through the intestinal wall, goes directly to the liver through the portal vein system and gets metabolized there before reaching the target organ. This is avoided by giving the drugs by other routes (e.g. intramuscular, intravenous).

Fundoscopy Examining the back of the eye using an ophthalmoscope.

Half-life The time taken for the plasma concentration of a drug to fall by half after the administration of the drug is stopped.

Hepatomegaly An abnormally enlarged liver.

Hypersensitivity An exaggerated response by the immune system to a foreign substance.

Isoenzymes Enzymes that perform the same function but have different sets of amino acids. These enzymes may have different physical properties.

Jugular venous pressure The indirect, observed pressure measurement of the venous system. It helps by giving useful clues that may aid diagnosis of heart and lung diseases.

Ligand A small molecule that binds to a specific site on a protein.

Lipolysis The breakdown of fats.

M$_{1/2/3/4}$ Muscarinic receptor subtypes; they mediate parasympathetic neurotransmission.

MAO (Monoamine oxidase) is a neuronal enzyme that metabolizes monoamines (noradrenaline, serotonin and dopamine). It has two main isoforms: MAO_A and MAO_B. Drugs may selectively target one isoenzyme or be non-selective.

Monoclonal antibodies Highly specific, purified antibodies that are derived from only one clone of cells and recognize only one antigen. They can be created to target a specific compound of interest and thus serve to detect specific characteristics of certain cells.

MRSA (Multiple drug resistant *Staphylococcus aureus*) is an increasingly dangerous bacterium that is resistant to many antibiotics.

Noradrenaline A neurotransmitter mediating sympathetic neurotransmission.

Na+/K+ATPase An energy dependent ion transporter.

Non-steroidal anti-inflammatory drug (NSAID) A drug used in the treatment of inflammation and mild pain.

Orthopnoea Breathlessness on lying flat.

Partial agonist A ligand that can activate a receptor, but cannot bring about a maximum response despite occupying all receptors.

Pathogenesis The cellular events, reactions and mechanisms resulting in the development of disease.

Peripheral nervous system (PNS) Comprises all nerves, with the exception of those in the brain and the spinal cord.

Pharmacodynamics The effects a drug will have on the body's organs and the relation between drug concentration and effect.

Pharmacokinetics The study of how compounds are absorbed, distributed, metabolized and eliminated by the body. In other words, the study of how the body acts on the drug.

Phosphorylation The addition of a phosphate group to a molecule, often causing activation, or sometimes deactivation, of proteins.

Receptor A molecule on the surface of a cell that serves as a recognition or binding site for antigens, antibodies, or other cellular or immunological components, resulting in a change in the activity of the cell.

Smoking pack years A measurement of a person's total cigarette smoking over a lifetime. It is calculated as the average number of packs smoked per day (where a pack is 20 cigarettes) multiplied by number of years. For example, somebody who smoked 10 cigarettes (half a pack) every day for 30 years would have a 15 pack year history: $0.5 \times 30 = 15$.

Systemic lupus erythematosus A chronic inflammatory connective tissue disease with features including skin rashes, joint pain and swelling, and inflammation of the kidneys and the fibrous tissue surrounding the heart (i.e. the pericardium).

Thrombocytopenia Reduced platelet numbers in the blood.

Torsades de pointes arrhythmia A potentially fatal form of ventricular tachycardia. On the electrocardiogram (ECG), it will present like ventricular tachycardia, but the QRS complexes will swing up and down around the baseline in a chaotic fashion.

PRINCIPLES OF PHARMACOLOGY

Introduction to pharmacology

Objectives

After reading this chapter, you will:

- Understand the principles by which drugs act in the body
- Know the main mechanisms by which drugs act and the features of different receptor systems
- Understand that the pharmacodynamics and pharmacokinetics of a drug determine the drug's effect on the body and the body's response to the drug
- Know the importance of drug interactions, adverse drug effects and their monitoring
- Have a basic knowledge of the drug development process.

MOLECULAR BASIS OF PHARMACOLOGY

What is pharmacology?

The word 'pharmacology' derives from the Greek word for drug, *pharmakon*. Pharmacology is the study of the actions, mechanisms, uses and adverse effects of drugs.

A drug is any natural or synthetic substance that alters the physiological state of a living organism. Drugs can be divided into two groups:

- Medicinal drugs: substances used for the prevention, treatment and diagnosis of disease.
- Non-medicinal drugs or social drugs: substances used for recreational purposes. Non-medicinal drugs include illegal mood-altering substances such as cannabis, heroin and cocaine as well as everyday substances such as caffeine, nicotine and alcohol.

Although drugs are intended to have a selective action, this is rarely achieved.

There is always a risk of adverse effects associated with the use of any drug, and each time a drug is used the prescriber should be happy that the benefits of giving the drug outweigh potential drawbacks, or adverse effects.

Drug names and classification

A single drug can have a variety of names (Fig. 1.1) and belong to many classes. Factors used for classifying drugs include their:

- Pharmacotherapeutic actions
- Pharmacological actions
- Molecular actions
- Chemical nature.

The generic name of a drug is that which appears in official national pharmacopoeias. When a drug company's patent expires, the marketing of the drug is open to any number of manufacturers. Although the generic name is retained, the variety of brand names inevitably increases.

How do drugs work?

Most drugs produce their effects by targeting specific cellular macromolecules. This may involve inhibition of transport systems or enzymes or, more commonly, action on receptors. Some drugs target non-mammalian tissue. For example, β-lactam antibiotics

Name	Description
Chemical	Describes the atomic/molecular structure of the drug. Usually long and complex, e.g. *N*-acetyl-*p*-aminophenol.
Generic	Name given to government-approved drugs sold on prescription or over the counter, e.g. paracetamol.
Proprietary	The brand name a particular company assigns to the drug product, indicated by ®, e.g. Calpol®.

Fig. 1.1 The main methods of naming drugs

are bactericidal and act by interfering with bacterial cell wall synthesis.

Certain drugs do not have conventional targets. For example, succimer is a chelating drug that is used to treat heavy metal poisoning. It binds to metals, rendering them inactive and more readily excretable. Such drugs work by means of their physicochemical properties and are said to have a non-specific mechanism of action. For this reason these drugs must be given in much higher doses (mg–g) than the more specific drugs.

Transport systems

Ion channels

Ion channels are pores located in the cell membrane that allow selective transfer of ions (charged species) in and out of the cell. Opening or closing of these channels, known as 'gating', occurs as a result of the channel proteins undergoing a change in shape. Gating is controlled either by transmitter substances or by the membrane potential (voltage-operated channels).

Some drugs modulate ion channel function directly by binding to a part of the channel protein itself, e.g. the blocking action of local anaesthetics on sodium channels. Other drugs interact with ion channels indirectly via a G-protein and other intermediates.

Carrier molecules

Transfer of ions and molecules against their concentration gradients is facilitated by carrier molecules located in the cell membrane. There are two types of carrier molecule:

- Energy-independent carriers are transporters (move one type of ion/molecule in one direction), symporters (move two or more ions/molecules) or antiporters (exchange one or more ions/molecules for one or more other ions/molecules).
- Energy-dependent carriers are termed pumps (e.g. the Na^+/K^+ ATPase pump).

Enzymes

Enzymes are protein catalysts that increase the rate of specific chemical reactions without undergoing any net change themselves during the reaction. All enzymes are potential targets for drugs. Drugs either act as a false substrate for the enzyme or inhibit the enzyme's activity directly by binding to other sites on the enzyme protein.

Certain drugs may require enzymatic modification. This degradation converts a drug from its inactive form (prodrug) to its active form.

Receptors

Receptors are the means through which most drugs produce their effects. A receptor is a specific protein molecule that is usually located in the cell membrane, although intracellular receptors and intranuclear receptors also exist, on which drugs and endogenous mediators act.

Agonist drugs mimic endogenous mediators and activate the receptor, whereas **antagonist** drugs bind to the receptor preventing receptor activation by endogenous mediators.

Synaptic transmitter substances and hormones, the body's chemical messengers, are natural ligands (i.e. molecules that bind with a molecular target) for receptors and have the following modes of action:

- Neurotransmitters are chemicals that are released from nerve terminals, diffuse across the synaptic cleft, and bind to pre- or postsynaptic receptors.
- Hormones are chemicals that, after being released into the bloodstream from specialized cells, can act at neighbouring or distant cells.

Each cell expresses only certain receptors, depending on the function of the cell. Receptor number and responsiveness to messengers can be modulated.

In many cases there is more than one receptor for each messenger, so that the messenger often has different pharmacological specificity and different functions according to where it binds (e.g. adrenaline is able to produce different effects in different tissues).

Using conventional molecular biology techniques it is now possible to clone receptors and express them in cultured cells, so allowing their properties to be studied. In particular, amino acid mutations can be reproduced so that the relation between protein structure and function can be evaluated.

There are four main types of receptor (Fig. 1.2). For changes that require an immediate response, such as removing a hand from boiling water, fast-acting mechanisms must be used, such as via ion channel linked receptors found in neurons.

Fig. 1.2 The four main types of receptor and their uses

Receptor type	Time for effect	Receptor example	Function example
Ion channel linked	Milliseconds	Nicotinic acetylcholine receptor	Removing hand from hot water
G-protein linked	Seconds	β-adrenergic receptor	Airway smooth muscle relaxation
Tyrosine kinase linked	Minutes	Insulin receptor	Glucose uptake into cells
DNA linked	Hours to days	Steroid receptor	Cellular proliferation

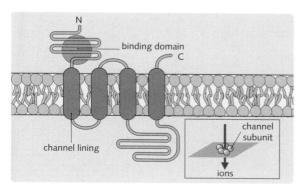

Fig. 1.3 General structure of the subunits of receptors directly linked to ion channels. (N, N-terminal; C, C-terminal.) (Redrawn from Page et al. 2002.)

Fig. 1.4 General structure of the subunits of receptors linked to G-proteins. (N, N-terminal; C, C-terminal.) (Redrawn from Page et al. 2002.)

Receptors directly linked to ion channels

Receptors that are directly linked to ion channels (Fig. 1.3) are mainly involved in fast synaptic neurotransmission. A classic example of a receptor linked directly to an ion channel is the nicotinic acetylcholine receptor (nicAChR). The nicAChR consists of five subunits – two α, one β, one γ and one δ – each of molecular weight 40–58 kDa and of great sequence homology.

The nicAChRs possess several characteristics:

- Acetylcholine (ACh) must bind to the N-terminal of both α subunits in order to activate the receptor.
- The whole receptor oligomer incorporates 20 transmembrane segments arranged around a central aqueous channel. One of the transmembrane helices (M_2) from each of the subunits is believed to form the lining of the channel.
- The receptor shows marked similarities with the two other receptors for fast transmission, namely the γ-aminobutyric acid (GABA)$_A$ and glycine receptors.

G-protein linked receptors

G-protein linked receptors (Fig. 1.4) are involved in relatively fast transduction. Muscarinic ACh, adrenergic, dopamine, serotonin and opiate receptors are all examples of G-protein linked receptors.

Molecular structure of the receptor

Most of the G-protein linked receptors consist of a single polypeptide chain of 400–500 residues and have seven transmembrane-spanning α helices. The third intracellular loop of the receptor is larger than the other loops and interacts with the G-protein.

The ligand-binding domain is buried within the membrane on one or more of the α helical segments. This is unlike ion channel coupled receptors, where the ligand binds to the extracellular N-terminal region – an area easily accessible to small hydrophobic molecules.

G-proteins

Figure 1.5 illustrated the mechanism of G-protein linked receptors:

Fig. 1.5 Mechanism of action: G-protein linked receptors. (α, β, γ, subunits of G-protein; cAMP, cyclic adenosine monophosphate; ATP, adenosine triphosphate; G, guanosine; GDP, GTP, guanosine di- and triphosphate; p, phosphate.) (Redrawn from Page et al. 2002.)

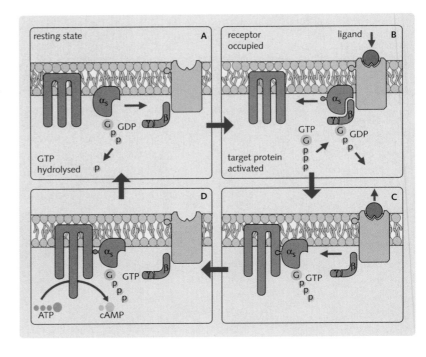

- In the resting state the G-protein is unattached to the receptor and is a trimer consisting of α, β, and γ subunits (Fig. 1.5A).
- The occupation of the receptor by an agonist produces a conformational change, causing its affinity for the trimer to increase. Subsequent association of the trimer with the receptor results in the dissociation of bound guanosine diphosphate (GDP) from the α subunit. Guanosine triphosphate (GTP) replaces GDP in the cleft thus activating the G-protein and causing the α subunit to dissociate from the $\beta\gamma$ dimer (Fig. 1.5B).
- α-GTP represents the active form of the G-protein (although this is not always the case: in the heart, potassium channels are activated by the $\beta\gamma$ dimer and recent research has shown that the γ subunit alone may play a role in activation). This component diffuses in the plane of the membrane where it is free to interact with downstream effectors such as enzymes and ion channels. The $\beta\gamma$ dimer remains associated with the membrane owing to its hydrophobicity (Fig. 1.5C).
- The cycle is completed when the α subunit, which has enzymic activity, hydrolyses the

bound GTP to GDP. The GDP-bound α subunit dissociates from the effector and recombines with the $\beta\gamma$ dimer (Fig. 1.5D).

This whole process results in an amplification effect because the binding of an agonist to the receptor can cause the activation of numerous G-proteins which in turn can each, via their association with the effector, produce many molecules of product.

Targets for G-proteins

G-proteins interact with either ion channels or second messengers.

Ion channels

G-proteins may activate ion channels directly, e.g. muscarinic receptors in the heart are linked to potassium channels which open directly on inter-action with the G-protein, causing a slowing down of the heart rate.

Second messengers

Three second-messenger systems exist as targets of G-proteins (Fig. 1.6).

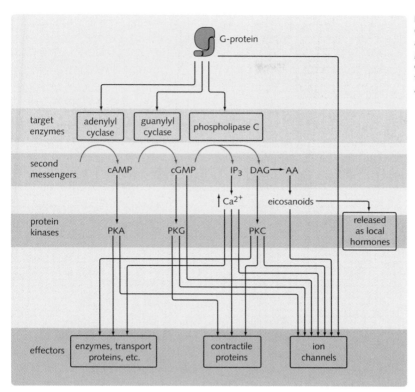

Fig. 1.6 Second-messenger targets of G-proteins and their effects. (cAMP, cyclic adenosine monophosphate; cGMP, cyclic guanosine monophosphate; DAG, diacylglycerol; IP_3, inositol (1,4,5) triphosphate; PK, protein kinase; AA, arachidonic acid.)

Adenylyl cyclase/cAMP system

Many types of G-protein exist. This is probably attributable to the variability of the α subunit. G_s and G_i/G_o cause stimulation and inhibition, respectively, of the target enzyme adenylyl cyclase. This explains why muscarinic ACh receptors (G_i/G_o linked) and β-adrenoreceptors (G_s linked) located in the heart produce opposite effects.

The bacterial toxins cholera and pertussis can be used in order to determine which G-protein is involved in a particular situation. Each has enzymic action on a conjugation reaction with the α subunit, such that:

- Cholera affects G_s causing continued activation of adenylyl cyclase. This explains why infection with cholera toxin results in uncontrolled fluid secretion from the gastrointestinal tract.
- Pertussis affects G_i and G_o causing continued inactivation of adenylyl cyclase. This explains why infection with *Bordetella pertussis* causes a 'whooping' cough, characteristic of this infection, as the airways are constricted, and the larynx experiences muscular spasms.

Adenylyl cyclase (stimulated via G_s) catalyses the conversion of ATP to cyclic cAMP within cells. The cAMP produced in turn causes activation of certain protein kinases, enzymes that phosphorylate serine and threonine residues in various proteins, thereby producing either activation or inactivation of these proteins. This can lead to:

- Increased lipolysis through activation of hormone-sensitive lipase
- Reduced glycogen synthesis through inactivation of glycogen synthase
- Increased glycogen breakdown through the activation of phosphorylase kinase and therefore conversion of inactive phosphorylase b to active phosphorylase a.

Activation of $β_1$-adrenergic receptors found in cardiac muscle results in activation of cAMP-dependent protein kinase A, which phosphorylates and opens voltage-operated calcium channels. This increases calcium levels in the cells and results in an increased rate and force of contraction.

Activation of $β_2$-adrenergic receptors found in smooth muscle causes activation of protein kinase and therefore phosphorylation of myosin light-chain kinase. This results in activation of the contractile machinery in smooth muscle.

Receptors linked to G_i inhibit adenylyl cyclase and reduce cAMP production. Examples of these receptors are the M_2 and M_4 muscarinic, the opioid, the 5-HT_1 (hydroxytryptamine) and the α_2-adrenoreceptors.

Phospholipase C/inositol phosphate system

Activation of M_1, M_3, 5-HT_2, peptide and α_1-adrenoreceptors, via G_q, cause activation of phospholipase C, a membrane-bound enzyme, which increases the rate of degradation of phosphatidylinositol (4,5) bisphosphate into diacylglycerol (DAG) and inositol (1,4,5) triphosphate (IP_3). DAG and IP_3 act as second messengers.

IP_3 binds to the membrane of the endoplasmic reticulum, opening calcium channels and increasing the concentration of calcium within the cell by 10–100-fold. Increased calcium levels may result in smooth muscle contraction, increased secretion from exocrine glands, increased hormone or transmitter release, or increased force and rate of contraction of the heart.

DAG, which remains associated with the membrane owing to its hydrophobicity, causes protein kinase C to move from the cytosol to the membrane where DAG can regulate the activity of the latter. There are at least six types of protein kinase C, with 50 or more targets including:

- Release of hormones and neurotransmitters
- Smooth muscle contraction
- Inflammation
- Ion transport
- Tumour promotion.

Guanylyl cyclase system

Guanylyl cyclase catalyses the conversion of GTP to cGMP. This cGMP goes on to cause activation of protein kinase G which in turn phosphorylates contractile proteins and ion channels.

Transmembrane guanylyl cyclase activity is exhibited by the atrial natriuretic peptide receptor upon the binding of atrial natriuretic peptide. Cytoplasmic guanylyl cyclase activity is exhibited when bradykinin activates receptors on the membrane of endothelial cells to generate nitric oxide, which then acts as a second messenger to activate guanylyl cyclase within the cell.

Sodium nitroprusside is a nitrovasodilator that relaxes the smooth muscle of arteries and veins by increasing cGMP production. Because both central venous pressure and arterial pressure drop, there is little change in cardiac output. Sodium nitroprusside is used for angina and hypertension.

Tyrosine kinase linked receptors

Tyrosine kinase linked receptors are involved in the regulation of growth and differentiation, and responses to metabolic signals. The response time of enzyme-initiated transduction is slow (minutes). Examples include the receptors for insulin, platelet-derived growth factor and epidermal growth factor.

Activation of tyrosine kinase receptors results in autophosphorylation of tyrosine residues leading to the activation of pathways involving protein kinases.

DNA linked receptors

Corticosteroids, thyroid hormone, retinoic acid, and vitamin D are all molecules with receptors that are linked so as to interact with DNA. The receptors are located intracellularly and so agonists must pass through the cell membrane in order to reach the receptor. Receptor–agonist complexes are then transported to the nucleus. Once in the nucleus the complex can bind to specific DNA sequences and so alter the expression of specific genes. As a result, secondary transduction involving an increase or decrease in the synthesis of various proteins occurs. The process is much slower than for other receptor–ligand interactions, and the effects usually last longer.

> Drugs, like naturally occurring chemical mediators, act on receptors located in the cell membrane, in the cytoplasm of the cell, or in the cells nucleus, to bring about a cellular, and eventually organ or tissue response.

DRUG–RECEPTOR INTERACTIONS

Most drugs produce their effects by acting through specific protein molecules called receptors.

Receptors respond to endogenous chemicals in the body that are either synaptic transmitter substances (e.g. ACh, noradrenaline) or hormones (endocrine, e.g. insulin; or local mediators, e.g. histamine). These chemicals or drugs will do one of the following:

- Activate receptors and produce a subsequent response (agonists)
- Associate with receptors but not cause activation (antagonists). Antagonists reduce the chance of transmitters or agonists binding to the receptor and thereby oppose their action by effectively diluting or removing the receptors from the system.

Electrostatic forces initially attract a drug to a receptor. If the shape of the drug corresponds to that of the binding site of the receptor, then it will be held there temporarily by weak bonds or, in the case of irreversible antagonists, permanently by stronger covalent bonds. The number of bonds, and the complementariness of fit, between drug and receptor determines the affinity of the drug for that receptor. The greater the number of bonds and the greater degree of complementariness of fit, the higher the affinity.

The affinity is defined by the dissociation constant which is given the symbol K_d. The lower the K_d, the higher the affinity. K_d values in the nanomolar range represent drugs (D) with a high affinity for their receptor (R):

$$D + R \underset{k_{-1}}{\overset{k_{+1}}{\rightleftharpoons}} DR$$

The rate at which the forward reaction occurs depends on the drug concentration [D] and the receptor concentration [R]:

Forward rate = K_{+1} [D][R]

The rate at which the backward reaction occurs mainly depends on the interaction between the drug and the receptor [DR]:

Backward rate = K_{-1} [DR]

$K_d = K_{-1}/K_{+1}$

K_a is the association constant and is used to quantify affinity. It can be defined as the concentration of drug that produces 50% of the maximum response at equilibrium, in the absence of receptor reserve (p. 10):

$K_a = 1/K_d$

Drugs with a high affinity stay bound to their receptor for a relatively long time and are said to have a slow off-rate. This means that at any time the probability that any given receptor will be occupied by the drug is high.

The ability of a drug to combine with one type of receptor is termed specificity. Although no drug is truly specific, most exhibit relatively selective action on one type of receptor.

Agonists

Agonists (A) bind to the receptor (R) and the chemical energy released on binding induces a conformational change that sets off a chain of biochemical events within the cell, leading to a response (AR*). The equation for this is:

$$A + R \xrightarrow{(1)} AR \xrightarrow{(2)} AR^*$$

where
(1) – affinity dependent
(2) – efficacy dependent.

Partial agonists cannot bring about the same maximum response as full agonists, even if their affinity for the receptor is the same (Figs 1.7 and 1.8).

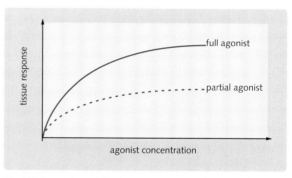

Fig. 1.7 Comparison of the dose–response curve for a partial agonist and a full agonist. (From *Medical Pharmacology at a Glance*, 2nd edition. Courtesy of Blackwell Scientific Publications.)

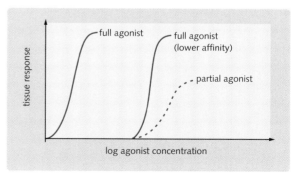

Fig. 1.8 Comparison of the log dose–response curve for a partial agonist and a full agonist. (From *Medical Pharmacology at a Glance*, 2nd edition. Courtesy of Blackwell Scientific Publications.)

The ability of agonists, once bound, to activate receptors is termed efficacy, such that:

- Full agonists have high efficacy and are able to produce a maximum response while occupying only a small percentage of the receptors available.
- Partial agonists have low efficacy and are unable to elicit the maximum response even if they are occupying all the available receptors.

Antagonists

Antagonists bind to receptors but do not activate them, do not induce a conformational change and thus have no efficacy. However, because antagonists occupy the receptor, they prevent agonists from binding and therefore block their action.

Two types of antagonist exist: competitive and non-competitive.

Competitive antagonists

Competitive antagonists bind to receptors reversibly and effectively produce a dilution of the receptors, such that:

- A parallel shift is produced to the right of the agonist dose–response curve (Fig. 1.9).
- The maximum response is not depressed. This reflects the fact that the antagonist's effect can be overcome by increasing the dose of agonist, i.e. the block is surmountable. Increasing the concentration of agonist increases the probability of the agonist taking the place of an antagonist leaving the receptor.
- The size of the shift in the agonist dose–response curve produced by the antagonist reflects the

affinity of the antagonist for the receptor. High-affinity antagonists stay bound to the receptor for a relatively long period of time allowing the agonist little chance to take the antagonist's place.

This concept can be quantified in terms of the dose ratio. The dose ratio is the ratio of the concentration of agonist producing a given response in the presence and absence of a certain concentration of antagonist, e.g. a dose ratio of 3 tells us that three times as much agonist was required to produce a given response in the presence of the antagonist than it did in its absence.

A 22-year-old man is admitted to hospital with signs of respiratory depression, drowsiness, bradycardia and confusion. His girlfriend tells the medical team that he uses heroin and an overdose is therefore suspected. Heroin act as an agonist, activating the opioid receptors. Naloxone is a competitive antagonist at those receptors and so is administered as treatment. Minutes later the man's condition improves and his respiratory rate rises to normal. Careful titration of the naloxone dose should allow treatment of respiratory depression without provoking acute withdrawal signs.

Non-competitive antagonists

Non-competitive antagonists are also known as irreversible antagonists. Their presence:

- Also produces a parallel shift to the right of the agonist dose–response curve (see Fig. 1.9).
- Depresses the maximum response, reflecting the fact that the antagonist's effect cannot be overcome by the addition of greater doses of agonist. At low concentrations, however, a parallel shift may occur without a reduced maximum response. This tells us that not all of the receptors need be occupied to elicit a maximum response, because irreversible antagonists effectively remove receptors, and there must be a number of spare receptors.

Receptor reserve

Although on a log scale the relation between the concentration of agonist and the response produces a symmetrical sigmoid curve, rarely does a 50%

Fig. 1.9 Comparison of the log dose–response curves for competitive and non-competitive (irreversible) antagonists. (From *Medical Pharmacology at a Glance*, 2nd edition. Courtesy of Blackwell Scientific Publications.)

response correspond to 50% receptor occupancy. This is because there are spare receptors.

This excess of receptors is known as receptor reserve and serves to sharpen the sensitivity of the cell to small changes in agonist concentration. The low efficacy of partial agonists can be overcome in tissues with a large receptor reserve and in these circumstances partial agonists may act as full agonists.

Potency

Potency relates to the concentration of a drug needed to elicit a response. The EC_{50}, where EC stands for effective concentration, is a number used to quantify potency. EC_{50} is the concentration producing 50% of the maximum response. Thus, the lower the EC_{50}, the more potent the drug.

Where agonists are concerned, potency is related to both affinity and efficacy.

Pharmacokinetic variables also affect potency. For example, the acidic pH of the stomach may breakdown a drug that has been found to be very potent in a test tube. This means that, if given as a tablet, it would have very little potency and would be ineffective.

> The kinetic equations simply demonstrate how drugs act, and how they differ from one another. You are unlikely to be asked about them, though try to work through them as they aid in the building of a good foundation in the subject.

PHARMACOKINETICS

Pharmacology can be divided into two disciplines. These are:

- **Pharmacokinetics** – which considers drug disposition and the way the body affects the drug with time, i.e. the factors that determine its absorption, distribution, metabolism and excretion.
- **Pharmacodynamics** – which deals with the effect of the drug on the body.

Compliance

Compliance on the patient's behalf is very important as far as taking drugs is concerned. For some drugs to be effective (e.g. antibiotics), they must be taken at regular intervals and for a certain period of time. For certain forms of treatment, patients may even need to come to hospital, in which case transport, work and having young children around might be a problem.

Compliance tends to be more of a problem in paediatric practice because it involves both parents and the child: the parent must remember to give the medicine and follow directions accurately; the child must cooperate and not spit out or spill the medicine. Also, elderly patients' capacity to understand and remember to take their medicines must be ascertained, as well as their physical ability to carry out the task. For example, an elderly patient with arthritis may struggle to administer medicines unaided.

Practical dosage forms are important in achieving compliance. Many tablets are now sugar coated, making them easier to take, and a large number of the drugs manufactured for children are in the form of elixirs or suspensions, which may be available in a variety of different flavours, making their administration less of a problem.

The route of administration of a drug may affect compliance. Taking a drug orally, for example, is more simple than injecting it.

The dosing schedule is also an important aspect of compliance. The easier this is to follow, and the less frequently a drug needs to be taken or administered, the more likely it is to achieve compliance.

Routes of administration

Topical

Topical drugs are applied where they are needed, giving them the advantage that they do not have to cross any barriers or membranes. Examples include skin ointments; ear, nose or eye drops; and aerosols inhaled in the treatment of asthma.

Enteral

Enteral administration means that the drug reaches its target via the gut. It is the least predictable route of administration, owing to metabolism by the liver, chemical breakdown and the possible binding to food. Drugs must cross several barriers, which may or may not be a problem according to their physicochemical properties, such as charge and size. However:

- Most drugs are administered orally unless the drug is unstable, or is rapidly inactivated in the gastrointestinal tract, or if its efficacy of absorption from the gastrointestinal tract is uncertain owing to metabolism by the liver or the intestines, vomiting or a disease that may affect drug absorption.
- Absorption of drugs via the buccal or sublingual route avoids the portal circulation and is therefore valuable when administering drugs subject to a high degree of first-pass metabolism (which is unavoidable if taken orally). It is also useful for potent drugs with a non-disagreeable taste, such as sublingual nitroglycerin given to relieve acute attacks of angina.
- Administration of drugs rectally, such as in the form of suppositories, means that there is less first-pass metabolism by the liver because the venous return from the lower gastrointestinal tract is less than that from the upper gastrointestinal tract. It has the disadvantage, however, of being inconsistent.
- Antacids have their effect in the stomach and may be considered as being topical.

Parenteral

Parenteral administration means that the drug is administered in a manner that avoids the gut. The protein drug insulin, for example, is destroyed by the acidity of the stomach and the digestive enzymes within the gut and must therefore be injected, usually subcutaneously.

Intravenous injection of drugs has several advantages:

- It is the most direct route of administration. The drug enters the bloodstream directly and bypasses absorption barriers.
- A drug is distributed in a large volume and acts rapidly.

For drugs that must be given continuously by infusion, or for drugs that damage tissues, this is an important method of administration.

Alternative parenteral routes of administration include subcutaneous, intramuscular, epidural or intrathecal injections, and transdermal patches, such as are used in angina.

The rate of drug absorption from the site of the injection can be decreased by binding the drug to a vehicle or co-administering a vasoconstrictor, such as adrenaline, to reduce blood flow to the site.

Drug absorption

Bioavailability takes into account both absorption and metabolism and describes the proportion of the drug that passes into the systemic circulation. This will, of course, be 100% after an intravenous injection, but following oral administration it will depend on the drug, the individual, and the circumstances under which the drug is given.

Drugs must cross membranes to enter cells or to transfer between body compartments, therefore, drug absorption will be affected by both chemical and physiological factors.

Cell membranes

Cell membranes are composed of lipid bi-layers and thus absorption is usually proportional to the lipid solubility of the drug. Unionized molecules (B) are far more soluble than those that are ionized (BH^+) and surrounded by a 'shell' of water.

$$B + H^+ \rightleftharpoons BH^+$$

Size

Small size is another factor that favours absorption. Most drugs are small molecules (molecular weight <1000) that are able to diffuse across membranes in their uncharged state.

pH

Since most drugs are either weak bases, weak acids or amphoteric, the pH of the environment in which they dissolve, as well as the pK_a value of the drug, will be important in determining the fraction in the unionized form that is in solution and able to diffuse across cell membranes. The pK_a of a drug is defined as the pH at which 50% of the molecules in solution are in the ionized form, and is characterized by the Henderson–Hasselbalch equation:

For acidic molecules:

$$HA \rightleftharpoons H^+ + A^-$$
$$pK_a = pH + \log [HA]/[A^-]$$

For basic molecules:

$$BH^+ \rightleftharpoons B + H^+$$
$$pK_a = pH + \log [BH^+]/[B]$$

Drugs will tend to exist in the ionized form when exposed to an environment with a pH opposite to their own state. Therefore, acids become increasingly ionized with increasing pH (i.e. basic).

It is useful to consider three important body compartments – plasma (pH = 7.4), stomach (pH = 2.0) and urine (pH = 8.0) – in relation to drugs. Thus:

- Aspirin is a weak acid (pK_a = 3.5) and its absorption will therefore be favoured in the stomach, where it is uncharged, and not in the plasma or the urine, where it is highly charged; aspirin in high doses may even damage the stomach.
- Morphine is a weak base (pK_a = 8.0) that is highly charged in the stomach, quite charged in the plasma, and half charged in the urine. Morphine is able to cross the blood–brain barrier but is poorly and erratically absorbed from the stomach and intestines, and metabolized by the liver, and must therefore be given by injection or delayed-release capsules. Some drugs, such as quaternary ammonium compounds (e.g. suxamethonium, tubocurarine), are always charged, and must therefore be injected.

Drug distribution

Once drugs have reached the circulation, they are distributed around the body. As most drugs have a very small molecular size, they are able to leave the circulation by capillary filtration to act on the tissues.

The half-life of a drug ($t_{1/2}$) is the time taken for the plasma concentration of that drug to fall to half of its original value. Bulk transfer in the blood is very quick. Drugs:

- Exist either dissolved in blood or bound to plasma proteins such as albumin. Albumin is the most important circulating protein for binding many acidic drugs.
- That are basic tend to be bound to a globulin fraction that increases with age. A drug that is bound is confined to the vascular system and is unable to exert its actions; this becomes a problem if more than 80% of the drug is bound.

- Interact and one drug may displace another. For example, aspirin can displace the benzodiazepine diazepam from albumin.

The apparent volume of distribution (V_d) is the calculated pharmacokinetic space into which a drug is distributed.

$$V_d = \frac{\text{dose administered}}{\text{initial apparent plasma concentration}}$$

V_d values:

- That amount to less than a certain body compartment volume indicate that the drug is contained within that compartment. For example, when the volume of distribution is less than 5 L, it is likely that the drug is restricted to the vasculature.
- Less than 15 L imply that the drug is restricted to the extracellular fluid.
- Greater than 15 L suggest distribution within the total body water. Some drugs (usually basic) have a volume of distribution that exceeds body weight, in which case tissue binding is occurring. These drugs tend to be contained outside the circulation and may accumulate in certain tissues. Very lipid-soluble substances, such as thiopental, can build-up in fat; lead accumulates in bone; and mepacrine, an anti-malarial drug, has a concentration in the liver 200 times that in the plasma because it binds to nucleic acids. Some drugs are even actively transported into certain organs.

Highly lipid soluble drugs such as thiopental will accumulate in fat, and as such, its half-life will be much longer in obese than in thinner patients.

Drug metabolism

Before being excreted from the body, most drugs are metabolized. A small number of drugs exist in their fully ionized form at physiological pH (7.4) and, owing to this highly polar nature are metabolized to only a minor extent, if at all. The sequential metabolic reactions that occur have been categorized as phases 1 and 2.

Sites of metabolism

The liver is the major site of drug metabolism although most tissues are able to metabolize specific drugs. Other sites of metabolism include the kidney, the lung, and the gastrointestinal tract.

Orally administered drugs, which are usually absorbed in the small intestine, reach the liver via the portal circulation. At this stage, or within the small intestine, the drugs may be extensively metabolized; this is known as first-pass metabolism and means that considerably less drug reaches the systemic circulation than enters the portal vein. This causes problems because it means that higher doses of drug must be given and, owing to individual variation in the degree of first-pass metabolism, the effects of the drug can be unpredictable. Drugs that are subject to a high degree of first-pass metabolism, such as the local anaesthetic lidocaine, cannot be given orally and must be administered by some other route.

Phase 1 metabolic reactions

Phase 1 metabolic reactions include oxidation, reduction and hydrolysis. These reactions introduce a functional group, such as OH^- or NH_2, which increases the polarity of the drug molecule and provides a site for phase 2 reactions.

Oxidation

Oxidations are the most common type of reaction and are catalysed by an enzyme system known as the microsomal mixed function oxidase system, which is located on the smooth endoplasmic reticulum. The enzyme system forms small vesicles known as microsomes when the tissue is homogenized.

Cytochrome P_{450}:

- Is the most important enzyme, although other enzymes are involved. This enzyme is a haemoprotein that requires the presence of oxygen, reduced nicotinamide adenine dinucleotide phosphate (NADPH) and NADPH cytochrome P_{450} reductase in order to function.
- Exists in several hundred isoforms, some of which are constitutive, whereas others are synthesized in response to specific signals. The substrate specificity of this enzyme depends on the isoform but tends to be low, meaning that a whole variety of drugs can be oxidized.

Although oxidative reactions usually result in inactivation of the drug, sometimes a metabolite is produced that is pharmacologically active and may have a duration of action exceeding that of the original drug. In these cases the drug is known as a prodrug, e.g. codeine which is demethylated to morphine.

Reduction

Reduction reactions also involve microsomal enzymes but are much less common than oxidation reactions. Examples of drugs subject to reduction include prednisone, which is given as a prodrug and reduced to the active glucocorticoid prednisolone, and warfarin, an anticoagulant, which is inactivated by the transformation of a ketone group to a hydroxyl group.

Hydrolysis

Hydrolysis is not restricted to the liver and occurs in a variety of tissues. Aspirin is spontaneously hydrolysed to salicylic acid in moisture.

Phase 2 metabolic reactions

Drug molecules that possess a suitable site that was either present before phase 1 or is the result of a phase 1 reaction, are susceptible to phase 2 reactions. Phase 2 reactions involve conjugation, the attachment of a large chemical group to a functional group on the drug molecule. Conjugation results in the drug being more hydrophilic and thus more easily excreted from the body. In conjugation:

- It is mainly the liver that is involved, although conjugation can occur in a wide variety of tissues.
- Chemical groups involved are endogenous activated moieties such as glucuronic acid, sulphate, methyl, acetyl and glutathione.
- The conjugating enzymes exist in many isoforms and show relative substrate and metabolite specificity.

Unlike the products of phase 1 reactions, the conjugate is almost invariably inactive. An important exception is morphine, which is converted to morphine 6-glucuronide, which has an analgesic effect lasting longer than that of its parent molecule.

Factors affecting metabolism

Enzyme induction is the increased synthesis or decreased degradation of enzymes and occurs as a result of the presence of an exogenous substance. For example:

- Some drugs are able to increase the activity of certain isoenzyme forms of cytochrome P_{450} and

Fig. 1.10 Examples of drugs that induce or inhibit drug-metabolizing enzymes

Drugs modifying enzyme action	Drugs whose metabolism is affected
Enzymes induction	
Phenobarbital and other barbiturates	Warfarin
Rifampicin	Oral contraceptives
Phenytoin	Corticosteroids
Ethanol	Ciclosporin
Carbamazepine	
Enzyme inhibition	
Allopurinol	Azathioprine
Chloramphenicol	Phenytoin
Corticosteroids	Various drugs—TCA, cyclophosphamide
Cimetidine	Many drugs—amiodarone, phenytoin, pethidine
MAO inhibitors	Pethidine
Erythromycin	Ciclosporin
Ciprofloxacin	Theophylline

MAO, monoamine oxidase; TCA, tricyclic antidepressant
Adapted from Rang et al. Pharmacology, 4th edition, Churchill Livingstone

thus increase their own metabolism, as well as that of other drugs.

- Smokers can show increased metabolism of certain drugs because of the induction of cytochrome P_{448} by a constituent in tobacco smoke.
- In contrast, some drugs inhibit microsomal enzyme activity and therefore increase their own activity as well as that of other drugs.

Figure 1.10 gives some examples of enzyme-inducing agents, and the drugs whose metabolism is affected. Competition for a metabolic enzyme may occur between two drugs, in which case there is a decreased metabolism of one or both drugs. This is known as inhibition.

Enzymes that metabolize drugs are affected by many aspects of diet, such as the ratio of protein to carbohydrate, flavonoids contained in vegetables, and polycyclic aromatic hydrocarbons found in barbecued foods.

Paracetamol poisoning

Paracetamol is a classic example of a drug that can be lethal at high doses (two to three times the maximum therapeutic dose), owing to the accumulation of its metabolites.

In phase 2 of the metabolic process, paracetamol is conjugated with glucuronic acid and sulphate. When high doses of paracetamol are ingested, these pathways become saturated and the drug is metabolized by the mixed function oxidases. This results in the formation of the toxic metabolite N-acetyl-p-benzoquinone which is inactivated by glutathione. However, when glutathione is depleted, this toxic metabolite reacts with nucleophilic constituents in the cell leading to necrosis in the liver and kidneys.

N-acetylcysteine or methionine can be administered in cases of paracetamol overdose, because these increase liver glutathione formation and the conjugation reactions, respectively.

Drug excretion

Drugs are excreted from the body in a variety of different ways. Excretion can occur by the kidneys into urine, by the gastrointestinal tract into bile and faeces, and by the lungs into exhaled air. Drugs may also leave the body through breast milk and sweat. The most important routes for drug excretion are through the urine and faeces.

The volume of plasma cleared of drug per unit time is known as the clearance.

Renal excretion

Glomerular filtration, tubular reabsorption (passive and active), and tubular secretion all determine the extent to which a drug will be excreted by the kidneys.

Glomerular capillaries allow the passage of molecules with a molecular weight <20 000. The glomerular filtrate thus contains most of the substances in plasma except proteins. In the glomerular capillaries:

- The negative charge of the corpuscular membrane also repels negatively charged molecules, including plasma proteins.
- Drugs that bind to plasma proteins such as albumin will not be filtered.

Most of the drug in the blood does not pass into the glomerular filtrate, but passes into the peritubular capillaries of the proximal tubule where, depending on its nature, it may be transported into the lumen of the tubule by either of two transport mechanisms. One transport mechanism deals with acidic molecules, the other with basic molecules. In the peritubular capillaries:

- Tubular secretion is responsible for most of the drug excretion carried out by the kidneys and, unlike glomerular filtration, allows the clearance of drugs bound to plasma proteins. Competition between drugs that share the same transport mechanism may occur, in which case the excretion of these drugs will be reduced. Probenecid is a drug that was designed to compete with penicillin for excretion and therefore increase the duration of action of penicillin.
- Reabsorption of a drug will depend upon the fraction of molecules in the ionized state, which is in turn dependent on the pH of the urine. Intoxification with aspirin (weak acid, $pK_a = 3.5$) can be treated by administering bicarbonate which makes the urine more alkaline; this ionizes aspirin and renders it less prone to reabsorption.
- Renal disease will affect the excretion of certain drugs. The extent to which excretion is impaired can be deduced by measuring 24-hour creatinine clearance.

Gastrointestinal excretion

Some drug conjugates are excreted into the bile and subsequently released into the intestines where they are hydrolysed back to the parent compound and reabsorbed. This 'enterohepatic circulation' prolongs the effect of the drug.

The liver is the main site of drug inactivation, and the kidneys and gastrointestinal tract the main site for drug excretion – disease of these organs will alter a drug's pharmacokinetics.

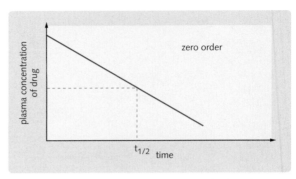

Fig. 1.11 Plasma drug concentration versus time plot for a drug displaying zero-order kinetics. ($t_{1/2}$, half-life.)

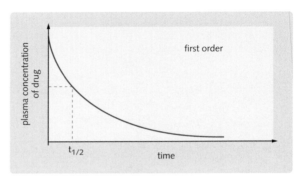

Fig. 1.12 Plasma drug concentration versus time plot for a drug displaying first-order kinetics. ($t_{1/2}$, half-life.)

Mathematical aspects of pharmacokinetics

Kinetic order

Two types of kinetics, related to the plasma concentration of a drug, describe the rate at which a drug leaves the body:

- Zero-order kinetics (Fig. 1.11) describes a decrease in drug levels in the body that is independent of the plasma concentration, and the rate is held constant by a limiting factor, such as a co-factor of enzyme availability. When the plasma concentration is plotted against time, the decrease is a straight line. Alcohol is an example of a drug that displays zero-order kinetics.
- First-order kinetics (Fig. 1.12) is displayed by most drugs. It describes a decrease in drug levels in the body that is dependent on the plasma concentration, as the concentration of the

Fig. 1.13 Log plasma drug concentration versus time plot compatible with the one-compartment open pharmacokinetic model for drug disposition after a parenteral dose, assuming first-order kinetics. (K_{el}, elimination rate constant; C_o initial drug concentration; $t_{1/2}$, half-life.)

Fig. 1.14 Log plasma drug concentration versus time plot for a drug compatible with the one-compartment open pharmacokinetic model for drug disposition after an oral dose. (K_{el}, elimination rate constant; C_o initial drug concentration.) (Redrawn from Page et al. 2002.)

substrate (drug) is the rate limiting factor. When the plasma concentration is plotted against time, the decrease is exponential.

One-compartment model

The one-compartment model usually gives an adequate clinical approximation of drug concentration by considering the body to be a single compartment. Within this single compartment a drug is absorbed, immediately distributed, and subsequently eliminated by metabolism and excretion.

If the volume of the compartment is V_d and the dose administered D, then the initial drug concentration, C_o, will be:

$$C_o = D/V_d$$

The time taken for the plasma drug concentration to fall to half of its original value is the half-life of that drug. The decline in concentration may be exponential, but this situation expresses itself graphically as a straight line when the log plasma concentration is plotted against the time after intravenous dose (Fig. 1.13).

Half-life is related to the elimination rate constant (K_{el}) by the following equation:

$$t_{1/2} \times K_{el} = \text{natural log 2 (ln 2)}$$

Half-life is related to V_d, but does not determine the ability of the body to remove the drug from the circulation, since both V_d and half-life change in the same direction. The body's ability to remove a drug

from the blood is termed clearance (Cl_p) and is constant for individual drugs:

$$Cl_p = V_d \times K_{el}$$

If the drug is not administered parenterally, plotting the log plasma drug concentration against time will require the consideration of both absorption and elimination from the compartment (Fig. 1.14).

The one-compartment model is widely used to determine the dose of drug to be administered. The two-compartment model, which is also used and can be more accurate. It expands on the model by considering the body as two compartments and so allows some consideration of drug distribution.

Model-independent approach

For drugs displaying first-order kinetics, the level of the drug in the body increases until it is equal to the level excreted, at which point steady-state is reached (Fig. 1.15), such that:

- The time to reach steady-state is usually equal to four to five half-lives.
- The amount of drug in the body at steady-state will depend upon the frequency of drug administration – the greater the frequency, the greater the amount of drug and the less the variation between peak and trough plasma concentrations. If the frequency of administration is greater than the half-life, then accumulation of the drug will occur.

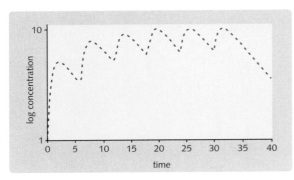

Fig. 1.15 Log plasma drug concentration versus time plot for a drug administered by mouth every 6 hours when its terminal disposition half-life is 6 hours.

The loading dose can be calculated according to the desired plasma concentration at steady-state (C_{ss}) and the volume of distribution (V_d) of the drug:

$$\text{Loading dose (mg/kg)} = V_d \text{ (L/kg)} \times C_{ss} \text{ (mg/L)}$$

DRUG INTERACTIONS AND ADVERSE EFFECTS

Drug interactions

Drugs interact in a number of ways that may produce unwanted effects. Two types of interactions exist: pharmacodynamic and pharmacokinetic.

Pharmacodynamic interactions

Pharmacodynamic interactions involve a direct conflict between the effects of drugs. This conflict results in the effect of one of the two drugs being enhanced or reduced. For example:

- Propranolol, a β-adrenoceptor antagonist given for angina and hypertension, will reduce the effect of salbutamol, a β$_2$-adrenoceptor agonist given for the treatment of asthma. The administration of β-blockers to asthmatics should therefore be avoided, or undertaken with caution.
- Administration of monoamine oxidase inhibitors, which inhibit the metabolism of catecholamines, enhances the effects of drugs such as ephedrine. This enhancement causes the release of noradrenaline from stores in the nerve terminal and is known as 'potentiation'.

Pharmacokinetic interactions

Absorption, distribution, metabolism and excretion all affect the pharmacokinetic properties of drugs. Thus any drug that interferes with these processes will be altering the effect of other drugs. For example:

- If administered with diuretics, non-steroidal anti-inflammatory drugs (NSAIDs) will reduce the antihypertensive action of these drugs. NSAIDs bring about this effect by reducing prostaglandin synthesis in the kidney, thus impairing renal blood flow and consequently decreasing the excretion of waste and sodium. This results in an increased blood volume and a rise in blood pressure.
- Enzyme induction, which occurs as a result of the administration of certain drugs, can affect the metabolism of other drugs served by that enzyme (see Fig. 1.10).

In some cases, however, drugs are used together so that their interaction can bring about the desired effect.

- For example, carbidopa is a drug used in conjunction with levodopa (L-dopa) in the treatment of Parkinson's disease. L-dopa, which is converted to dopamine in the body can cross the blood–brain barrier. Carbidopa prevents the conversion of L-dopa to dopamine, however, it cannot cross the blood–brain barrier and so acts to reduce the peripheral side-effects while still allowing the desired effects of the drug.

Mr Abbas is a 66-year-old man, who has been on metoprolol, a β-blocker, since being diagnosed with hypertension. He had a myocardial infarction (heart attack) 2 days ago and has now developed ventricular tachycardia (a type of cardiac arrhythmia). His management included receiving amiodarone, which is a class III antiarrhythmic agent.

It is vital to note that both the metoprolol and amiodarone slow the heart. This additive effect can be clinically desirable. However, as well as this dual effect, it is important the medical team is aware that amiodarone inhibits the cytochrome P_{450} enzymes responsible for breaking down metoprolol. Meaning, in the presence of amiodarone, the plasma concentration of metoprolol is higher than normally expected (Fig. 1.16). This should be taken into account when deciding the drug dosage so that excessively slow beating of the heart and conduction block of heart impulses does not occur.

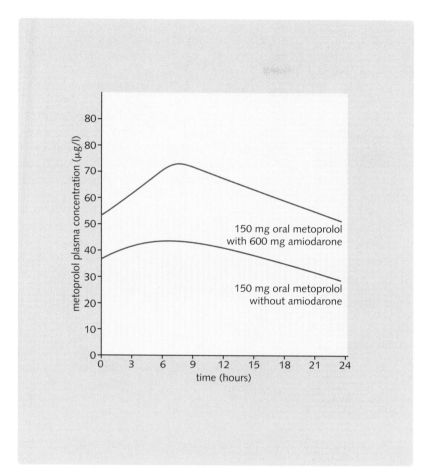

Fig. 1.16 Metoprolol plasma concentration against time, with and without amiodarone. (Adapted from Werner et al. 2004. Effect of amiodarone on the plasma levels of metoprolol. *Am J Cardiol* 94:1319–1321.)

Within the figure:
150 mg oral metoprolol with 600 mg amiodarone
150 mg oral metoprolol without amiodarone

y-axis: metoprolol plasma concentration (μg/l)
x-axis: time (hours)

Adverse effects

As well as interacting with one another and with their target tissue, drugs will also interact with other tissues and organs and alter their function. No drug is without side-effects, although the severity and frequency of these will vary from drug to drug and from person to person.

The liver and the kidneys are susceptible to the adverse effects of drugs, as these are the sites of drug metabolism and excretion. Some drugs cause hepatotoxicity or nephrotoxicity.

Those who are more prone to the adverse effects of drugs, include:

- Pregnant women, who must be careful about taking drugs as certain drugs are teratogenic, i.e. cause fetal malformations (e.g. thalidomide taken in the 1960s for morning sickness).
- Breastfeeding women, who must also be careful about which drugs they take, as many drugs can be passed on in the breast milk to the developing infant.
- Patients with an underlying illness other than the one being treated, such as liver or kidney disease. These illnesses will result in decreased metabolism and excretion of the drug and will produce the side-effects of an increased dose of the same drug.
- Elderly people, who tend to take a large number of drugs, greatly increasing the risk of drug interactions and the associated side-effects. In addition, elderly patients have a reduced renal clearance, and a nervous system that is more sensitive to drugs. The dose of drug initially given is usually 50% of the adult dose, and certain drugs are contraindicated.
- Patients with genetic enzyme defects, such as glucose 6-phosphate dehydrogenase deficiency. The deficiency will result in haemolysis if an oxidant drug, e.g. aspirin, is taken.

Certain drugs are carcinogenic, i.e. induce cancer. Genotoxic carcinogens cause mutations, either directly (primary carcinogens) or through their metabolites (secondary carcinogens). Epigenetic carcinogens, such as phorbol esters, do not induce mutations themselves, but increase the likelihood that a mutagen will do so.

Allergic reactions to certain drugs are common, occurring in 2–25% of cases. Most of these are not serious, e.g. skin reactions; however, rarely, reactions such as anaphylactic shock (type 1 hypersensitivity) occur that may be lethal, unless treated with intravenous adrenaline. The most common allergic reaction is to penicillin, which produces anaphylactic shock in approximately 1:50 000 people.

> Adverse reaction and allergy to a drug are different. Adverse reactions can be minor irritations or upset; an allergic reaction can be life-threatening.

Some drugs, e.g. the vasodilator hydralazine, induce autoimmune reactions similar to systemic lupus erythematosus. Stopping the drug usually puts an end to this reaction, although in some cases glucocorticoid therapy may be needed.

DRUG HISTORY AND DRUG DEVELOPMENT

Drug history

A patient's drug history is a crucial component of the clerking process, as drug effects account for a significant proportion of hospital admissions, and potential drug interactions and adverse events are crucial to foresee.

A complete list of the names and doses of prescribed drugs taken by the patient (noting the proprietary or trade name and the generic or chemical name, e.g. Viagra® and sildenafil, respectively), and any other medications or supplements they may have bought themselves over the counter at a pharmacy should be documented. Women often forget the contraceptive pill and hormone replacement therapy, and should be sensitively questioned about these. NSAIDs and paracetamol are often taken by the bucket load in patients with arthritis, and again these should be specifically asked about. Make sure to note how often the drugs were taken, and at what times.

If presented with numerous bottles and packets of tablets, it is important to ensure that they all belong to the patient, and not the partner of the patient, or to someone else; the effects could be devastating. Ask the patient if they were taking all their medicines as prescribed – it is not unusual for people to alter their dosages without consulting a doctor!

Occasionally it is useful to know what drugs have been taken in the recent and distant past, for example, monoamine oxidase inhibitors should be stopped or at least 3 weeks prior to starting a different antidepressant therapy, and the cytotoxic drug bleomycin can cause lung fibrosis years later.

Previous adverse reaction to drugs, and to non-drug products such as latex, is essential to ascertain. Explore what happened to the patient, and what was done about it. A simple upset stomach and loose stools just for one day after taking penicillin previously is an acceptable side-effect, and is not grounds for choosing another antibiotic when treating a penicillin-sensitive infection in the future. Widespread cutaneous rash, and difficulty breathing which required adrenaline and hospital admission is a genuinely worrying adverse effect of a penicillin, and any such drug should be clearly avoided in the future as this was an allergic drug reaction. Allergy to drugs should be clearly marked in the patient's notes and drug charts.

Family history of adverse drug reactions is usually confined to the anaesthetic history, where the concern is largely in relation to the muscle relaxing drugs, particularly suxamethonium.

Asking a patient about recreational or illicit drug use is occasionally important, though on the whole patients find it uncomfortable to talk about, and usually this adds little to the overall drug history.

Knowledge about any hepatic or renal disease, and general health problems is important when it comes to management and prescribing, as are specific considerations, such as not prescribing aspirin in peptic ulcer disease, or oestrogen to patients with oestrogen-dependent cancers. These aspects are usually brought to light in the rest of the history taking.

kinetics and pharmacodynamics, efficacy, dose–response relationship and safety (Fig. 1.17).

Phase 4 can be regarded as an ongoing phase, where drugs are monitored once licensed for general use. By this stage, the efficacy and dose–response relationship are known, although the side-effect profile is often incomplete, and information is gathered on these 'adverse reactions' which are due to, or likely due to new drugs.

In the UK this is known as the yellow card scheme. The *British National Formulary* (*BNF*) contains detachable yellow cards, which medical staff complete, documenting adverse drug reactions in their patients, which can then be forwarded to the Medicines Control Agency. The Medicines Control Agency collates these data, and uses them for surveillance of unacceptably common or severe adverse effects. The data are publicized in future copies of the *BNF*, or used in the reassessment of certain drug licences.

The salient points of the drug history are:

- current and previous drugs and their doses
- adverse drug reactions and allergies
- family history of allergies
- recreational drug use
- existing renal or hepatic and general disease.

Drug development

Hundreds of thousands of substances have been produced by the pharmaceutical industry over the past 50 years, though very few ever get past preclinical screening, and fewer than 10% of these survive clinical assessment.

There are four clinical stages a potential drug goes through as part of the assessment of its pharmaco-

Fig. 1.17 The five stages of drug development and monitoring

Phase	Main aims/means of investigation	Subjects
Preclincal	• Pharmacology • Toxicology	• *In vitro* • In laboratory animals
Phase 1	• Clinical pharmacology and toxicology • Drug metabolism and bioavailability • Evaluate safety	• Healthy individuals and/or patients
Phase 2	• Initial treatment studies • Evaluate efficacy	• Small numbers of patients
Phase 3	• Large randomized controlled trials • Comparing new to old treatments • Evaluate safety and efficacy	• Large numbers of patients
Phase 4	• Post-marketing surveillance • Long-term safety and rare events • Yellow card scheme	• All patients prescribed the drug

CLINICAL PHARMACOLOGY

Cardiovascular system 25

Respiratory system 55

Peripheral nervous system 65

Central nervous system 81

Endocrine and reproductive systems 119

Kidney and urinary system 143

Gastrointestinal system 153

Pain and anaesthesia 167

Inflammation, allergic diseases and
immunosuppression 183

Infectious diseases 201

Cancer 227

Cardiovascular system

2

Objectives

After reading this chapter, you will:

- Be able to describe the functions of the heart and blood
- Know which drugs affect heart function and circulating blood, and understand how they do so
- Be aware of any indications, contraindications and adverse drug reactions.

THE HEART

Basic concepts

The heart as a pump

The heart functions as a pump, which together with the vascular system supplies the tissues with blood containing oxygen and nutrients, and removes waste products.

The flow of blood around the body is as follows (Fig. 2.1):

- Deoxygenated blood from body tissues reaches the right atrium through the systemic veins (the superior and inferior venae cavae).

- Blood flows into the right ventricle, which then pumps the deoxygenated blood via the pulmonary circulation to the lungs, where the blood becomes oxygenated before reaching the left atrium.
- Blood flows from the left atrium into the left ventricle, from where it is pumped into the systemic circulation via the aorta, to supply the tissues of the body.

Cardiac rate and rhythm

The sinoatrial node (SAN), located in the roof of the right atrium near the entrance of the superior vena cava, and the atrioventricular node (AVN), located at the base of the right atrium, possess a

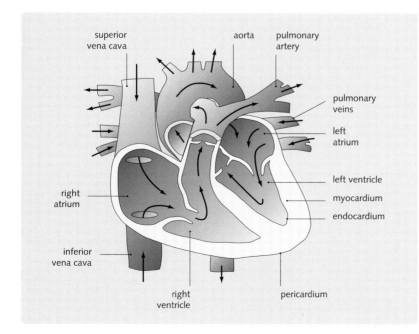

Fig. 2.1 Blood flow through the heart chambers. (Redrawn from Page et al. 2002.)

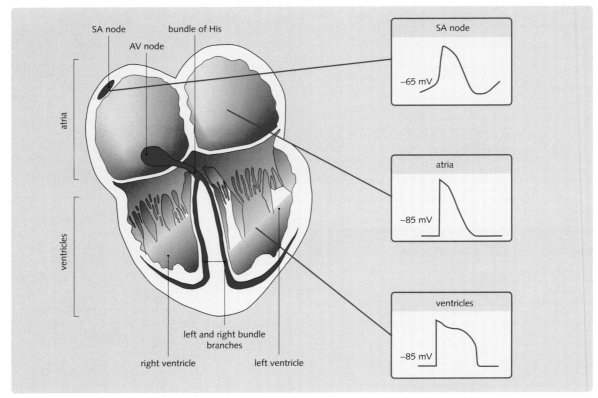

Fig. 2.2 Regional variation in action potential configuration throughout the heart. (AV, atrioventricular; SA, sinoatrial.) (Redrawn from Page et al. 2002.)

spontaneous intrinsic rhythm. The SAN discharges at a frequency higher than other regions of the heart (80 impulses/minute). Thus it is the pacemaker for the heart, and as such determines the heart rate.

The action potential generated by the SAN spreads throughout both atria, reaching the AVN, from which it enters the interventricular septum by means of the bundle of His. The bundle of His splits into left and right branches making contact with the Purkinje fibres, which conduct the impulse throughout the ventricles, causing them to contract (Fig. 2.2).

Cardiac action potential

The shape of the action potential is characteristic of the location of its origin (i.e. whether from nodal tissue, the atria or the ventricles) (Fig. 2.2).

Non-nodal cells

The resting membrane potential across the ventricular cell membrane is approximately –85 mV; this is because the resting membrane is more permeable to potassium than to other ions. Four phases occurring at the ventricular cell membrane are (Fig. 2.3):

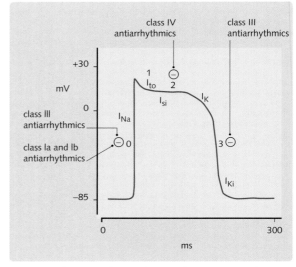

Fig. 2.3 Configuration of a typical ventricular action potential showing the ionic currents, the phases and where class I, III and IV antiarrhythmic drugs act. (0, 1, 2 and 3, phases of the action potential; I_{Na}, fast inward Na^+ current; I_{si}, slow inward Ca^{2+} current; I_{to}, transient outward K^+ current; I_K, delayed rectifier K^+ current; I_{Ki}, inward rectifier K^+ current.) (Redrawn from Page et al. 2002.)

- Phase 0 or depolarization – Depolarization occurs when the membrane potential reaches a critical value of –60 mV. The upstroke of the action potential is due to the transient opening of voltage-gated sodium channels, allowing sodium ions into the cell. In addition, potassium conductance falls to very low levels.
- Phase 1 or partial repolarization – Partial repolarization occurs as a result of the inactivation of the sodium current, and a transient outward potassium current.
- Phase 2 or plateau phase – The membrane remains depolarized at a plateau of approximately 0 mV. This is due to the activation of a voltage-dependent slow inward calcium current, conducting positive charge into the cell, and a delayed rectifier potassium current conducting positive charge out of the cell.
- Phase 3 or repolarization – Repolarization is due to the inactivation of the calcium current and an increase in potassium conductance.

Nodal cells

The resting membrane potential of nodal cells is approximately –60 mV.

In nodal cells, there is no fast sodium current. Instead, the action potential is initiated by an inward calcium current, and because calcium spikes conduct slowly, there is a delay of approximately 0.1 seconds between atrial and ventricular contraction.

Nodal cells have a phase known as phase 4 or the pacemaker potential. This phase involves a gradual depolarization that occurs during diastole and is known as the f current (I_f, funny). The f current is activated by hyperpolarization at –45 mV, and consists of sodium and calcium ions entering the cell (Fig. 2.4).

Autonomic control of the heart

Both the parasympathetic and sympathetic nervous systems influence the heart, though parasympathetic activity predominates and explains why the heart rate is lower than the inherent firing frequency of the SAN.

The sympathetic nervous system mediates its effects through the cardiac nerve, and activation of β_1 adrenoceptors. These are linked to adenylyl cyclase and their activation causes increased levels of cyclic adenosine monophosphate (cAMP), and a subsequent increase in intracellular calcium levels.

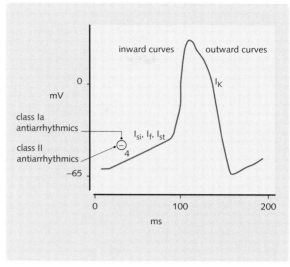

Fig. 2.4 Configuration of a typical sinoatrial node action potential showing the ionic currents, the phases, and where class Ia and II antiarrhythmic drugs act. (4, phase of the action potential; I_{si}, an inward current carried by Ca^{2+} ions; I_f, a 'funny' current carried by Na^+ and Ca^{2+} ions; I_{st}, the sustained inward Na^+ current; I_K, the delayed rectifier current which is an outward K^+ current.) (Redrawn from Page et al. 2002.)

The parasympathetic nervous system mediates its effects through the vagus nerve, and activation of M_2 receptors. These are also linked to adenylyl cyclase, but their activation causes decreased levels of cAMP, and a subsequent decrease in intracellular calcium levels.

The effects of the sympathetic and parasympathetic nervous systems on the heart are summarized in Figure 2.5.

Cardiac contractility

Myocardial contraction is the result of calcium entry through L-type channels, giving rise to an increase in cytosolic calcium (Fig. 2.6).

The calcium is derived from two sources:

- The sarcoplasmic reticulum within the cell
- The extracellular medium.

Extracellular calcium enters the cell, triggering larger amounts of calcium to be released from the sarcoplasmic reticulum, a process known as calcium-induced calcium release.

During contraction, the intracellular levels of calcium rise to levels 10 000 times greater than those at rest. Calcium binds to troponin C, thus

Fig. 2.5 Effects of the sympathetic and parasympathetic systems on the heart

	Sympathetic	Parasympathetic
Heart rate	Increased	Decreased
Force of contraction	Increased	Decreased
Automaticity	Increased	Reduced
AV node conduction	Facilitated	Inhibited
Cardiac efficiency	Reduced	Increased

AV, atrioventricular

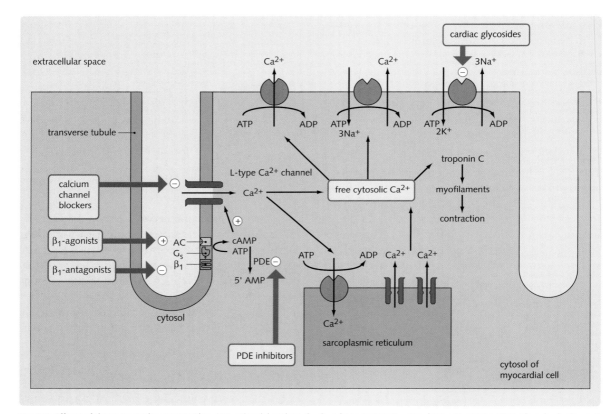

Fig. 2.6 Effects of drugs on cardiac contractility. (AC, adenylyl cyclase; β_1, β_1-adrenoceptor; G_s, stimulatory G-protein; PDE, phosphodiesterase.)

modifying the position of actin and myosin filaments, and allowing the cell to contract. Contraction ceases only once calcium has been removed from the cytoplasm. This occurs through two mechanisms:

- Calcium is pumped out of the cell via the electrogenic Na^+/Ca^{2+} exchanger, which pumps one calcium ion out for every three sodium ions in.

- Calcium is re-sequestered into sarcoplasmic reticulum stores by a Ca^{2+} ATPase pump.

Cardiac dysfunction

Congestive cardiac failure

Congestive cardiac failure (CCF) is the combined failure of both the left and right sides of the heart.

Fig. 2.7 Causes and symptoms/signs of acute and chronic cardiac failure (CF)

Causes		Symptoms/signs	
Acute CF	Chronic CF	Acute CF	Chronic CF
Myocardial infarction	Systemic hypertension	Tachycardia	Exertional dyspnoea
Acute valvular lesion	Myocardial infarction	Hypotension	Systemic oedema
	Valvular lesions	Dyspnoea	Cardiomegaly
	Cardiomyopathies	Pulmonary oedema	Fatigue
		Systemic oedema	Orthopnoea

Fig. 2.8 Characteristics of right and left ventricular failure

Right ventricular failure	Left ventricular failure
Reduced cardiac output	Reduced cardiac output
Hypotension	Hypotension
Peripheral oedema	Pulmonary oedema
Raised jugular venous pressure	Dyspnoea
Hepatomegaly	Fatigue
Ascites	

The incidence of cardiac failure in the UK is between 1 and 5 per 1000 per year, and doubles for each decade of life after the age of 45; over 100 000 hospital admissions annually are directly related to cardiac failure.

CCF occurs when the cardiac output does not meet the needs of the tissues. This is thought to be due to defective excitation–contraction coupling, with progressive systolic and diastolic ventricular dysfunction. Some of the causes and symptoms and signs of acute and chronic cardiac failure are given in Figure 2.7. The characteristics of left and right ventricular failure are listed in Figure 2.8.

The body attempts to compensate for the effects of CCF by two processes – extrinsic and intrinsic.

Extrinsic neurohumoral reflexes

Extrinsic neurohumoral reflexes aim to maintain cardiac output and blood pressure such that hypotension → activation of baroreceptors (receptors responding to changes in pressure) → increased sympathetic activity → increased heart rate and vasoconstriction → increased cardiac contractility and vascular tone → increased arterial pressure.

However, the greater the resistance (arterial pressure) against which the heart must pump, the greater the reduction in both the ejection fraction and the perfusion of the tissues.

The reduced perfusion of the kidneys activates the renin–angiotensin system (RAS), leading to renin secretion and subsequent elevation of plasma angiotensin II and aldosterone levels (see Fig. 2.13 later). Angiotensin II causes peripheral vasoconstriction and aldosterone increases sodium retention, leading to increased water retention, oedema and an increased preload.

Intrinsic cardiac compensation

The increased cardiac preload leads to incomplete emptying of the ventricles and an increase in end-diastolic pressure. The heart eventually fails, owing to the massive increase in myocardial energy requirements.

Arrhythmias

The most common cause of sudden death in developed countries is arrhythmia, and it usually results from underlying cardiovascular pathology such as atherosclerosis.

Myocardial ischaemia is one of the most important causes of arrhythmias, and occurs when a coronary artery becomes occluded, thus preventing sufficient blood from reaching the myocardium. Accumulation of endogenous biological mediators, including potassium, cAMP, thromboxane A_2 and free radicals, is believed to initiate arrhythmias.

Reperfusion after coronary occlusion is necessary for tissue recovery and prevention of myocardial necrosis, but spontaneous resumption of coronary flow is often itself a cause of arrhythmia.

Arrhythmias have been defined according to their appearance on the electrocardiogram (ECG) by the

Lambeth Conventions. These include:

- Ventricular – premature beats, tachycardia, fibrillation and torsades de pointes.
- Atrial – premature beats, tachycardia, flutter and fibrillation.

The two main mechanisms by which cardiac rhythm becomes dysfunctional are:

- Abnormal impulse generation (automatic or triggered).
- Abnormal impulse conduction.

Abnormal impulse generation

Automatic: Automatic abnormal impulse generation is likely to cause sinus and atrial tachycardia, and ventricular premature beats. It can be:

- Enhanced: pathological conditions, such as ischaemia, may effect nodal and conducting tissue so their inherent pacemaker frequency is greater than that of the SAN. Ischaemia causes partial depolarization of tissues (owing to a decrease in the activity of the electrogenic sodium pump) and catecholamine release, thus enhancing the automaticity of the slow pacemakers (AVN, Purkinje fibres, bundle of His) and often giving rise to an ectopic focus triggering the development of a premature beat.
- Abnormal: a premature beat may also develop in atrial or ventricular tissue, which are not normally automatic.

Triggered: Forms of triggered abnormal impulse generation are:

- Early after-depolarizations (EADs), which are likely to cause torsade de pointes and reperfusion-induced arrhythmias. EADs are triggered during repolarization, i.e. phase 2 or 3, of a previously normal impulse. They may result from a decrease in the delayed rectifier K^+ current and are associated with abnormally long action potentials. They are therefore more likely to occur during bradycardia and class III antiarrhythmic drug treatment.
- Delayed after-depolarizations (DADs) are triggered once the action potential has ended, i.e. during phase 4, of a previously normal impulse. DADs usually result from cellular calcium overload, associated with ischaemia, reperfusion and cardiac glycoside intoxication.

Abnormal impulse conduction

Heart block: Heart block is likely to cause ventricular premature beats and results from damage to nodal tissue (most commonly the AVN) caused by conditions such as infarction. AV block may be first, second or third degree, manifesting itself from slowed conduction to complete block of conduction, where the atria and ventricles beat independently.

Re-entry: Re-entry is likely to cause ventricular and atrial tachycardia and fibrillation, atrial flutter and Wolff–Parkinson–White syndrome. Re-entry is of two types, circus movement and reflection.

- In circus movement, an impulse re-excites an area of the myocardium, recently excited, after the refractory period has ended. This usually occurs in a ring of tissue in which a unidirectional block is present, preventing anterograde conduction of the impulse, but allowing retrograde conduction of the same impulse. This results in its continuous circulation, termed circus movement. The time taken for the impulse to propagate around the ring must exceed the refractory period; thus, administration of drugs that prolong the refractory period will interrupt the circuit and terminate re-entry.
- Reflection occurs in non-branching bundles within which electrical dissociation has taken place. Owing to this electrical dissociation, an impulse can return over the same bundle.

Mrs Fibbs, a 70-year-old retired financier with a history of mitral stenosis, presented with palpitations and dyspnoea. On examination, she had an irregularly irregular pulse, diagnostic of atrial fibrillation. This was confirmed on ECG by absent P waves and irregular QRS complexes. Digoxin was given to slow the heart rate. Her management also included anticoagulation by warfarin, since she is over 65 and her atrial fibrillation puts her at increased risk of embolic stroke.

Angina pectoris

Angina is associated with acute myocardial ischaemia, and results from underlying cardiovascular pathology. When coronary flow does not meet the metabolic needs of the heart, a radiating chest pain results. This is angina pectoris.

Stable or classic angina is due to fixed stenosis of the coronary arteries, and is brought on by exercise and stress. Unstable angina or crescendo angina can occur suddenly at rest, and becomes progressively worse, with an increase in the number and severity of attacks. The following conditions can all cause unstable angina:

- Coronary atherosclerosis
- Coronary artery spasm
- Transient platelet aggregation and coronary thrombosis
- Endothelial injury causing the accumulation of vasoconstrictor substances
- Coronary vasoconstriction following adrenergic stimulation.

Variant angina or Prinzmetal's angina occurs at rest, at the same time each day, and is usually due to coronary artery spasm. It is characterized by an elevated ST segment on the ECG during chest pain, and may be accompanied by ventricular arrhythmias.

Treatment of cardiac dysfunction

Drugs used in heart failure

Cardiac glycosides

Examples of cardiac glycosides include digoxin and digitoxin.

Cardiac glycosides possess an aglycone steroid nucleus, conveying the pharmacological activity of these compounds; an unsaturated lactone ring, conveying cardiotonic activity; and sugar moieties, able to modulate potency and pharmacokinetic distribution.

Although the positive inotropic actions of cardiac glycosides shift the Frank–Starling ventricular function curve to a more favourable position (Fig. 2.9), thus improving the symptoms of CCF, there is no evidence that they have a beneficial effect on the long-term prognosis of patients with CCF.

Mechanism of action: Cardiac glycosides act by inhibiting the membrane Na^+/K^+ ATPase pump (see Fig. 2.6). This increases intracellular Na^+ concentration, thus reducing the sodium gradient across the membrane and decreasing the amount of calcium pumped out of the cell by the Na^+/Ca^{2+} exchanger during diastole. Consequently, the intracellular calcium concentration rises, thus increasing the force of cardiac contraction and maintaining normal blood pressure.

In addition, cardiac glycosides alter the electrical activity of the heart, both directly and indirectly. At therapeutic doses they indirectly decrease the heart rate, slow AV conductance and shorten the atrial action potential by stimulating vagal activity. This is useful in atrial fibrillation. At toxic doses they indirectly increase the sympathetic activity of the heart, and cause arrhythmias, including heart block. The direct effects are mainly due to loss of intracellular potassium, and are most pronounced at high doses. The resting membrane potential is reduced, causing enhanced automaticity, slowed cardiac conduction, and increased AVN refractory period.

The increased cytosolic calcium concentration may reach toxic levels thereby saturating the sarcoplasmic reticulum sequestration mechanism and causing oscillations in calcium owing to calcium-induced calcium release. This results in oscillatory afterpotentials and subsequent arrhythmias.

Fig. 2.9 The Frank-Starling curve, positive inotropes, and congestive cardiac failure (CCF). Normal cardiac output is determined by the pressure in the left ventricle at end-diastole. In CCF, the set point for cardiac output is reduced and cardiac output falls (1). Compensatory neurohumoral responses become activated which increase end-diastolic pressure and improve cardiac output; however, this can give rise to backward failure (2). Positive inotropic agents increase cardiac output (3). The improved cardiac output reduces the drive for a high end-diastolic pressure, and decompensation occurs to a new set point (4).

31

In addition, cardiac glycosides have a direct effect on α-adrenoceptors, causing vasoconstriction and a consequent increase in peripheral vascular resistance, which is further enhanced by a centrally mediated increase in sympathetic tone.

Route of administration: Oral.

Indications: Heart failure, supraventricular arrhythmias.

Contraindications: Heart block, hypokalaemia associated with the use of diuretics (the lack of competition from potassium potentiates the effects of cardiac glycosides on the Na^+/K^+ ATPase pump).

Adverse effects: Arrhythmias, anorexia, nausea and vomiting, visual disturbances, abdominal pain and diarrhoea.

Therapeutic notes: The cardiac glycosides have a very narrow therapeutic window, and toxicity is therefore relatively common. If this occurs, the drug should be withdrawn and, if necessary, potassium supplements and antiarrhythmic drugs administered. For severe intoxication, antibodies specific to cardiac glycosides are available.

Phosphodiesterase inhibitors

Examples of phosphodiesterase (PDE) inhibitors include enoximone and milrinone. These have been developed as a result of the many adverse effects and problems associated with cardiac glycosides. There is no evidence that these improve the mortality rate.

Mechanism of action: The type III PDE isoenzyme is found in myocardial and vascular smooth muscle.

Phosphodiesterase is responsible for the degradation of cAMP; thus, inhibiting this enzyme raises cAMP levels and causes an increase in myocardial contractility and vasodilatation (Fig. 2.6). Cardiac output is increased, and pulmonary wedge pressure and total peripheral resistance are reduced, without much change in heart rate or blood pressure.

Route of administration: Intravenous.

Indications: PDE inhibitors are given for severe acute heart failure that is resistant to other drugs.

Adverse effects: Nausea and vomiting, arrhythmias, liver dysfunction, abdominal pain, hypersensitivity.

β-Adrenoceptor agonists

Examples of β-adrenoceptor agonists (p. 43) include dobutamine and dopamine. They are used intravenously in CCF emergencies (see Fig. 2.6).

Drugs with proven mortality benefits in cardiac failure should be remembered. They are β adrenoceptor antagonists, angiotensin-converting enzyme (ACE) inhibitors, nitrates with hydralazine and spironolactone.

Diuretics

The diuretics used in CCF are:

- Thiazides
- Loop diuretics
- Spironolactone.

Diuretics inhibit sodium and water retention by the kidneys, and so reduce oedema due to heart failure. Venous pressure and thus cardiac preload are reduced, increasing the efficiency of the heart as a pump (see Ch. 7). Spironolactone appears to have a beneficial effect in cardiac failure at doses lower than it would be expected to function as a diuretic.

Angiotensin-converting-enzyme inhibitors

For details of angiotensin converting enzyme (ACE) inhibitors see p. 39.

Nitrates

See antianginal drugs (p. 35).

Vasodilating drugs

Hydralazine is discussed on page 40.

Antiarrhythmic drugs

Antiarrhythmic drugs are classified according to a system devised by Vaughan Williams in 1970, and later modified by Harrison. A summary of the effects of the different classes of drug is given in Figure 2.10.

Class I

All class I drugs block the voltage-dependent sodium channels in a dose-dependent manner. Their action resembles that of local anaesthetics (Ch. 9).

All class I drugs have the following effects:

- They prolong the effective refractory period (terminate re-entry).
- They convert unidirectional block to bidirectional block (prevent re-entry).

Class Ia

Examples of class Ia drugs include quinidine, procainamide and disopyramide.

Fig. 2.10 Effects of the antiarrhythmic drugs

Class	Example	Myocardial contractility	AV conduction	AP duration	Effective refractory period
Ia	Procainamide	↓	↓	↑	↑
Ib	Lidocaine	–	–	↓	↑↑
Ic	Flecainide	↓↓	↓↓	–	–
II	Propanolol	↓↓	–/↓	–	–
III	Amiodarone	–	↑	↑↑↑	↑↑↑
IV	Verapamil	↓↓↓	↓↓	↓↓	–

AP, action potential; AV, atrioventricular
The number of arrows indicates the degree of the effect caused

Class Ia drugs affect atrial muscle, ventricular muscle, the bundle of His, the Purkinje fibres and the AVN.

Mechanism of action: Class Ia drugs block voltage-dependent sodium channels in their open (activated) or refractory (inactivated) state (see Figs 2.3 and 2.4). Their effects are to slow phase 0 (increasing the effective refractory period) and phase 4 (reducing automaticity), and to prolong action potential duration.

Route of administration: Oral, intravenous. Consult the *British National Formulary* (*BNF*).

Indications: Ventricular, supraventricular arrhythmias.

Contraindications: Heart block, sinus node dysfunction, cardiogenic shock, severe uncompensated heart failure. Procainamide should not be given to patients with systemic lupus erythematosus.

Adverse effects: Arrhythmias, nausea and vomiting, hypersensitivity, thrombocytopenia and agranulocytosis. Procainamide can cause a lupus-like syndrome, and disopyramide causes hypotension.

Class Ib
Examples of class Ib drugs include lidocaine, mexiletine and phenytoin.

Mechanism of action: Class Ib drugs exert their effects in several ways (see Fig. 2.3). These include:

- Blocking voltage-dependent sodium channels in their refractory (inactivated) state, i.e. when depolarized, as occurs in ischaemia.
- Binding to open channels during phase 0, and dissociating by the next beat, if the rhythm is normal, but abolishing premature beats.
- Decreasing action potential duration.
- Increasing the effective refractory period.

Route of administration: Lidocaine is administered intravenously, and mexiletine and phenytoin either orally or intravenously.

Indications: Ventricular arrhythmias following myocardial infarction. Phenytoin is used in epilepsy (Ch. 5).

Contraindications: Class Ib drugs should not be given to patients with sinoatrial disorders, AV block and porphyria.

Adverse effects: Hypotension, bradycardia, drowsiness and confusion, convulsions and paraesthesia (pins and needles).
Lidocaine may cause dizziness and respiratory depression; mexiletine may cause nausea and vomiting, constipation, arrhythmias and hepatitis; and phenytoin may cause nausea and vomiting and peripheral neuropathy.

Class Ic
Flecainide is the only drug used from class Ic.

Mechanism of action: Flecainide blocks sodium channels in a fashion similar to the class Ia and Ib drugs, but shows no preference for refractory channels. Class Ic drugs therefore result in a general reduction in the excitability of the myocardium.

Route of administration: Oral, intravenous.

Indications: Ventricular tachyarrhythmias.

Contraindications: Heart failure, history of myocardial infarction.

Adverse effects: Dizziness, visual disturbances, arrhythmias.

Class II

Examples of class II drugs include propranolol, atenolol and pindolol (see Figs 2.4 and 2.6).

Class II drugs are β-adrenoceptor antagonists (atenolol is $β_1$ selective) (p. 35). They have been shown to prevent sudden death after myocardial infarction by 50% (although this is believed to be due to prevention of cardiac rupture as opposed to prevention of ventricular fibrillation).

Class III

Examples of class III drugs include bretylium, amiodarone, sotalol and ibutilide.

Mechanism of action: All class III drugs used clinically are potassium-channel blockers. They prolong cardiac action potential duration (increased QT interval on the ECG), and prolong the effective refractory period (see Fig. 2.3).

Amiodarone also blocks sodium and calcium channels, i.e. slows phase 0 and 3, and blocks α- and β-adrenoceptors. Sotalol is a β-adrenoceptor antagonist with class III activity.

Route of administration: Bretylium is administered intravenously while amiodarone and sotalol are administered orally or intravenously.

Indications: Class III drugs are given for ventricular and supraventricular arrhythmias.

Contraindications: Bretylium should not be given to patients with phaeochromocytoma while amiodarone should not be given to those with AV block, sinus bradycardia or thyroid dysfunction.

For contraindications regarding sotalol, see under β-blockers (p. 35).

Adverse effects: Class III drugs can cause arrhythmias, especially torsades de pointes. Bretylium may cause hypotension, nausea and vomiting, whereas amiodarone may cause thyroid dysfunction, liver damage, pulmonary disorders, photosensitivity and neuropathy.

For adverse effects regarding sotalol see under β-blockers (p. 35).

Class IV

Examples of class IV drugs include verapamil and diltiazem (see Figs 2.3 and 2.6).

Class IV drugs are calcium antagonists that shorten phase 2 of the action potential, thus decreasing action potential duration. They are particularly effective in nodal cells, where calcium spikes initiate conduction.

Details of the drugs are given in the section on antianginal drugs (p. 35).

Other antiarrhythmics

The cardiac glycosides (p. 31) and adenosine are agents used in arrhythmias, but which do not fit into the four classes described.

Adenosine

Adenosine is produced endogenously, and acts upon many tissues, including the lungs, afferent nerves and platelets.

Mechanism of action: Adenosine acts at A_1 receptors in cardiac conducting tissue and causes myocyte hyperpolarization. This acts to slow the rate of rise of an action potential, and brings about delay in conduction.

Route of administration: Intravenous.

Indications: Paroxysmal supraventricular tachycardia. Aid diagnosis of broad and narrow complex supraventricular tachycardia.

Contraindications: Second- or third-degree heart block, sick sinus syndrome.

Adverse effects: Transient facial flushing, chest pain, dyspnoea, bronchospasm. Side-effects are very short lived, often lasting less than 30 seconds.

Adrenaline

Adrenaline (epinephrine) is a sympathomimetic agent used in cardiac arrest and in the management of anaphylaxis. Adrenaline is discussed on page 43.

The drugs used in stable angina pectoris are β-adrenoceptor antagonists, nitrates, calcium antagonists, antiplatelets and potassium-channel activators.

Antianginal drugs

Acute attacks of angina are treated with:

- Sublingual nitrates.

In the hospital setting, acute anginal pain is treated with an opiate (Ch. 9).

Stable angina is treated with:

- Long-acting nitrates
- Antiplatelets
- β-adrenoceptor antagonists
- Calcium antagonists
- Potassium-channel activators.

Unstable angina is a medical emergency, and requires hospital admission. Unstable angina is treated with:

- Antiplatelets (aspirin, clopidogrel, dipyridamole and the glycoprotein IIb/IIIa inhibitors, p. 51).
- Heparin/low-molecular-weight heparin (page 5).
- Standard antianginal drug regimen.

Organic nitrates

The organic nitrates, glyceryl trinitrate (GTN), isosorbide mononitrate (ISMN) and isosorbide dinitrate (ISDN) can relieve angina within minutes.

Mechanism of action: Most nitrates are prodrugs, decomposing to form nitric oxide (NO), which activates guanylyl cyclase, thereby increasing the levels of cyclic guanosine monophosphate (cGMP). Protein kinase G is activated and contractile proteins are phosphorylated. Dilatation of the systemic veins decreases preload and thus the oxygen demand of the heart, while dilatation of the coronary arteries increases blood flow and oxygen delivery to the myocardium.

Route of administration: Sublingual, oral (modified release), transcutaneous patches. GTN can be given by intravenous infusion.

Indications: Organic nitrates are given for the prophylaxis and treatment of angina, and in left ventricular failure.

Contraindications: Organic nitrates should not be given to patients with hypersensitivity to nitrates, or those with hypotension and hypovolaemia

Adverse effects: Postural hypotension, tachycardia, headache, flushing and dizziness.

Therapeutic notes: To avoid nitrate tolerance, a drug-free period of approximately 8 hours is needed.

β-Adrenoceptor antagonists (β-blockers)

Examples of β-blockers include propranolol, atenolol, bisoprolol and metoprolol.

β-adrenoceptors are found in many tissues, though the β_1-adrenoceptor is found predominantly in the heart, and the β_2-adrenoceptor is found mainly in the smooth muscle of the vasculature (see p. 74). Some overlap does exist.

Different β-blockers have different affinity for the two types of adrenoceptor. Propanolol is non-selective, having equal affinity for both the β_1- and β_2-adrenoceptors. Atenolol, bisoprolol and meto-prolol have greater affinity for the β_1-adrenoceptor, and are therefore more 'cardiac-specific'. Some β-blockers even appear to have partial agonistic effects at β-adrenoceptors, as well as antagonistic effects.

Mechanism of action: The aim of using β-adrenoceptor antagonists in cardiac disease is to block β-adrenoceptors in the heart. This has the effect of causing a fall in heart rate (slowing of phase 4, Fig. 2.4), in systolic blood pressure, in cardiac contractile activity and in myocardial oxygen demand.

Route of administration: Oral, intravenous.

Indications: Angina, post-myocardial infraction, arrhythmias, hypertension, thyrotoxicosis, glaucoma, anxiety.

Contraindications: Non-selective β-blockers (e.g. propranolol) must not be given to asthmatic patients. At high doses β_1-adrenoceptor antagonists lose their selectivity, and should be used with caution in those with asthma. Other contraindications for β-blockers include bradycardia, hypotension, AV block and CCF.

Adverse effects: Bronchospasm, fatigue and insomnia, dizziness, cold extremities (β_2-adrenoceptor effect), bradycardia, heart block, hypotension and decreased glucose tolerance in diabetic patients.

Calcium-channel blockers (CCBs)

There are two types of CCBs. Examples of rate-limiting CCBs: verapamil and diltiazem. Examples of dihy-dropyridine CCBs are nifedipine (short acting), felodipine (long acting) and amlodipine (long acting)

Mechanism of action: Rate-limiting CCBs block L-type calcium channels found in the heart and in the vascular smooth muscle, thereby reducing calcium entry into cardiac and vascular cells (Figs 2.3 and 2.6, and Fig. 2.12 later). This decrease in intracellular calcium reduces cardiac contractility and causes vasodilatation, which results in several effects: reduced preload due to the reduced venous pressure; reduced afterload due to the reduced arteriolar pressure; increased coronary blood flow; reduced cardiac contractility and thus reduced myocardial oxygen consumption; and a decreased heart rate. High doses of these drugs affect AV nodal conduction.

Dihydropyridines blocks L-type calcium channels in vascular cells. They do not affect cardiac contractility, or AVN conduction, and the beneficial effects are due to increased coronary flow and peripheral vasodilatation.

Route of administration: Oral.

Indications: Calcium-channel blockers are used for the prophylaxis and treatment of angina and hypertension. Dihydropyridines are especially useful in angina associated with coronary vasospasm, with the long-acting dihydropyridines being particularly useful for hypertension management. Verapamil and diltiazem are given for supraventricular arrhythmias, and nifedipine for Raynaud's syndrome (peripheral vasoconstriction).

Contraindications: Calcium-channel blockers should not be given to patients in cardiogenic shock.

Dihydropyridines are contraindicated in advanced aortic stenosis, and verapamil and diltiazem should not be given to patients in severe heart failure (owing to their negative inotropic action), to those taking β-blockers (risk of AV block and impaired cardiac output), and those with severe bradycardia.

Adverse effects: Verapamil and diltiazem may cause hypotension, rash, bradycardia, CCF, heart block and constipation.

Dihydropyridines may cause hypotension, rash, tachycardia, peripheral oedema, and flushing and dizziness.

There are three classes of calcium-channel blockers. Two of them act mostly on the heart (verapamil and diltiazem) and the other acts mostly on peripheral vascular tone (nifedipine). Concurrent use of a β-adrenoceptor antagonist and a calcium-channel blocker could result in profound bradycardia.

Potassium-channel activators

Nicorandil is the only licensed drug in this class.

Mechanism of action: Nicorandil acts to activate the potassium channels of the vascular smooth muscle. Once activated, potassium flows out of the cells, causing hyperpolarization of the cell membrane. The hyperpolarized membrane inhibits the influx of calcium, and therefore inhibits contraction – the overall effect is relaxation of the smooth muscle and vasodilatation (Fig. 2.12).

Route of administration: Oral.

Indications: Prophylaxis of angina.

Contraindications: Cardiogenic shock, left ventricular failure, hypotension.

Adverse effects: Headache, cutaneous vasodilatation, nausea and vomiting.

Figure 2.11 summarises the main drug classes used in angina, cardiac failure and arrhythmias.

Fig. 2.11 Classes of drugs used to treat angina, cardiac failure, and arrhythmias

Angina	Heart failure	Arrhythmias
Organic nitrates	Cardiac glycosides	Na⁺-channel blockers (Class I)
β₁-adrenoceptor antagonists	Phosphodiesterase inhibitors	β₁-adrenoceptor antagonists (Class II)
Ca²⁺ antagonists	β₁-adrenoceptor agonists	K⁺-channel blockers (Class III)
Antiplatelets	Diuretics	Ca²⁺ antagonists (Class IV)
Potassium-channel activators	ACE inhibitors	Cardiac glycosides
	Nitrates	Adenosine
	Vasodilating drugs	

The overall aim of symptom management in angina is to: dilate coronary arteries to allow maximal myocardial perfusion; to decrease the heart rate to minimize oxygen demands of the myocardium, and lengthen diastole when cardiac perfusion occurs, and to prevent platelets from aggregating and forming platelet plugs. In addition to this, reversible risk factors need to be addressed to limit the progression of the disease.

THE CIRCULATION

Control of vascular tone

α-Adrenoceptor activation

α-Adrenoceptor activation (Fig. 2.12) causes contraction of vascular smooth muscle through the activation of phospholipase C (PLC). The resulting increased levels of IP_3 cause the release of calcium from the endoplasmic reticulum, thus increasing calcium levels. Calcium then binds to calmodulin, thus activating myosin light-chain kinase (MLCK) and allowing contraction.

β₂-Adrenoceptor activation

$β_2$-Adrenoceptor activation (Fig. 2.12) causes relaxation of vascular smooth muscle through the activation of adenylyl cyclase. The resulting increased levels of cAMP activate protein kinase A, which phosphorylates and inactivates MLCK.

M₃-receptor activation

M_3-receptor activation causes relaxation of vascular smooth muscle through the release of endothelium-derived relaxing factor (EDRF), which is believed to be NO (Fig. 2.12). Guanylyl cyclase is activated by NO, thus increasing the levels of cGMP and activating protein kinase G. Protein kinase G inhibits contraction by phosphorylating contractile proteins.

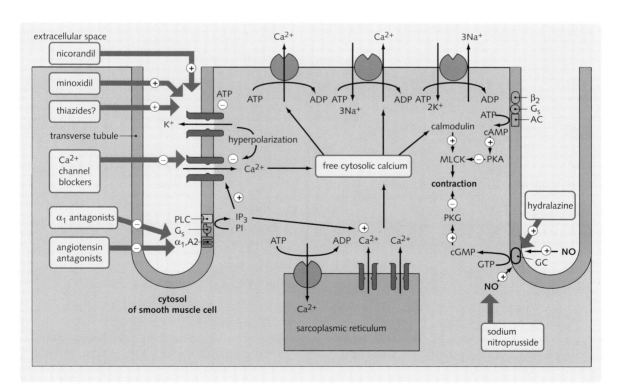

Fig. 2.12 Drugs affecting vascular tone. (AC, adenyl cyclase; $α_1$, $α_1$-adrenoceptor; A2, angiotensin II; $β_2$, $β_2$-adrenoceptor; GC, guanylyl cyclase; GS, stimulatory G-protein; IP_3, inositol triphosphate; MLCK, myosin light-chain kinase; NO, nitric oxide; PLC, phospholipase C; PI, phosphatidylinositol; PKA, protein kinase A; PKG, protein kinase G.)

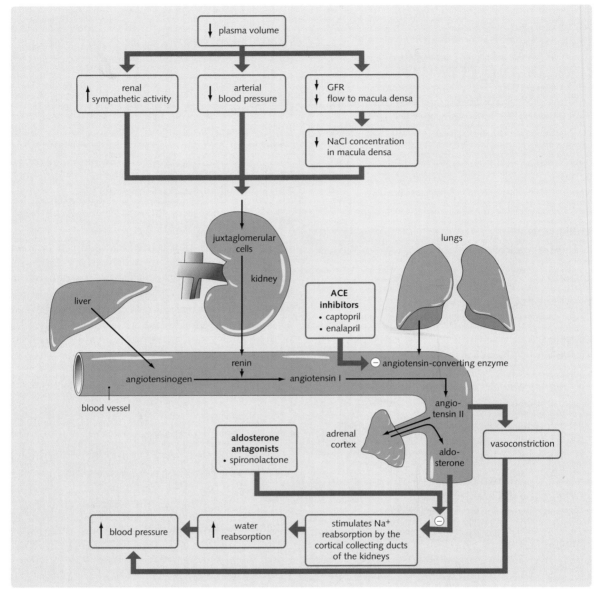

Fig. 2.13 Renin–angiotensin system and ACE inhibitors. (GFR, glomerular filtration rate.)

Renin–angiotensin system

A decrease in plasma volume results in the activation of the renin–angiotensin system (RAS) (Ch. 7), which is summarized in Figure 2.13.

Angiotensin-converting enzyme (ACE) catalyses the production of angiotensin II. The effects of angiotensin II are:

- Potent vasoconstriction (40 times as potent as noradrenaline)

- Release of noradrenaline
- Stimulates the secretion of aldosterone.

ACE also catalyses the inactivation of bradykinin, which is an endogenous vasodilator.

Aldosterone is a steroid that induces the synthesis of sodium channels and Na^+/K^+ ATPase pumps in the luminal membrane of the cortical collecting ducts. This results in a greater amount of sodium and consequently water being reabsorbed, thus increasing the blood volume and pressure.

Certain renal diseases and renal artery occlusion will cause activation of the RAS and result in the development of hypertension.

Hypertension

Normal blood pressure is generally regarded as 120/80 mmHg (systolic pressure/diastolic pressure). Hypertension is defined as a diastolic arterial pressure greater than 90 mmHg, or a systolic arterial pressure greater than 140 mmHg. The condition can be fatal if left untreated, as it greatly increases the risk of thrombosis, stroke and renal failure.

Three factors determine blood pressure:

- Blood volume
- Cardiac output
- Peripheral vascular resistance.

'Primary' or 'essential' hypertension accounts for 90–95% of all cases of hypertension. This has no known cause, but is associated with:

- Age (40+)
- Obesity
- Physical inactivity
- Smoking and alcohol consumption
- Genetic predisposition.

'Secondary hypertension' accounts for the remaining 5–10% of cases of hypertension. The cause is usually one of the following:

- Renal disease, which activates the RAS
- Endocrine disease, e.g. phaeochromocytoma, steroid-secreting tumour of the adrenal cortex, adrenaline-secreting tumour of the adrenal medulla.

Treatment of hypertension

The treatment of hypertension is aimed at various targets; these are summarized in Fig. 2.14.

Vasodilators

Angiotensin-converting enzyme (ACE) inhibitors

Captopril, enalapril, lisinopril and ramipril are examples of ACE inhibitors.

Mechanism of action: ACE inhibitors cause inhibition of ACE with consequent reduced angiotensin II and aldosterone levels (Fig. 2.13), and increased bradykinin levels. This therefore causes vasodilatation with a consequent reduction in peripheral resistance, little change in heart rate and cardiac output and reduced sodium retention.

Route of administration: Oral.

Indications: Hypertension, heart failure and renal dysfunction (especially in diabetic patients to slow progression of diabetic or reduced renal functional nephropathy).

Contraindications: Pregnancy, renovascular disease, aortic stenosis.

Adverse effects: Characteristic cough, hypotension, dizziness and headache, diarrhoea, muscle cramps.

Therapeutic notes: First-dose hypotension is relatively common, and should ideally be given just before bed.

Angiotensin-II receptor antagonists

Losartan and valsartan are examples of angiotensin-II receptor antagonists.

Mr Gill is a 41-year-old African Caribbean, who presents to his GP with increasing frequency of headaches. He has noticed recent visual disturbances as well. His GP notes he smokes about 15 cigarettes per day, undertakes very little exercise and mainly eats fast foods. Urine dipstick was immediately carried out and revealed significant proteinuria. On questioning, Mr Gill denies any family history of diabetes and a random blood glucose test gave a score of 4.7, within the normal range. However, his resting blood pressure was found to be 210/140, which is severely elevated and indicative of malignant hypertension. Fundoscopy

also revealed hypertensive changes (silver wiring and cotton wool spots). He is admitted for immediate treatment.

He was given the long-acting calcium-channel blocker, amlodipine. Two days later, bendroflumethiazide (a thiazide diuretic) was also added to his management. These two drug classes have been shown to be particularly effective in African Caribbeans with hypertension because of their effect on salt sensitivity and volume expansion. He is also advised to stop smoking, eat a healthier salt-restricted diet and do more exercise.

Fig. 2.14 Advantages and disadvantages of drugs used in hypertension with respect to associated conditions

	Diuretics	β-Blocker	ACE inhibitor/angiotensin II receptor antagonist	Calcium-channel blockers	α-Blocker
Diabetes	Care[a]	Care[a]	Yes	Yes	Yes
Gout	No	Yes	Yes	Yes	Yes
Dyslipidaemia	Care[b]	Care[b]	Yes	Yes	Yes
Ischaemic heart disease	Yes	Yes	Yes	Yes	Yes
Heart failure	Yes	Care[c]	Yes	Care[d]	Yes
Asthma	Yes	No	Yes	Yes	Yes
Peripheral vascular disease	Yes	Care	Care[e]	Yes	Yes
Renal artery stenosis	Yes	Care	No	Yes	Yes
Pregnancy	Caution	Not in late pregnancy	No	No	Caution

[a]Diuretics may aggravate diabetes: β-blockers worsen glucose intolerance and mask symptoms of hypoglycaemia.
[b]Both diuretics and β-blockers disturb the lipid profile.
[c]There is some evidence for beneficial effects of some β-blockers when used cautiously in heart failure.
[d]Verapamil and diltiazem may exacerbate heart failure, although amlodipine appears to be safe.
[e]Patients with peripheral vascular disease may also have renal artery stenosis; therefore ACE inhibitors should be used cautiously.
Reproduced from Kumar and Clark, Clinical Medicine, 4th edn. WB Saunders 1998

Mechanism of action: Angiotensin-II receptor antagonists cause inhibition at the angiotensin-II receptor (see Fig. 2.12), resulting in vasodilatation with a consequent reduction in peripheral resistance.

Route of administration: Oral.

Indications: Hypertension.

Contraindications: Pregnancy, breastfeeding. Caution in renal artery stenosis and aortic stenosis.

Adverse effects: Cough (less common than with ACE inhibitors), orthostatic hypotension, dizziness, headache and fatigue, hyperkalaemia and rash.

Calcium antagonists
Nifedipine has more effect upon vascular tone than diltiazem or verapamil, which are more cardioselective (Fig. 2.12, p. 37).

α₁-Adrenoceptor antagonists
Prazosin and doxazosin are examples of α₁-adrenoceptor antagonists.

Mechanism of action: α_1-Adrenoceptor antagonists cause inhibition of α_1-adrenoceptor-mediated vasoconstriction – thus reducing peripheral resistance and venous pressure (Fig. 2.12). They also lower plasma low-density lipoprotein (LDL) cholesterol levels, very-low-density lipoprotein (VLDL) levels, and triglyceride (TGA) levels, and increase high-density lipoprotein (HDL) cholesterol levels, thus reducing the risk of coronary artery disease.

Route of administration: Oral.

Indications: Hypertension (especially in patients with CCF), prostate hyperplasia (reduced bladder and prostate resistance), coronary artery disease.

Contraindications: Prazosin should not be given to people with CCF due to aortic stenosis.

Adverse effects: Postural hypotension, dizziness, headache and fatigue, weakness, palpitations, nausea.

Hydralazine
Hydralazine is a second- or third-line drug for the treatment of mild to moderate hypertension.

Mechanism of action: Hydralazine effects are unclear, though it appears to interfere with the action of inositol triphosphate in vascular smooth muscle, thereby reducing peripheral resistance and blood pressure (Fig. 2.12).

Route of administration: Oral, intravenous.

Indications: Moderate to severe hypertension. Also used in conjunction with β-blockers and thiazides in hypertensive emergencies, and in hypertensive pregnant women.

Contraindications: Idiopathic systemic lupus erythematosus, severe tachycardia.

Adverse effects: Tachycardia, fluid retention, nausea and vomiting, headache.

Minoxidil

Owing to its adverse effects, minoxidil is the drug of last resort in the long-term treatment of hypertension.

Mechanism of action: Minoxidil activates vascular smooth muscle ATP-sensitive potassium channels, resulting in hyperpolarization of the cell membrane and consequent reduced calcium entry through L-type channels (see Fig. 2.12). The overall effect is inhibition of smooth muscle contraction, and subsequent vasodilatation.

Route of administration: Oral for hypertension; topical cream for baldness.

Indications: Severe hypertension, baldness.

Contraindications: Phaeochromocytoma, porphyria.

Adverse effects: Hirsutism (limits use in women), sodium and water retention, tachycardia, cardiotoxicity.

Therapeutic notes: Though unrelated chemically, the drug diazoxide acts in a similar fashion to minoxidil, and activates potassium channels, resulting in vasodilatation.

Sodium nitroprusside

Mechanism of action: Sodium nitroprusside is a prodrug that spontaneously decomposes into NO inside smooth muscle cells. NO activates guanylyl cyclase, thus increasing intracellular cGMP levels, and causing vasodilatation (Fig. 2.12).

Route of administration: Intravenous.

Indications: Sodium nitroprusside is given in hypertensive crises, and for controlled hypotension in surgery, and in heart failure.

Contraindications: Sodium nitroprusside should not be given to patients with severe hepatic impairment, vitamin B_{12} deficiency, Leber's optic atrophy.

Adverse effects: Headache and dizziness, nausea, abdominal pain, palpitations, retrosternal discomfort.

Therapeutic notes: Sodium nitroprusside is broken down in the body to thiocyanate, which has a half-life of only a few minutes, though prolonged exposure to nitroprusside and thiocyanate can result in thiocyanate toxicity (weakness, nausea and inhibition of thyroid function).

The commoner adverse effects of the vasodilating drugs are hypotension and headache, both of which directly result from reducing peripheral vascular resistance.

Diuretic drugs

Diuretics used in hypertension include:

- Thiazides
- Loop diuretics
- Potassium-sparing diuretics.

See Chapter 7 for details of each of these drugs.

Mechanism of action: The antihypertensive action of diuretic drugs does not seem to correlate with their diuretic activity: loop diuretics are powerful diuretics but only moderate antihypertensives while thiazides are moderate diuretics but powerful antihypertensives.

It has recently been suggested that the anti-hypertensive effects of diuretics (especially the thiazides) are not necessarily due to their diuretic effect, but rather may be due to activation of ATP-regulated potassium channels in resistance arterioles, with a mechanism of action similar to that of nicorandil (p. 36) and minoxidil. This causes hyperpolarization, and thus inhibition of calcium entry into vascular smooth muscle cells with consequent vasodilatation and reduced peripheral vascular resistance (Fig. 2.12).

Centrally acting antihypertensive drugs

Clonidine, methyldopa and moxonidine are examples of centrally acting antihypertensive drugs. These agents are second- or third-line drugs in the treatment of hypertension

Mechanism of action: Centrally acting antihypertensive drugs are α_2-adrenoceptor agonists. The activation of presynaptic α_2-adrenoceptors causes inhibition of noradrenaline release and consequent vasodilatation. The activation of postsynaptic α_2-adrenoceptors causes vasoconstriction, although presynaptic effects dominate.

Centrally acting anti-hypertensive drugs reduce the activity of the vasomotor centre in the brain, causing reduced sympathetic activity and subsequent vasodilatation. They also reduce heart rate and cardiac output.

Route of administration: Oral. Clonidine can be given by intravenous infusion.

Indications: Hypertensive patients when first-line antihypertensive agents are ineffective or contraindicated. Methyldopa is safe for hypertension in pregnancy, asthmatic patients and those with heart failure.

Contraindications: Methyldopa should not be given to people with depression, liver disease or phaeochromocytoma.

Adverse effects: Dry mouth, sedation, orthostatic hypotension, male sexual dysfunction, galactorrhoea. Methyldopa can cause diffuse parenchymal liver injury, fever and, rarely, haemolytic anaemia. Clonidine can cause a withdrawal hypertensive crisis on stopping treatment.

Phaeochromocytoma

Phaeochromocytoma is a rare endocrine tumour, most commonly of the adrenal gland. These tumours can secrete adrenaline and various intermediates in its biosynthesis. These vasoactive compounds result in the clinical signs and symptoms of phaeochromocytomas, which include facial flushing, sweating, breathlessness, anxiety, tachycardia and paroxysmal hypertension.

Medical management of phaeochromocytoma-induced hypertension relies on the powerful α-adrenoceptor antagonist phenoxybenzamine. α-Adrenoceptor blockade reduces peripheral vascular resistance and lowers blood pressure. The use of β-adrenoceptor antagonists is dangerous, as tumour-secreted sympathomimetics act unopposed on α-adrenoceptors, increasing both peripheral vascular resistance and blood pressure.

Phenoxybenzamine

Mechanism of action: Phenoxybenzamine antagonises α-adrenoceptors in the vascular smooth muscles, resulting in vasodilatation.

Route of administration: Oral, intravenous.

Indications: Hypertensive episodes in phaeochromocytoma.

Contraindications: History of cerebrovascular events, post-myocardial infarction.

Adverse effects: Postural hypotension, tachycardia, nasal congestion.

Therapeutic notes: Phentolamine is another powerful α-adrenoceptor antagonist which can be used in phaeochromocytoma, though has a much shorter half-life, and is commonly used prior to, and during surgery to excise the tumour.

Vasoconstrictors and the management of shock

Shock

Shock is a state of circulatory collapse, characterized by an arterial blood pressure unable to maintain adequate tissue perfusion. Shock is a life-threatening condition.

The body responds inappropriately to shock, releasing mediators such as histamine, prostaglandins, bradykinin and serotonin, which cause capillary dilatation and increased capillary permeability. This further reduces blood pressure and cardiac output.

Signs of shock include:

- Very low arterial blood pressure
- A weak, rapid pulse
- Cold, pale, sweaty skin
- Rapid breathing
- Dry mouth
- Reduced urine output
- Anxiousness.

Causes of shock include:

- Haemorrhage
- Burns
- Dehydration
- Severe vomiting or diarrhoea
- Bacterial septicaemia
- Myocardial infarction
- Pulmonary embolism.

Types of shock include:

- Hypovolemic – caused by a reduction in the circulating blood volume.
- Cardiogenic – reduced cardiac output due to 'pump failure'.
- Septic – caused by massive vasodilatation.
- Anaphylactic – a severe allergic reaction, in which there is a massive generalized release of vasodilating mediators.
- Spinal – disruption of neuronal control on vascular tone and cardiac output.

Management of shock

The medical management of shock ultimately depends upon its underlying cause, e.g. if a child is shocked due to chronic diarrhoea and vomiting, fluid and electrolyte replacement is most appropriate management.

The following drugs are useful in restoring blood pressure and tissue perfusion, but on the whole do not address the underlying cause of the different types of shock.

Sympathomimetic amines

Examples of sympathomimetic amines include adrenaline, noradrenaline, phenylephrine and ephedrine.

Sympathomimetic amines raise blood pressure at the expense of vital organs such as the kidneys, and raise peripheral resistance, which is already high in patients with shock.

Mechanism of action: Adrenaline and noradrenaline are agonists at both α- and β-adrenoceptors, and phenylephrine is an α_1-adrenoceptor agonist. Ephedrine is a β-adrenoceptor agonist and causes noradrenaline release. These drugs work either by activating α-adrenoceptors which then activate phospholipase C, causing vasoconstriction and a consequent increase in arterial blood pressure, or by activating β-adrenoceptors which then activate adenylyl cyclase, causing an increased heart rate, increased cardiac contractility and vasodilatation.

Route of administration: Parenterally, commonly intravenously.

Indications: Shock, acute hypotension and reversal of hypotension caused by spinal or epidural anaesthesia. Adrenaline is used in cardiac arrest and anaphylaxis.

Contraindications: Sympathomimetic amines should not be given in pregnancy or in people who have hypertension.

Adverse effects: Tachycardia, anxiety, insomnia, arrhythmias, dry mouth, cold extremities.

Therapeutic notes: In a cardiac arrest, adrenaline is used at a concentration of 1 mg/10 mL (1:10 000) intravenously, whereas in anaphylaxis, adrenaline is used at a concentration of 1 mg/1 mL (1:1000) intramuscularly.

Dopamine and dobutamine

Mechanism of action: Dopamine is a precursor of noradrenaline. It activates dopamine receptors and α- and β-adrenoceptors. When administered by intravenous infusion, dopamine acts on:

- Dopamine receptors, causing vasodilatation in the kidneys at low doses
- α_1-adrenoceptors, causing vasoconstriction in other vasculature
- β_1-adrenoceptors, causing positive inotropic and chronotropic effects.

Dobutamine has no effect on dopaminergic receptors, but does activate β_1-adrenoceptors.

If renal perfusion is not impaired, dobutamine and dopamine are a more appropriate means of treating shock than α-adrenoceptor agonists. This form of treatment maintains renal perfusion, and inhibits the activation of the RAS.

Route of administration: Intravenous.

Indications: CCF (emergencies only), cardiogenic shock, septic shock, hypovolaemic shock, cardiomyopathy, cardiac surgery.

Contraindications: Tachyarrhythmias; dopamine is contraindicated in people with phaeochromocytoma.

Adverse effects: Tachycardia and hypertension; dopamine causes nausea and vomiting and hypotension.

Therapeutic notes: Although low doses of dopamine cause vasodilatation, high doses cause vasoconstriction and may exacerbate heart failure.

Vasopressin (ADH) and desmopressin

Vasopressin (antidiuretic hormone; ADH), and desmopressin are examples of antidiuretic peptides.

Vasopressin is short acting ($t_{1/2}$ = 10 minutes) while desmopressin is longer acting ($t_{1/2}$ = 75 minutes).

Mechanism of action: Antidiuretic peptides activate V_1 receptors on smooth muscle cells, which stimulate phospholipase C, causing contraction. They also activate V_2 receptors on the tubular cells of the kidneys, which stimulate adenylyl cyclase and thereby increase the permeability of these cells to water, and reduce sodium and water excretion. Vasopressin has a much greater affinity for V_2 receptors than V_1 receptors whereas desmopressin is selective for V_1 receptors.

Route of administration: Oral, intravenous, intranasal.

Indications: Pituitary diabetes insipidus. The antidiuretic peptides are no longer used in the management of shock, though their pharmacology is both academically interesting and a potential target for future drugs.

Contraindications: Vascular disease, chronic nephritis.

Adverse effects: Fluid retention, nausea, pallor, abdominal cramps, belching. They may induce anginal attacks (due to coronary vasoconstriction).

Corticosteroids

The use of corticosteroids in septic shock, remains controversial, though they are also given by intravenous injection in the treatment of anaphylactic shock as an adjunct to adrenaline (Ch. 6).

It is possible to distinguish between the types of shock clinically:

- Hypovolaemic – low jugular venous pressure (JVP), cool, clammy peripheries, confusion/restlessness.
- Cardiogenic – raised JVP, cool, clammy peripheries, anxiousness/agitation.
- Septic – warm, sweaty peripheries, pyrexia, nausea.
- Anaphylactic – warm peripheries, ? ureterica, nausea.
- Spinal – history of trauma or spinal anaesthesia.
- Tachycardia, hypotension and tachypnoea will feature in all types of shock.

Lipoprotein circulation and atherosclerosis

Lipoproteins provide a means of transporting lipids (cholesterol, triglycerides and phospholipids), which are insoluble in the blood, around the body.

Four classes of lipoproteins exist. These differ in size, density, constituent lipids and type of surface protein (apoprotein). These lipoproteins are:

- High-density lipoproteins (HDL)
- Low-density lipoproteins (LDL)
- Very-low-density lipoproteins (VLDL)
- Chylomicrons.

Lipid transport in the blood is via two pathways, exogenous and endogenous, which are summarized in Fig. 2.15.

In the exogenous pathway (numbers refer to those in Fig. 2.15):

1. Diet-derived lipid breakdown leads to the formation of chylomicrons.
2. Lipoprotein lipase (LPL), found in the endothelium of extrahepatic tissues, hydrolyses the triglycerides in chylomicrons to glycerol and free fatty acids (FFAs), for use by the tissues.
3. The chylomicron remnant is taken up by the liver.
4. The liver secretes cholesterol and bile acids into the gut, creating an enterohepatic circulation.

In the endogenous pathway (numbers refer to those in Fig. 2.15):

1. The liver secretes VLDLs, the components of which may be derived either endogenously or from the diet.
2. Lipoprotein lipase (LPL), found in the endothelium of extrahepatic tissues, hydrolyses triglycerides in the VLDLs to glycerol and FFAs, for use by the tissues, and leaves LDL.
3. LDL is then taken up by the liver and extrahepatic tissues.
4. HDL is secreted by the liver into the plasma, where it is modified by lecithin cholesterol acyltransferase (LCAT) and uptake of cholesterol from the tissues. LCAT transfers cholesterol esters to LDLs and VLDLs.

Hyperlipidaemias

Hyperlipidaemias are characterized by markedly elevated plasma triglycerides, cholesterol, and lipoprotein concentrations.

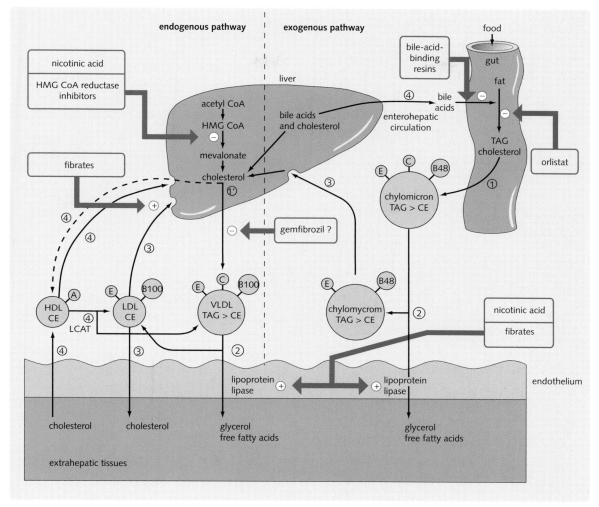

Fig. 2.15 Endogenous and exogenous pathways of lipid transport. (CE, cholesterol ester; HDL, high density lipoprotein; LCAT, lecithin cholesterol acyltransferase; TAG, triacylglycerol; VLDL, very low density lipoproteins; numbers refer to steps in pathways, see p. 44.)

Cholesterol is deposited in various tissues:

- Deposition in arterial plaques results in atherosclerosis, which leads to heart attacks, strokes and peripheral vascular disease.
- Deposition in tendons and skin results in xanthomas.

Primary

Primary hyperlipidaemias are genetic, and numerous types exist.

Secondary

Secondary hyperlipidaemias are the consequences of other conditions such as:

- Diabetes
- Liver disease
- Nephrotic syndrome
- Renal failure
- Alcoholism
- Hypothyroidism
- Oestrogen administration.

Treatment (lipid-lowering drugs)

HMG CoA reductase inhibitors ('statins')

Atorvastatin, pravastatin and simvastatin are examples of 3-hydroxy-3-methylglutaryl co-enzyme A (HMG CoA) reductase inhibitors. These drugs have been shown to reduce blood cholesterol by up to 35% in some patients.

HMG CoA reductase inhibitors can reduce the risk of dying from a coronary event by up to nearly half.

Mechanism of action: Statins reversibly inhibit the enzyme HMG CoA reductase, which catalyses the rate-limiting step in the synthesis of cholesterol: HMG CoA → mevalonic acid → cholesterol (Fig. 2.15). The decrease in cholesterol synthesis also increases the number of LDL receptors, thus decreasing LDL levels.

Route of administration: Oral.

Indications: Hyperlipidaemia resistant to dietary control, as part of secondary prevention in patients with serum cholesterol greater than 5.5 mmol/L (though this value will vary depending upon local policy).

Contraindications: Pregnancy, breastfeeding, liver disease.

Adverse effects: Reversible myositis (rare), constipation or diarrhoea, abdominal pain and flatulence, nausea and headache, fatigue, insomnia, rash.

Fibrates
Fibrates include bezafibrate, ciprofibrate and gemfibrozil. These are broad-spectrum lipid-modulating agents that are ineffective in patients with elevated cholesterol but normal triglyceride concentrations.

Mechanism of action: Fibrates work in several ways, as follows: stimulation of lipoprotein lipase (Fig. 2.15), thus reducing the triglyceride content of VLDLs and chylomicrons; stimulation of hepatic LDL clearance, by increasing hepatic LDL uptake (Fig. 2.15); reduction of plasma triglyceride, LDL, and VLDL concentrations; and increase of HDL-cholesterol concentration (except bezafibrate). Gemfibrozil decreases lipolysis and may decrease VLDL secretion.

Route of administration: Oral.

Indications: Hyperlipidaemia unresponsive to dietary control.

Contraindications: Gallbladder disease, severe renal or hepatic impairment, hypoalbuminaemia, pregnancy, breastfeeding.

Adverse effects: Side-effects of fibrates include:

- Myositis-like syndrome (especially if renal function is impaired)
- Gastrointestinal disturbances
- Dermatitis, pruritus, rash and urticaria
- Impotence
- Headache, dizziness, blurred vision.

> Changing a patient's diet alone can lower serum cholesterol, and should be the first-line treatment option in mild to moderate hyperlipidaemia.

Nicotinic acid
The side-effects of nicotinic acid limit its use in the treatment of hyperlipidaemias. Nicotinic acid has been shown to reduce the incidence of coronary artery disease.

Mechanism of action: Nicotinic acid has the following effects: it inhibits cholesterol synthesis (Fig. 2.15), thereby decreasing VLDL and thus LDL production; it stimulates lipoprotein lipase, thus reducing the triglyceride content of VLDLs and chylomicrons; it increases HDL-cholesterol; it increases the levels of tissue plasminogen activator (p. 48); and it decreases the levels of plasma fibrinogen (p. 48).

Route of administration: Oral.

Indications: Hyperlipidaemias unresponsive to other measures.

Contraindications: Pregnancy, breastfeeding.

Adverse effects: Flushing, dizziness, headache, palpitations, nausea and vomiting, pruritus.

Bile acid binding resins
Colestyramine and colestipol have been shown to decrease the rate of mortality from coronary artery disease.

Mechanism of action: Basic anion exchange resins act by binding bile acids in the intestine (Fig. 2.15), thus preventing their reabsorption and promoting hepatic conversion of cholesterol into bile acids. This increases hepatic LDL receptor activity, thus increasing the breakdown of LDL-cholesterol. Plasma LDL-cholesterol is therefore lowered.

Route of administration: Oral.

Indications: Bile acid binding resins are especially useful when elevated cholesterol is due to a high low-density lipoprotein concentration.

Colestyramine is used in the primary prevention of coronary heart disease in men aged 35–59 years with primary hypercholesterolaemia. It also relieves pruritus associated with partial biliary obstruction and primary biliary cirrhosis.

Contraindications: Complete biliary obstruction.

Adverse effects: Bile acid binding resins are not absorbed, and therefore have very few systemic side-effects. Side-effects include nausea and vomiting, constipation, heartburn, abdominal pain and flatulence, and aggravation of hypertriglyceridaemia. They may interfere with the absorption of fat-soluble vitamins and certain drugs.

Therapeutic regimen: To avoid interference with their absorption, other drugs should not be taken within 1 hour before or 3–4 hours after colestyramine or colestipol administration.

Other lipid-lowering drugs
Fish oils rich in omega-3 marine triglycerides can be useful in the treatment of severe hypertriglyceridaemia, though may sometimes worsen hypercholesteraemia. They role in clinical practice remains to be thoroughly ascertained.

Ispaghula husk is taken orally, and is presumed to act by binding bile acids, preventing their reabsorption, and is potentially useful in patients with hypercholesterolaemia but not hypertriglyceridaemia.

HAEMOSTASIS AND THROMBOSIS

Basic concepts

Haemostasis is the cessation of bleeding from damaged blood vessels. If haemostasis is defective or unable to cope with blood loss from larger vessels, blood may accumulate in the tissues. This accumulated blood is called a haematoma.

Three stages are involved in haemostasis. These are:

- Blood vessel constriction
- Formation of a platelet plug
- Formation of a clot.

Blood vessel constriction

The first response to a severed blood vessel is contraction of the smooth muscle of the vessel. This is mediated by the release of thromboxane A_2 and other substances from platelets.

Blood vessel constriction slows the flow of blood through the vessel, thus reducing the pressure, and pushes opposing surfaces of the vessel together. In very small vessels this results in permanent closure of the vessel, but in most cases blood vessel constriction is insufficient for this to occur.

Platelet plug formation

Exposure to the collagen underlying the vessel endothelium, as occurs during vessel injury, allows platelets to adhere to the collagen by binding to von Willebrand's factor. This factor, secreted by the platelets and endothelium, binds to the exposed collagen; platelets then bind to this complex.

Release of ADP, serotonin, thromboxane A_2 and other substances by the platelets causes the latter to aggregate, while fibrin acts to bind them together. The synthesis and release of prostacyclin by the intact endothelium inhibits platelet aggregation and acts to limit the extent of the platelet plug.

Intact endothelial cells also produce NO, a potent vasodilator and inhibitor of platelet aggregation.

Clot formation

Blood coagulation is the conversion of liquid blood into a solid gel, known as a clot. A clot:

- Consists of a meshwork of fibrin within which blood cells are trapped
- Functions to reinforce the platelet plug.

Fibrin is formed from its precursor fibrinogen, through the action of an enzyme called thrombin.

The formation of thrombin occurs via two distinct pathways, the intrinsic and the extrinsic pathways, which together are known as the coagulation cascade. Both pathways involve the conversion of inactive factors into active enzymes, which then go on to catalyse the conversion of other factors into enzymes, and so on (Fig. 2.16).

The extrinsic pathway is thus termed because the component needed for its initiation is contained outside the blood. Tissue factor binds factor VII on exposure of blood to subendothelial cells, and converts it to its active form, VIIa. This enzyme then catalyses the activation of factors X and IX.

Fig. 2.16 Effects of heparin, vitamin K and fibrinolytic drugs on the coagulation cascade. (Factor III, factor/tissue thromboplastin.)

The intrinsic pathway is thus termed because its components are contained in the blood. It merges with the extrinsic pathway at the step prior to thrombin activation.

The thrombin formed stimulates the activation of factors XI, VIII and V, and thus acts as a form of positive feedback.

Three naturally occurring anticoagulants limit the extent of clot formation. These are:

- Tissue factor pathway inhibitor, which binds to the tissue factor–VIIa complex, and inhibits its actions
- Protein C, which is activated by thrombin, and inactivates factors VII and V
- Antithrombin III, which is activated by heparin, and inactivates thrombin and other factors.

Fibrinolysis

The fibrinolytic or thrombolytic system functions to dissolve a clot once repair of the vessel is under way.

Plasmin digests fibrin. It is formed from plasminogen through the action of plasminogen activators, the best example of which is tissue plasminogen activator (tPA).

Thrombosis

Thrombosis is the pathological formation of a clot known as a thrombus, which may cause occlusion within blood vessels or the heart, and result in death. Thrombosis causes:

- Arterial occlusion – which may lead to myocardial infarction, stroke and peripheral ischaemia.

- Venous occlusion – which may lead to deep venous thrombosis and pulmonary embolism.

Mr Patel is 50 years old with a body mass index of 31, who presented to casualty with central crushing chest pain, shortness of breath and sweating. He is a longstanding smoker with a 60-pack year history and his younger brother recently died from a stroke associated with significant vascular disease. ECG showed ST segment elevation (a recognized ECG pattern), which combined with the history is highly suggestive of myocardial infarction.

He was given oxygen, aspirin (antithrombotic agent) to prevent further platelet aggregation, morphine for pain relief and the anti-ischaemic vasodilating spray (glyceryl trinitrate). To decrease ischaemia, he was then given atenolol intravenously, which acts by decreasing cardiac workload and therefore oxygen demand as well as causing vasodilatation. He was also given the thrombolytic streptokinase to dissolve any clots that may have caused the myocardial infarction.

Arterial thrombi form because of endothelial injury, which is in turn the result of underlying arterial wall pathology, such as atherosclerosis.

Venous and atrial thrombi tend to form as a result of blood stasis, allowing the build-up of platelets and fibrin. People with hypercoagulability, due to a lack of one or more of the naturally occurring anticoagulants, are particularly susceptible.

Arterial thrombi consist mainly of platelets, whereas venous thrombi consist mainly of fibrin.

Management of disorders of haemostasis

Bleeding disorders

Hereditary bleeding disorders are rare. Haemophilia is a genetic disorder in which excessive bleeding occurs, owing to the absence of factor VIII (haemophilia A) or IX (haemophilia B). Von Willebrand's disease is characterized by abnormal bruising and mucosal bleeding.

Acquired bleeding disorders may be due to liver disease, vitamin K deficiency, or anticoagulant drugs.

Caution should be taken when using the following drugs in patients with thromboembolic disease.

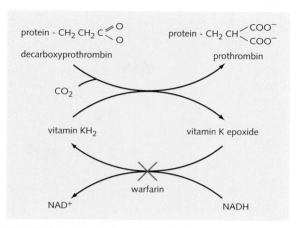

Fig. 2.17 Role of vitamin K in prothrombin formation. Warfarin inhibits the reduction of vitamin K epoxide.

Vitamin K

Mechanism of action: Vitamin K is needed for the post-transcriptional γ-carboxylation of glutamic acid residues of prothrombin (factor II) and clotting factors VII, IX and X by the liver (Fig. 2.17). Vitamin K is also necessary for normal calcification of bone.

Route of administration: Oral, intramuscular, intravenous.

Indications: Vitamin K is used as an antidote to the effects of oral anticoagulants, and in patients with biliary obstruction or liver disease, where Vitamin K deficiency may be a problem. It is also used after prolonged treatment with antibiotics that inhibit the formation of vitamin K by intestinal bacteria, and as prophylaxis against hypoprothrombinaemia in the newborn.

Adverse effects: Side-effects of vitamin K include haemolytic anaemia and hyperbilirubinaemia in the newborn.

Protamine

Mechanism of action: Protamine is a strongly basic protein, which forms an inactive complex with heparin, and as such is used in patients in whom heparin treatment has resulted in haemorrhage. High doses of protamine appear to have anticoagulant effects through an unknown mechanism.

Route of administration: Intravenous.

Indications: Haemorrhage secondary to heparinization.

Adverse effects: Nausea, vomiting, flushing, hypotension.

Clotting factors
Deficient clotting factors can be replaced by the administration of fresh plasma. Factors VIII and IX are available as freeze-dried concentrates.

Mechanism of action: All clotting factors are necessary for normal blood coagulation.

Route of administration: Intravenous.

Indications: Haemophilia; antidote to the effects of oral anticoagulants.

Adverse effects: Allergic reactions, including fevers and chills.

Desmopressin
Desmopressin is a synthetic analogue of vasopressin.

Mechanism of action: Desmopressin causes the release of factor VIII. Desmopressin is also used in diabetes insipidus, as it has antidiuretic effects.

Route of administration: Parenteral.

Indications: Desmopressin is given for mild factor VIII deficiency, and in the treatment of diabetes insipidus.

Adverse effects: Fluid retention, hyponatraemia, and headache, nausea and vomiting.

The liver is important in coagulation as it is the site at which many of the clotting factors are produced.
  It also produces bile salts necessary for the absorption of vitamin K, which is needed by the liver to produce prothrombin and clotting factors VII, IX and X.

Anticoagulants

Vitamin K antagonists
Warfarin, nicoumalone and phenindione are examples of vitamin K antagonists.

Mechanism of action: Vitamin K antagonists block the reduction of vitamin K epoxide, which is necessary for its action as a co-factor in the synthesis of factors II, VII, IX and X (see Fig. 2.16).

Route of administration: Oral.

Indications: Prophylaxis and treatment of deep vein thrombosis and pulmonary embolism, the prophylaxis of embolization in atrial fibrillation and rheumatic disease, and in patients with prosthetic heart valves.

Contraindications: Cerebral thrombosis, peripheral arterial occlusion, peptic ulcers, hypertension, pregnancy.

Adverse effects: Haemorrhage.

Therapeutic notes: The onset of action of vitamin K antagonists takes several hours, owing to the time needed for the degradation of factors that have already been carboxylated ($t_{1/2}$: VII = 6 hours, IX = 24 hours, X = 40 hours, II = 60 hours).

Heparin and the low-molecular-weight heparins (LMWHs)
Mechanism of action: Heparin activates antithrombin III, which limits blood clotting by inactivating thrombin and factor X. Heparin also inhibits platelet aggregation, possibly as a result of inhibiting thrombin. LMWHs are simply fragments of heparin which exhibit very similar activity to heparin. LMWHs are used more frequently because their dosing is more predictable and less frequent.

Route of administration: Intravenous, subcutaneous.

Indications: Treatment of deep vein thrombosis and pulmonary embolism; prophylaxis against postoperative deep vein thrombosis and pulmonary embolism in high-risk patients; myocardial infarction.

Contraindications: Heparin should not be given to patients with haemophilia, thrombocytopenia or peptic ulcers.

Adverse effects: Haemorrhage (treated by stopping therapy or administering a heparin antagonist such as protamine sulphate), skin necrosis, thrombocytopenia, hypersensitivity reactions.

Therapeutic regimen: Heparin is given intravenously by intravenous infusion, or 12-hourly by the subcutaneous route. LMWHs are given as a once-daily subcutaneous injection.

Therapeutic notes: Heparin has an immediate onset and can therefore be used in emergencies.

Hirudins

Mechanism of action: Derived from the medical leech, hirudin, or rather its recombinant derivatives, desirudin and lepirudin, inactivate thrombin.

Route of administration: Subcutaneous, intravenous.

Indications: Desirudin is used in patients with type II (immune) heparin-induced thrombocytopenia. Desirudin is used for prophylaxis of deep-vein thrombosis in patients undergoing hip and knee replacement.

Contraindications: Active bleeding, renal or hepatic impairment.

Adverse effects: Haemorrhage, hypersensitivity reactions.

Antiplatelet agents

Aspirin

Aspirin is acetylsalicylic acid, and originally derived from the willow tree.

Mechanism of action: Aspirin blocks the synthesis of thromboxane A_2 from arachidonic acid in platelets, by acetylating and thus inhibiting the enzyme cyclooxygenase. Thromboxane A_2 stimulates phospholipase C, thus increasing calcium levels and causing platelet aggregation. Aspirin also blocks the synthesis of prostacyclin from endothelial cells, which inhibits platelet aggregation. However, this effect is short lived because endothelial cells, unlike platelets, can synthesize new cyclooxygenase (Fig. 2.18).

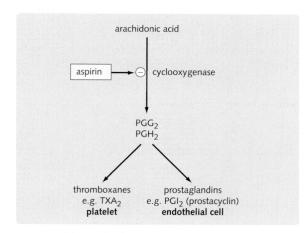

Fig. 2.18 Inhibition of cyclooxygenase by aspirin, leading to a reduction in the formation of thromboxane and prostacyclin. (PG, prostaglandin; PGI_2, prostacyclin; T_xA_2, thromboxane A_2.)

Route of administration: Oral.

Indications: Prevention and treatment of myocardial infarction and ischaemic stroke. Aspirin is also used as an analgesic and an anti-inflammatory agent (Ch. 10).

Contraindications: Children under 12 years of age (risk of Reye's syndrome), during breastfeeding, haemophilia, peptic ulcers or known hypersensitivity reactions.

Adverse effects: Bronchospasm, gastrointestinal haemorrhage.

Therapeutic regimen: Aspirin at 150 mg daily after myocardial infarction has been shown to decrease mortality significantly. Given on alternate days, aspirin may reduce the incidence of primary myocardial infarction.

Dipyridamole

Mechanism of action: Dipyridamole causes inhibition of the phosphodiesterase enzyme that hydrolyses cAMP. Increased cAMP levels result in decreased calcium levels and inhibition of platelet aggregation.

Route of administration: Oral.

Indications: Dipyridamole is used in conjunction with warfarin and other oral anticoagulants in the prophylaxis against thrombosis associated with prosthetic heart valves.

Adverse effects: Hypotension, nausea, diarrhoea, headache.

Clopidogrel

Mechanism of action: Clopidogrel inhibits activation of the glycoprotein IIb/IIIa receptor on the surface of platelets, which is required for aggregation to occur.

Route of administration: Oral.

Indications: Secondary prevention of cardiovascular and cerebrovascular events.

Adverse effects: Haemorrhage, abdominal discomfort, nausea and vomiting.

Therapeutic notes: If a patient is truly allergic to aspirin, clopidogrel can be used in its place.

Ticlopidine acts in a similar fashion to clopidogrel.

Glycoprotein IIb/IIIa inhibitors

Abciximab is the main drug currently in this class.

Mechanism of action: Abciximab is an antibody fragment directed towards the glycoprotein IIb/IIIa (GPIIb/IIIa) receptor of platelets. Binding and inactivation of the GPIIb/IIIa receptor prevents platelet aggregation.

Route of administration: Intravenous.

Indications: Prevention of ischaemic cardiac complications in patients undergoing percutaneous coronary intervention; short-term prevention of myocardial infarction in patients with unstable angina.

Contraindications: Active bleeding.

Adverse effects: Haemorrhage, nausea, vomiting, hypotension.

Therapeutic notes: Tirofiban and eptifibatide also act by inhibiting the GPIIb/IIIa receptor, though are peptide fragments. As peptides, these agents are potentially antigenic, and should only be used once.

Fibrinolytic agents

Streptokinase
Mechanism of action: Streptokinase forms a complex with, and activates, plasminogen into plasmin, a fibrinolytic enzyme.

Route of administration: Intravenous.

Indications: Life-threatening venous thrombosis, pulmonary embolism, arterial thromboembolism, acute myocardial infarction.

Contraindications: Recent haemorrhage, trauma, surgery, bleeding diathesis, aortic dissection, coma, history of cerebrovascular disease. Consult *BNF* for comprehensive list of contraindications.

Adverse effects: Nausea and vomiting, bleeding.

Therapeutic regimen: Streptokinase is commonly used in conjunction with antiplatelet and antico-agulant drugs.

Streptokinase is derived from haemolytic streptococci, and is thus antigenic. Repeated administration of streptokinase could result in an anaphylaxis-like reaction. If repeated fibrinolytic therapy is needed, the non-antigenic tissue-type plasminogen activators should be employed.

Tissue-type plasminogen activators (tPAs)
Alteplase and reteplase are examples of tPAs.

Mechanism of action: tPAs are tissue-type plasminogen activators.

Route of administration: Intravenous.

Indications: Myocardial infarction, pulmonary embolism.

Contraindications: As for streptokinase.

Adverse effects: Nausea and vomiting, bleeding.

While the administration of a fibrinolytic drug could improve the life expectancy of someone suffering from an acute myocardial infarction, it could also have disastrous effects. There are stringent criteria for administering or not administering fibrinolytic drugs. You should learn these.

Antifibrinolytic agents

Tranexamic acid
Mechanism of action: Tranexamic acid is antifibri-nolytic, inhibiting plasminogen activation and therefore preventing fibrinolysis.

Route of administration: Oral, intravenous.

Indications: Tranexamic acid agents is used for gastrointestinal haemorrhage and conditions in which there is haemorrhage or risk of haemorrhage, e.g. haemophilia, menorrhagia and dental extraction.

Contraindications: Thromboembolic disease.

Adverse effects: Nausea and vomiting, diarrhoea. Thromboembolic events are rare.

Aprotinin
Mechanism of action: Aprotinin inhibits the proteolytic enzymes plasmin and kallikrein, thus inhibiting fibrinolysis.

Route of administration: Intravenous.

Indications: Aprotinin is used when there is a risk of blood loss after open heart surgery, and in hyperplasminaemia.

Adverse effects: Allergy, localized thrombophlebitis.

Etamsylate
Mechanism of action: Etamsylate corrects abnormal platelet adhesion.

Route of administration: Oral, intravenous.

Indications: Etamsylate is used to reduce capillary bleeding and periventricular haemorrhage in premature infants.

Contraindications: Porphyria.

Adverse effects: Nausea, headache, rashes.

THE BLOOD AND FLUID REPLACEMENT

Anaemia

Anaemia is a common problem throughout the world. In the young it is commonly due to nutritional deficiencies (vitamin B_{12}, folate and iron), in fertile women menstrual loss accounts for most cases, and in the elderly, malignancy and renal failure are the commoner causes.

Iron
Ferrous sulphate, ferrous fumarate and ferrous gluconate are the commoner iron salt preparations.

Mechanism of action: Dietary supplementation of iron increases serum iron and stored iron in the liver and bone. Adequate iron is necessary for normal erythropoiesis, as well as for numerous iron-containing proteins.

Route of administration: Oral. Parenteral preparations of iron exist, but are seldom used.

Indications: Iron-deficiency anaemia.

Contraindications: Caution in pregnancy.

Adverse effects: Gastrointestinal irritation, nausea, epigastric pain, altered bowel habits.

Therapeutic notes: Iron overdose or chronic iron overload can be harmful, and either acquired, or inherited in the form of haemochromatosis. The iron-chelating agent desferrioxamine can be given parenterally, which allows iron to be excreted in the urine.

Vitamin B_{12}
Hydroxocobalamin and cyanocobalamin are vitamin B_{12} drug preparations.

Mechanism of action: Vitamin B_{12} is required for DNA synthesis and effective erythropoiesis.

Route of administration: Intramuscular, oral.

Indications: Pernicious anaemia, other macrocytic megaloblastic anaemias.

Contraindications: None.

Adverse effects: Itching, fever, chills, flushing, nausea.

Therapeutic notes: Initial treatment requires regular weekly injections, but once serum vitamin B_{12} is normalized, injections should be given at 3-monthly intervals.

Folate
Folic acid is the form folate is administered.

Mechanism of action: Folate is required for DNA synthesis and effective erythropoiesis.

Route of administration: Oral.

Indications: Macrocytic megaloblastic anaemias, prevention of neural tube defects in pregnancy.

Contraindications: None.

Adverse effects: None.

Therapeutic notes: Since the introduction of folate acid supplements for pregnant women, the rate of neural tube defects in newborn babies has fallen markedly.

Erythropoietin
Epoetin is a recombinant erythropoietin. Erythropoietin is synthesized in the kidney in response to a fall in the oxygen tension of the blood passing through it.

Mechanism of action: Erythropoietin acts upon the bone marrow to stimulate stem cells to divide, to produce cells of the red cell lineage.

Route of administration: Parenteral.

Indications: Anaemia of chronic renal failure, anaemia following cancer chemotherapy, prior to autologous blood donation.

Contraindications: Uncontrolled hypertension.

Adverse effects: Dose-dependant increase in blood pressure and platelet count, influenza-like symptoms.

Therapeutic notes: Erythropoietin often features in the news, as an increased haemoglobin concentration most probably improves an athletes performance, making this drug a potential drug of 'misuse' in sport.

Myeloproliferative disorders

The pharmacological management of the myeloproliferative disorders is outside the remit of this text, although it relies on cytotoxic drugs. Information on these agents should be learnt from a haematology or general medical textbook.

Fluid replacement

Fluid replacement should ideally be achieved orally, though this is often not practical. Intravenous administration of fluids is commonplace in hospital.

- Intravenous fluids are given for many reasons. In trauma they are used to replace blood loss, in septicaemia they are used to raise blood pressure and tissue perfusion, in the unconscious they are used to replace water and electrolytes lost in the urine and via insensible routes.
- There are many types of intravenous fluid. The commoner fluids given intravenously are blood, the crystalloids (sodium chloride (normal saline) and dextrose saline), and the colloids (dextrans and gelatin). Each has its role to play in the management of various conditions. Supplements can be added to intravenous fluids to provide the patient with all their requirements.
- The art of fluid replacement, and fluid management is best learnt from an anaesthetics or general medical textbook. The names and compositions of the various intravenous fluids can be obtained from the *BNF*.

Respiratory system

Objectives

After reading this chapter, you will:

- Be able to describe the characteristics of the main diseases of the respiratory system and their pharmacological management
- Know the main drug categories, their mechanism of action, when they are and are not used, and their adverse effects.

BASIC CONCEPTS

Respiration is the process of exchange of oxygen and carbon dioxide between an organism and its external environment. This principally involves the lungs (see Fig. 3.1 for the whole respiratory system), which possess the largest surface area in the body in contact with the external environment. It is, therefore, expected that the respiratory system has some defences to protect itself against foreign material. These defence mechanisms can be divided into physical (such as coughing or the mucociliary escalator, to remove foreign agents) and immunological (such as enzymes, pulmonary macrophages and lymphoid tissue, to 'disarm' foreign agents). These defence mechanisms can be launched inappropriately or may be insufficient to deal with the triggering agent and thus, disease may occur.

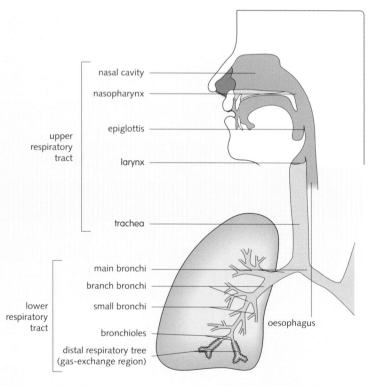

Fig. 3.1 A schematic diagram of the respiratory tract. (From: McGowan et al. *Respiratory System*, 2nd edition. Mosby, London, 2003.)

nasal cavity
nasopharynx
epiglottis
larynx
trachea

upper respiratory tract

main bronchi
branch bronchi
small bronchi
bronchioles
distal respiratory tree (gas-exchange region)
oesophagus

lower respiratory tract

OBSTRUCTIVE AIRWAYS DISEASES

Asthma

Asthma is a chronic inflammatory disease of the bronchiolar airways. It is characterized by recurrent reversible obstruction to airflow causing airflow limitation, airway hyperresponsiveness and inflammation of the bronchi. Asthma may be allergic (extrinsic) or non-allergic (intrinsic), although in practice this distinction makes little difference to the management.

In asthma, smooth muscle that surrounds the bronchi is hyperresponsive to stimuli, and underlying inflammatory changes are present in the airways. Asthmatic stimuli include inhaled allergens (e.g. pollen, animal dander), occupational allergens, and drugs or non-specific stimuli such as cold air, exercise, stress and pollution.

The stimuli cause asthmatic changes through several complex pathways (Fig. 3.2). The possible mechanisms of these pathways include the following:

- Immune reactions (type 1 hypersensitivity) and release of inflammatory mediators – the cross-linking of IgE by allergens causes mast cell degranulation, and release of histamine and powerful eosinophil and neutrophil chemotactic factors. The eosinophils, neutrophils and other inflammatory cells, release inflammatory mediators that cause a bronchial inflammatory reaction, tissue damage, and an increase in bronchial hyperresponsiveness. Bronchial inflammatory mediators include leukotrienes, prostaglandins, thromboxane, platelet-activating factor and eosinophilic major basic protein.
- An imbalance in airway smooth muscle tone involving the parasympathetic nerves (vagus), non-adrenergic non-cholinergic (NANC) nerves and circulating noradrenaline that act under normal circumstances to control airway diameter.
- Abnormal calcium flux across cell membranes, increasing smooth muscle contraction and mast cell degranulation.
- Leaky tight junctions between bronchial epithelial cells allowing allergen access.

The above result in symptoms of wheezing, breathlessness and sometimes cough. In many people the asthmatic attack consists of two phases – an immediate-phase response and a late-phase response.

Immediate-phase response

An immediate-phase response occurs on exposure to the eliciting stimulus. The response consists mainly of bronchospasm. Bronchodilators are effective in this early phase.

Late-phase response

Several hours later, the late-phase response occurs. This consists of bronchospasm, vasodilatation, oedema and mucus secretion caused by inflammatory mediators released from eosinophils, platelets and other cells, and neuropeptides released by axon reflexes. Anti-inflammatory drug action is necessary for the prevention and/or treatment of this phase (Fig. 3.2).

Children with asthma who are very young can have difficulty using inhalers or nebulizers, and it is therefore more effective to give them theophylline, as this can be given in tablet form. Zara is a 4-year-old girl, who is on theophylline for this very reason. Zara presents to accident and emergency (with her mother) in pain, distress and with pyrexia (a high temperature). She is found to have an infection. Should she be given erythromycin as normal? No! Theophylline plasma concentrations would increase because enzymes involved in its breakdown would be occupied with erythromycin as well. Theophylline has a very narrow therapeutic range and so small increases above the therapeutic dose can be toxic and even fatal.

Chronic obstructive pulmonary disease

Chronic obstructive pulmonary disease (COPD) is a chronic and progressive disease with fixed or poorly reversible airflow obstruction. It encompasses several disease components, namely, chronic bronchitis and bronchiolitis, consisting of inflammation and mucus hypersecretion and emphysema, involving destruction of alveolar walls. Long-term smoking is

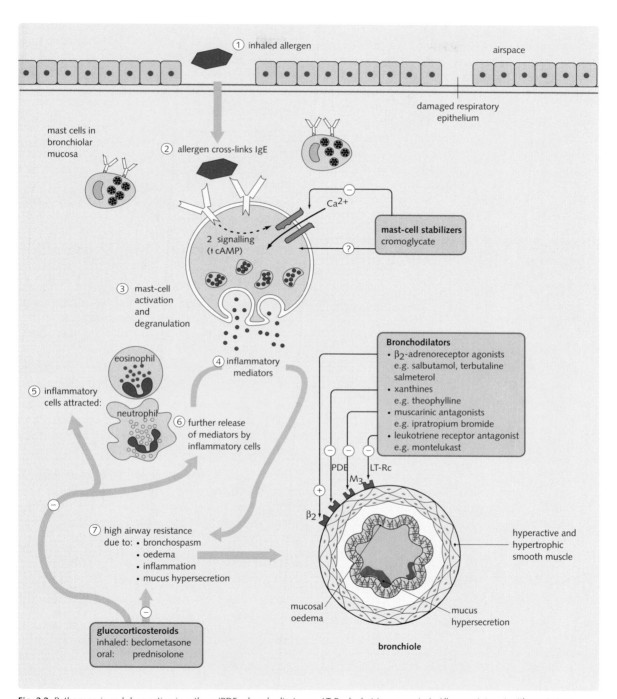

Fig. 3.2 Pathogenesis and drug action in asthma (PDE, phosphodiesterase; LT-Rc, leukotriene receptor). Allergens interact with respiratory mucosa (1), and trigger IgE-mediated mast cell response (2). Activation of mast cells causes them to degranulate (3) and release various proinflammatory mediators (4) which attract and recruit further inflammatory response cells (5). These cells also secrete mediators which amplifies the inflammatory response (6). The overall effect is narrowing of small airways (7) by bronchospasm, oedema and increased secretions.

the leading factor in the development of COPD. Cigarette smoke activates inflammatory cells (mainly macrophages and neutrophils), which can cause connective tissue damage in the lung parenchyma, resulting in emphysema and hypersecretion of mucus. α_1-Antitrypsin is a protease inhibitor, deficiency of which can result in decreased inhibition of proteases released by neutrophils, thus predisposing to destruction of lung tissue leading to emphysema. Other factors, such as atmospheric pollution can also have causal links.

Patients with COPD experience cough with the production of sputum, wheeze and breathlessness. Infective exacerbations can occur, giving purulent sputum.

Mrs Connors is a 62-year-old woman, who has been smoking approximately 15 cigarettes a day for the past 40 years. She presents with breathlessness and a 3-month history of cough, which is productive of sputum. After examination a diagnosis of COPD is made, concurrent with her presenting history. She is given Combivent® – a mixture of salbutamol (a β-agonist) and ipratropium bromide (an anticholinergic) – to relax the airways and increase the flow of air. In her case, she was not given a corticosteroid (such as fluticasone propionate) because her condition is currently mild, and it stabilized with the Combivent® treatment. In the future, as the disease progresses one may be added and she may also be put on long-term oxygen therapy. She is advised to have regular flu and pneumonia vaccinations to prevent exacerbation of her COPD.

Management of obstructive airways disease

Anti-asthmatic drugs include symptomatic bronchodilators (these are most effective in the immediate-phase response), and prophylactic or anti-inflammatory agents, which prevent and/or resolve the late-phase response. The step-wise management of asthma is summarized in Figure 3.3 and the stage-dependent treatment of COPD is shown in Figure 3.4. Most patients with COPD get some symptom relief from bronchodilators and anti-inflammatory agents in a fashion similar to people with asthma, yet the response of their airways to these drugs is much less marked, and there are no proved benefits for life expectancy. Long-term oxygen therapy does prolong survival in patients with COPD, however it must be undertaken with care in patients with carbon dioxide retention because it will reduce their hypoxic drive to breathe.

Bronchodilators

β₂-Adrenoceptor agonists

Examples of β_2-adrenoceptor agonists include salbutamol (short acting), formoterol (long acting) and salmeterol (long acting).

Mechanism of action: Airway smooth muscle does not have a sympathetic nervous supply, but it does contain β_2-adrenoceptors that respond to circulating adrenaline. The stimulation of β_2-adrenoceptors leads to a rise in intracellular cAMP levels and subsequent smooth muscle relaxation and bronchodilation.

- β_2-Adrenoceptor agonists may also help prevent the activation of mast cells, as a minor effect.
- Modern selective β_2-adrenoceptor agonists are potent bronchodilators and have very few β_1-stimulating properties (i.e. they do not affect the heart).

Route of administration: Inhaled.

Oral administration is reserved for children and people unable to use inhalers; intravenous administration for status asthmaticus.

Indications: β_2-Adrenoceptor agonists are used to relieve bronchospasm. They may be used alone in mild, occasional asthma, but are more commonly used in conjunction with other drugs, e.g. corticosteroids.

Contraindications: Caution in hyperthyroidism, cardiovascular disease, arrhythmias.

Adverse effects: Fine tremor, tachycardia, hypokalaemia after high doses.

Therapeutic notes: β_2-Adrenoceptor agonists treat the symptoms of asthma but not the underlying disease process. Salmeterol is a long-acting drug that can be administered twice daily. It is not suitable for relief of an acute attack.

Anticholinergics

Ipratropium bromide (short acting) and tiotropium (long acting) are examples of anticholinergic (antimuscarinic) drugs.

Fig. 3.3 Management of asthma in adults and children over the age of 5 years. Therapy should be started at step 1 and worked upwards until control of symptoms is achieved. Once symptoms have been controlled it may be possible to step down

Step 1	Inhaled short-acting β_2-agonist as required
Step 2	Inhaled short-acting β_2-agonist as required *Plus* *Either* regular standard-dose inhaled corticosteroid *Or* regular cromoglicate or nedocromil
Step 3	Inhaled short-acting β_2-agonist as required *Plus* *Either* regular high-dose inhaled corticosteroid *Or* regular standard-dose inhaled corticosteroid *plus* regular inhaled long-acting β_2-agonist

Step 4	Inhaled short-acting β_2-agonist as required
	    With
	Regular high-dose inhaled corticosteroid
	    Plus sequential therapeutic trial of one or more of:
	    Inhaled long-acting β_2-agonist
	    Modified-release oral theophylline
	    Inhaled ipratropium or, in adults, oxitropium
	    Modified-release oral β_2-agonist
	    High-dose inhaled bronchodilators
	    Cromoglicate or nedocromil

Step 5	Inhaled short-acting β_2-agonist as required
	    With
	Regular high-dose inhaled corticosteroid *and* one or more long-acting bronchodilators
	    Plus
	Regular prednisolone tablets

Stepping down	If control is achieved, stepwise reduction may be possible

Adapted from the British National Formulary, 41, March 2001

Fig. 3.4 Stage-dependent COPD treatment

Stage	0 (at risk)	I (mild)	II (moderate)	III (severe)	IV (very severe)
Characteristics	Normal spirometry; exposure to risk factors; chronic symptoms (cough, sputum production)	FEV_1/FVC <70% FEV_1 ≥80% predicted ± Chronic symptoms	FEV_1/FVC<70% 50% ≤FEV1 ≤80% predicted ± chronic symptoms	FEV_1/FVC<70% 30% ≤FEV_1 ≤50% ± chronic symptoms	FEV_1/FVC <70% FEV_1 <30% or FEV_1 <50% + chronic respiratory failure
Treatment	Avoidance of risk factor(s); influenza vaccination				
		Add short-acting bronchodilator when needed			
			Add regular treatment with one or more long-acting bronchodilators Add rehabilitation		
				Add inhaled glucocorticosteroids if repeated exacerbations	
					Add long-term oxygen therapy if chronic respiratory failure

FEV_1, forced expiratory volume in one second; FVC, forced vital capacity
Adapted from the GOLD Executive Summary (2005 Update)

Mechanism of action: Parasympathetic vagal fibres provide a bronchoconstrictor tone to the smooth muscle of the airways. They are activated by reflex on stimulation of sensory (irritant) receptors in the airway walls.

Muscarinic antagonists act by blocking muscarinic receptors, especially the M_3 subtype, which responds to this parasympathetic bronchoconstrictor tone.

Route of administration: Inhaled.

Indications: Anticholinergics are used as adjuncts to β_2-adrenoceptor agonists in the treatment of asthma.

Contraindications: Glaucoma, prostatic hypertrophy, pregnancy.

Adverse effects: Dry mouth may occur. Systemic anticholinergic effects are rare.

Therapeutic notes: Anticholinergics have a synergistic effect when administered with β_2-adrenoreceptor agonists in asthma.

Xanthines
Theophylline is an example of a xanthine.

Mechanism of action: The xanthines appear to increase cAMP levels in the bronchial smooth muscle cells by inhibiting phosphodiesterase, an enzyme which catalyses the hydrolysis of cAMP to AMP. Increased cAMP relaxes smooth muscle, causing bronchodilation.

Route of administration: Oral.
Aminophylline is the intravenous xanthine used in severe asthma attacks.

Indications: Xanthines are used in asthmatic children unable to use inhalers, and adults with predominantly nocturnal symptoms. They are administered intravenously in status asthmaticus.

Contraindications: Cardiac disease, hypertension, hepatic impairment.

Adverse effects: Nausea, vomiting, tremor, insomnia, tachycardia.

Therapeutic notes: Oral xanthines are formulated as sustained-release preparations. Xanthines often cause adverse effects, having a 'narrow therapeutic window', but are useful as oral drugs in preventing attacks for up to 12 hours.

Leukotriene receptor antagonists
Montelukast and zafirlukast are examples of leukotriene receptor antagonists.

Mechanism of action: The leukotriene receptor antagonists are believed to act at leukotriene receptors in the bronchiolar muscle, antagonising endogenous leukotrienes, thus causing bronchodilation.

Leukotrienes are thought to be partly responsible for airway narrowing which is sometimes observed with the use of non-steroidal anti-inflammatory drugs in asthmatic people (NSAIDs; see Ch. 9). The NSAIDs inhibit cyclooxygenase, and divert arachidonic acid breakdown via the lipoxygenase pathway, liberating leukotrienes among other mediators.

Route of administration: Oral.

Indications: Prophylaxis of asthma.

Contraindications: Elderly, pregnancy, Churg–Strauss syndrome.

Adverse effects: Gastrointestinal disturbance, dry mouth, headache.

Therapeutic notes: The leukotriene receptor antagonists are not yet widely used, though their potential as an agent in the combination therapy of asthma is becoming more widely accepted.

In an asthmatic emergency, when thinking what drugs to use, don't forget oxygen.

Prophylactic and anti-inflammatory drugs
Mast-cell stabilizers
Sodium cromoglicate and nedocromil sodium are examples of mast-cell stabilizers.

Mechanism of action: The exact modes of action of mast-cell stabilizers are unclear. These drugs appear to stabilize antigen-sensitized mast cells by reducing calcium influx and subsequent release of inflammatory mediators.

Route of administration: Inhaled.

Indications: Mast-cell stabilizers are useful in young patients (<20 years old) with marked allergic disease and moderate asthma.

Adverse effects: Cough, transient bronchospasm, throat irritation.

Therapeutic notes: Mast-cell stabilizers have a prophylactic action; they must be taken regularly for several weeks before any beneficial effects are noted. These drugs are therefore not of use in acute asthma attacks.

Anti-inflammatory glucocorticoids

Anti-inflammatory glucocorticoids include beclometasone, fluticasone, budesonide and prednisolone.

Mechanism of action: Corticosteroids depress the inflammatory response in bronchial mucosa and so diminish bronchial hyperresponsiveness. The specific effects include:

- Reduced mucosal oedema and mucus production
- Decreased local generation of prostaglandins and leukotrienes, with less inflammatory-cell activation
- Adrenoceptor up-regulation
- Long-term reduced T-cell cytokine production, and reduced eosinophil and mast-cell infiltration of bronchial mucosa.

For the intracellular events involved in corticosteroid action see Chapter 6.

Route of administration: Corticosteroids are usually delivered by metered-dose inhaler. Oral and intravenous administration is reserved for severe asthma and status asthmaticus.

Indications: Corticosteroids are used in patients with more than minimal symptoms, often in combination with β_2-agonists or drugs that block allergies (Fig. 3.3).

Contraindications: Caution in growing children and in those with systemic and local respiratory/ENT infections.

Adverse effects: Dysphonia, oral thrush and systemic penetration in high dosage. If given orally, cushingoid effects may occur (Ch. 6).

Therapeutic notes: The initial treatment of severe or refractory asthma may require oral corticosteroids. If possible, maintenance should be achieved with inhaled corticosteroids via a metered dose, to minimize side-effects. Inhaled corticosteroids are usually effective in 3–7 days, but must be taken regularly.

Use of inhalers, nebulizers and oxygen

In the treatment of asthma, inhalers and nebulizers are used to deliver drugs directly to the airways. This allows higher drug concentrations to be achieved locally, while minimizing systemic effects. Whatever device is used, less than 15% of the dose is deposited on the bronchial mucosa.

Inhalers

There are several types of inhaler: metered dose, breath-activated spray, breath-activated powder. They vary in cost, delivery efficiency and ease of use.

Spacer devices, used in conjunction with inhalers, improve drug delivery and are easy to use. Spacers are particularly effective in children.

Nebulizers

Nebulizers convert a solution of drug into an aerosol for inhalation. They are more efficient than inhalers and are used to deliver higher doses of drug. They are useful in status asthmaticus and for the acute hospital treatment of severe asthma.

The long-term use of nebulizers is limited by cost, convenience, and the danger of patient over-reliance.

Oxygen

High-flow oxygen should be given to any patient in respiratory distress unless they have COPD and a 'hypoxic drive'. In this situation, oxygen can be administered, but at a lower concentration.

Oxygen increases alveolar oxygen tension and decreases the work of breathing necessary to maintain arterial oxygen tension.

Allergic rhinitis

'Rhinitis' means an inflammatory response of the membrane lining the nose. 'Allergic rhinitis' means the inflammatory response is due to specific allergens causing a type 1 hypersensitivity reaction. Based on symptoms, it may be further classified as seasonal or perennial (throughout the year). The inflammation can cause swelling, blockages to airflow and overactivity of the mucous membrane glands, causing excessive mucus production. Allergic rhinitis is treated with antihistamine drugs or local steroid sprays (see Ch. 10). Decongestants can sometimes be helpful.

Decongestants

Nasal decongestion can occur acutely, or be a chronic disorder.

Decongestion relies on administration of agents which ultimately have sympathomimetic effects. This results in vasoconstriction of the mucosal blood vessels of the nose, and a reduction in oedema and secretions.

Ephedrine

This drug is the most commonly used decongestant.

Mechanism of action: Ephedrine's sympathomimetic activity results in vasoconstriction of nasal blood vessels, limiting oedema and nasal secretions.

Route of administration: Topical or oral.

Indications: Nasal congestion.

Contraindications: Caution in children.

Adverse effects: Local irritation, nausea, headache. Re-bound nasal congestion on withdrawal.

Therapeutic notes: Oral preparations are less effective than topical, and are contraindicated in diabetes, hypertension and hyperthyroidism.

RESPIRATORY STIMULANTS AND PULMONARY SURFACTANTS

Respiratory stimulants

Respiratory stimulants, or analeptic drugs, have a very limited place in the treatment of ventilatory failure in patients with chronic obstructive airways disease. They have largely been replaced by the use of ventilatory support.

Doxapram

This drug is an example of a respiratory stimulant.

Mechanism of action: Doxapram is used to improve both rate and depth of breathing. Doxapram is a central stimulant drug that acts on both carotid chemoreceptors and the respiratory centre in the brainstem to increase respiration.

Route of administration: Intravenous.

Indications: Acute respiratory failure.

Adverse effects: Perineal warmth, dizziness, sweating, increase in blood pressure and heart rate.

Therapeutic notes: Apart from naloxone and flumazenil, the respiratory stimulants are seldom employed in clinical practice.

Pulmonary surfactants

Pulmonary surfactants are used in the management of respiratory distress syndrome, which is most common amongst premature babies. Pulmonary surfactants act to decrease the surface tension of the alveoli, and allow ventilation to occur more easily. They are usually administered via endotracheal tubes directly into the pulmonary tree. Further information on these agents can be obtained from a neonatology text or the *British National Formulary* (*BNF*).

ANTITUSSIVES AND MUCOLYTICS

Antitussives

Antitussives are drugs that inhibit the cough reflex.

Cough is usually a valuable protective reflex mechanism for clearing foreign material and secretions from the airways. In some conditions, however, such as inflammation or neoplasia, the cough reflex may become inappropriately stimulated and in such cases antitussive drugs may be used.

Antitussives either reduce sensory receptor activation or work by an ill-defined mechanism, depressing a 'cough centre' in the brainstem.

Drugs that reduce receptor activation

Menthol vapour and topical local anaesthetics

Benzocaine is an example of a topical local anaesthetic.

Mechanism of action: Menthol vapour and topical local anaesthetics reduce the sensitivity of peripheral sensory 'cough receptors' in the pharynx and larynx to irritation.

Route of administration: Topical as a spray, lozenge or vapour.

Indications: Menthol vapour and topical local anaesthetics are used for unwanted cough.

Drugs that reduce the sensitivity of the 'cough centre'

Opioids (Ch. 9)

Opioids reduce the sensitivity of the 'cough centre'. Examples of these drugs include codeine and pholcodine.

Mechanism of action: Although not clearly understood, opioids seem to work via agonist action on opiate receptors, depressing a 'cough centre' in the brainstem.

Route of administration: Oral.

Indications: Opioids are used for inappropriate coughing.

Adverse effects: There are generally few side-effects of opioids at antitussive doses. Unlike pholcodine, codeine can cause constipation, and inhibition of mucociliary clearance.

Mucolytics

Mucolytics are drugs that reduce the viscosity of bronchial secretions. They are sometimes used when excess bronchial secretions need to be cleared.

Carbocisteine and mecysteine hydrochloride

These drugs act as mucolytics.

Mechanism of action: Carbocisteine and mecysteine hydrochloride reduce the viscosity of bronchial secretions by cleaving disulphide bonds cross-linking mucus glycoprotein molecules.

Route of administration: Oral.

Indications: Carbocisteine and mecysteine hydrochloride may be of benefit in some chronic obstructive airways disease, although there is no evidence supporting their use.

Therapeutic notes: A novel drug with 'mucolytic' properties is dornase alfa, a genetically engineered enzyme which cleaves extracellular DNA, and is used in cystic fibrosis, being administered by inhalation.

Peripheral nervous system

Objectives

After reading this chapter, you will:

- Have a good understanding of the peripheral nervous system and neurotransmitter action
- Know the different classes of drugs that are used in disorders of the peripheral nervous system and how their mechanisms of action result in beneficial and adverse effects.

NERVE CONDUCTION

Conduction of impulses through nerves occurs as an all-or-none event called the action potential. The action potential is caused by voltage-dependent opening of sodium and potassium channels in the cell membrane.

The sodium equilibrium potential (Eq Na$^+$) is +60 mV and the potassium equilibrium potential (Eq K$^+$) is –90 mV. Since a resting nerve has 50–75 more potassium channels open than sodium channels, the resting membrane potential is –70 mV.

Figure 4.1 shows the concentrations of sodium and potassium inside and outside a resting nerve. The Na$^+$/K$^+$ pump (Na$^+$/K$^+$ ATPase) is an energy-dependent pump that functions to maintain the concentration gradient of these two ionic species across the membrane. Three sodium ions are pumped out of the cell for every two potassium ions pumped in, and thus the excitability of the cell is retained. Figures 4.2 and 4.3 summarize the events that occur during a nerve action potential. During a nerve action potential:

- The rate of sodium entry into the nerve axon becomes greater than the rate of potassium out of the axon, at which point the membrane becomes depolarized (the loss of a electrical gradient across the membrane).
- Depolarization sets off a sodium-positive feedback whereby more voltage-gated sodium channels open and the membrane becomes more depolarized.

Fig. 4.1 Intracellular and extracellular sodium and potassium concentrations. The Na$^+$/K$^+$ ATPase pump maintains these concentration gradients across the cell membrane.

Fig. 4.2 Nerve action potential. For explanation of points 1–6, see Figure 4.3.

Fig. 4.3 State of sodium and potassium channels and membrane potential at different stages of the neuronal action potential

	Sodium channels	Potassium channels	Membrane potential
1	Closed resting	Closed resting	Resting (–70 mV)
2	Open	Closed resting	Depolarization (action potential upstroke)
3	More channels open	Closed resting	More depolarization
4	Channels close (inactive)	Special set of channels start opening	Peak of action potential reached
5	All inactivated	More channels open	Re-polarization
6	Closed resting	Channels close	Resting membrane potential re-established

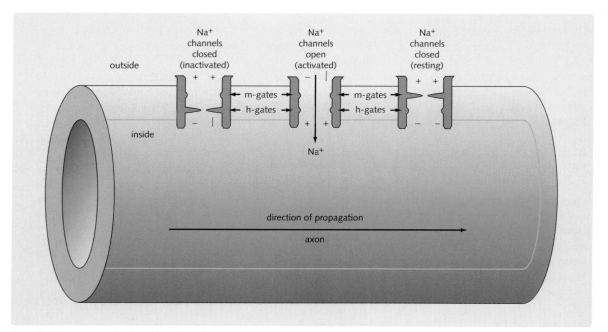

Fig. 4.4 Voltage-operated sodium channels in their inactivated, activated and resting states. The m-gates and h-gates open or close according to the state of the channel. In the resting sodium channel, the m-gates are held closed by the strongly negative (–70 mV) electrical gradient across the membrane. Once an action potential begins to propagate, the loss of the membrane potential causes the m-gates to open, allowing sodium into the cell, further propagating the action potential. After a very short time, a further conformational change causes the h-gates to close, inactivating the sodium channel. The membrane then re-polarizes, and once at –70 mV, the m-gates again close, and the h-gates open so the sodium channel is back in its resting state.

- A threshold, which is usually 15 mV greater than the resting membrane potential, must be reached if an action potential is to be generated.
- The membrane repolarizes when the sodium channels become inactivated; a special set of potassium channels open and potassium leaves the axon.

- The sodium channels eventually regain their resting excitable state and the Na$^+$/K$^+$ ATPase restores the membrane potential back to –70 mV.

Figure 4.4 shows the voltage-operated sodium channels in their inactivated, activated and resting states. Two types of gate exist within the channel, the m-gates and the h-gates. These gates are open or closed according to the state of the channel.

Sodium channel

The voltage-operated sodium channel is present in all excitable tissues. It is a transmembrane protein made up of four domains, each with six transmembrane regions. It is sensitive to membrane potential and selectively passes sodium ions.

Local anaesthetics block the sodium channel, and thus nerve conduction, by binding to the sixth transmembrane region of the fourth domain.

Size of the nerve fibre

Small nerve fibres are preferentially blocked because of their high surface-area to volume ratio. This results in a differential block whereby the small nociceptive (pain) and autonomic fibres are blocked but not the larger fibres responsible for the mediation of movement and touch.

SOMATIC NERVOUS SYSTEM

Neuromuscular junction

Physiology of transduction

Skeletal (voluntary) muscle is innervated by motor neurons, the axons of which are able to propagate action potentials at high velocities. The area of muscle that lies below the axon terminal is known as the motor end-plate, and the chemical synapse between the two is known as the neuromuscular junction (NMJ).

The axon terminal incorporates membrane-bound vesicles containing the neurotransmitter acetylcholine (ACh). Depolarization of the presynaptic terminal of the nerve by an action potential (generated by sodium influx) causes voltage-sensitive calcium channels to open, allowing calcium ions into the terminal. Normally, the level of calcium ions inside the nerves is very low – 10 000 times lower than the external concentration. This calcium influx results in the release of ACh by exocytosis from vesicles. ACh diffuses across to the muscle membrane where it binds to the nicotinic acetylcholine receptor (nicAChR) and/or is inactivated by acetylcholinesterase (Fig. 4.5). Several events then occur:

- During association, ACh binds to the nicAChR, which is an ion channel that allows cations into the muscle (mainly sodium but also potassium to a lesser extent).
- During the conformational change, the pore of the ion channel is open for 1 ms, during which approximately 20 000 sodium ions enter the cell. The resulting depolarization, called an end-plate potential (EPP), depolarizes the adjacent muscle fibre.
- If the cellular response is large enough, an action potential is generated in the rest of the muscle fibre (sodium influx), resulting in the opening of voltage-operated calcium channels, but this time the calcium influx mediates contraction.
- ACh is rapidly inactivated by an enzyme called acetylcholinesterase (AChE) which hydrolyses ACh into the inactive metabolites choline and acetic acid.
- In the synthesis of ACh, the choline generated is taken up by the nerve terminal where another enzyme, choline acetyl transferase (ChAT), converts it back to ACh to be reused.

The neuromuscular junction is a very important site for therapeutic manipulation. The electrical impulse from the neuron is converted into a chemical signal that mediates the effect–largely muscular contraction.

Nicotinic acetylcholine receptor

The nicAChR is made up of five subunits (two α, one β, one γ and one δ) that traverse the membrane and surround a central pore. All the subunits show high sequence identity. The binding site for ACh lies on the α subunits, therefore ACh must bind to both α subunits to open the channel.

Each subunit has four membrane-spanning regions (helices), i.e. each receptor has a total of 20. One of the transmembrane helices (M_2) from each subunit forms the lining of the channel pore.

Pharmacological targets

There are three major targets within the NMJ for clinically useful drugs (Fig. 4.6):

Fig. 4.5 Physiology of impulse transduction at the neuromuscular junction (NMJ) showing the site of action of drugs used in conjunction with the NMJ. (VOSC, voltage-operated sodium channel; VOCC, voltage-operated calcium channel; AChE, acetylcholinesterase; ChAT, choline acetyl transferase; vesamicol, an experimental drug.)

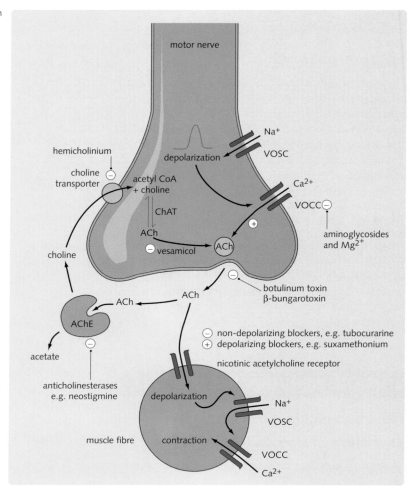

Fig. 4.6 Targets for clinically useful drugs at the neuromuscular junction. Myasthenia gravis is an autoimmune disease in which there is a decrease in the number of available receptors at the end-plate due to antibody binding. To allow normal neuromuscular function, drugs that increase the amount of acetylcholine in the cleft are given

Site	Action	Use
nicAChR	Block transmission	Neuromuscular blockers for surgery
AChE	Enhance transmission	Peripheral neuropathy, e.g. myasthenia gravis
Release	Block transmission	Spasms, e.g. squints, tics, tremors, etc.

AChE, acetylcholine esterase; nicAChR, nicotinic acetylcholine receptor

- Presynaptic release
- Nicotinic acetylcholine receptor
- Acetylcholinesterase.

Drugs affecting the neuromuscular junction

Presynaptic agents

Drugs inhibiting ACh synthesis: The rate-limiting step in the synthesis of ACh is the uptake of choline into the nerve terminal.

Hemicholinium is an analogue of choline that competitively blocks the choline transporter and causes a depletion of ACh stores. Because of the time taken for the stores to run down, the onset of this drug is slow. This, and the frequency-dependent

Fig. 4.7 Non-depolarizing blockers of postsynaptic receptors at the neuromuscular junction

| Drug | Approximate duration (mins) | Side effects | | | Elimination |
		Ganglion block	Histamine release	Other	
Tubocurarine	60–120	Partial	Sometimes	Hypersensitivity (rare)	Mainly hepatic
Pancuronium	40–60	X	Minimal	Block of muscarinic receptors in the heart → tachycardia	Mainly renal
Gallamine	15	X	X	Block of muscarinic receptors in the heart → tachycardia	Mainly renal: avoid in patients with renal disease
Alcuronium	20	X	X	Dose dependency	Mainly hepatic
Vecuronium	20–30	X	X		Mainly hepatic
Atracurium	15–30	X	Sometimes		Degradation in plasma at body pH (Hofmann elimination)

nature of the block (depletion of stores is related to release of ACh), means that it is not useful clinically. The block is reversed by the addition of choline.

Drugs inhibiting vesicular packaging of ACh: Vesamicol inhibits the active transport of ACh into storage vesicles and results in neuromuscular block.

Drugs inhibiting ACh release: Calcium entry into the nerve terminal is necessary for the release of ACh; thus, agents such as aminoglycoside antibiotics (e.g. streptomycin) that prevent this step will cause neuromuscular blockade. Muscle paralysis is occasionally a side-effect of aminoglycoside antibiotics, but it can be reversed by the administration of calcium salts.

Botulinum toxin is a neurotoxin produced by the anaerobic bacillus *Clostridium botulinum*. The toxin is very potent and it is believed to inhibit ACh release by inactivating actin, which is necessary for exocytosis. In botulism, a serious type of food poisoning caused by this toxin, victims experience progressive parasympathetic and motor paralysis. Botulinum toxin type A is sometimes used clinically in the treatment of excessive muscle contraction

disorders (dystonias) such as strabismus (squint), spasticity and tremors.

β-Bungarotoxin contained in snake venom acts in a similar manner to botulinum toxin.

Postsynaptic agents

Non-depolarizing blockers: These act as competitive antagonists by binding to the nicAChR but not activating it, and producing motor paralysis. Details of the most commonly used non-depolarizing blockers are given in Figure 4.7.

Approximately 80–90% of receptors must be blocked to prevent transmission, since the amount of ACh released by nerve terminal depolarization usually greatly exceeds that required to generate an action potential in the muscle. The drugs are all quaternary ammonium compounds and, therefore, do not cross the blood–brain barrier or the placenta. They are poorly absorbed orally and they must be administered by intravenous injection. 'Tetanic fade' (i.e. non-maintained muscle tension during brief nerve stimulation) is seen with some of these drugs. This can be explained by the blocking of presynaptic autoreceptors which usually maintain the release of ACh during repeated stimulation.

The block can be reversed by anticholinesterases and depolarizing drugs. It is also enhanced in patients with myasthenia gravis. The main side-effect from these drugs is hypotension caused by the blocking of ganglionic transmission. Histamine release from mast cells, resulting in bronchospasm, may be a problem in certain individuals (see Fig. 4.7).

Depolarizing (non-competitive) blockers: Depolarizing blockers initially activate receptors, causing depolarization, but in doing so block further activation.

Depolarizing blockers act on the motor end-plate in the same manner as ACh, i.e. they are agonists and increase the cation permeability of the end-plate. However, unlike ACh, which is released in brief spurts and rapidly hydrolysed, depolarizing blockers remain associated with the receptors long enough to cause a sustained depolarization and a resulting loss of electrical excitability (phase I).

Repeated or continuous administration of depolarizing blockers leads to the block becoming more characteristic of non-depolarizing drugs. This is known as phase II and is probably due to receptor desensitization, whereby the end-plate becomes less sensitive to ACh. The block starts to show tetanic fade and it is partly reversed by anticholinesterase drugs.

Suxamethonium is the only depolarizing blocker used clinically because of its rapid onset time and short duration of action (approximately 4 minutes). Suxamethonium is a quaternary ammonium compound, and it must be given by intravenous injection. It is rapidly hydrolysed by plasma cholinesterase, although certain people with a genetic variant of this enzyme may experience a neuromuscular block that may last for hours.

Depolarizing blockers have no effect in patients with myasthenia gravis, since these patients have a decreased number of receptors at the end-plate. In this instance, the blocking potency of depolarizing blockers is reduced.

The side-effects of depolarizing blockers include:

- Initial spasms, which occur prior to paralysis, often resulting in postoperative muscle pain.
- Muscarinic receptor activation resulting in bradycardia. Bradycardia can be prevented by the administration of atropine.
- Potassium release from muscle resulting in elevated plasma potassium levels. This is usually a problem only in the case of trauma.

Anticholinesterases

Anticholinesterases inhibit AChE and thus increase the amount of ACh in the synaptic cleft and enhance cholinergic transmission. Most of the anticholinesterases used are quaternary ammonium compounds and, therefore, they do not penetrate the blood–brain barrier.

Short-acting anticholinesterases include edrophonium. This is selective for the NMJ and clinically relevant in the diagnosis of myasthenia gravis. Edrophonium's duration of action is only 2–10 minutes because it binds by electrostatic forces (no covalent bonds) to the active site of the enzyme. It is therefore not used therapeutically.

Intermediate-acting anticholinesterases include neostigmine, pyridostigmine and physostigmine.

Neostigmine is used intravenously to reverse the effects of non-depolarizing blockers. Its duration of action is 2-4 hours, and it is used orally in the treatment of myasthenia gravis. Although neostigmine shows some selectivity for the NMJ, atropine is sometimes co-administered to block the muscarinic effects of the drug.

Pyridostigmine has a duration of action of 3–6 hours, and it is also used orally in the treatment of myasthenia gravis. It has few parasympathetic actions.

Physostigmine shows selectivity for the postganglionic parasympathetic junction. It is a tertiary amine and its use is, therefore, associated with central effects such as initial excitation followed by depression, and possibly respiratory depression and unconsciousness. The central effects can be antagonized by atropine. Physostigmine is used in the form of eye drops to constrict the pupil and contract the ciliary muscle in the treatment of glaucoma.

Most of the long-lasting or irreversible anticholinesterases are organophosphorus compounds. For example, sarin and tabun were developed as nerve gases, and parathion was developed as an insecticide, as well as for clinical use. These drugs have many adverse effects, such as bradycardia, hypotension, breathing problems, depolarizing neuromuscular block, central effects and possible death from peripheral nerve demyelination. Echothiophate shows selectivity for the postganglionic parasympathetic junction, and it is used in the treatment of glaucoma.

In the treatment of myasthenia gravis, prednisolone can be added to help manage symptoms, usually with azathioprine to allow a lower dose of the steroid.

Mrs Thumma, 34 years old, presented to her doctors with a 3-month history of early fatigue and muscle weakness. She finds it difficult to finish her meals as she gets tired chewing and has now lost 2 kg. She is otherwise a healthy non-smoker, who rarely drinks alcohol. Her husband has noticed her voice becoming quieter, especially towards the end of the day.

On examination, she looks well. Power in all muscle groups is grossly normal but weakens after repeated testing. Tone, coordination, reflexes and sensation are normal. She is referred to a neurologist, who orders more investigations. Serum acetylcholine receptor antibodies test positive. A CT scan of her thymus reveals an enlarged thymus gland.

She therefore has a thymectomy, histopathological examination of which revealed benign hyperplasia. She is also given the anticholinesterase pyridostigmine and an appointment for review.

AUTONOMIC NERVOUS SYSTEM

The autonomic nervous system comprises the sympathetic and parasympathetic systems, which generally have opposite effects on the body. It innervates all tissues, except skeletal muscle (Fig. 4.8). The axons of the autonomic nervous system arise from their cell body, located in the central nervous system (CNS), as preganglionic fibres. These synapse in the appropriate ganglion, and leave as postganglionic fibres, which reach the effector cells.

The neurotransmitter released by preganglionic fibres at autonomic ganglia, regardless of whether sympathetic or parasympathetic, is ACh. The ACh receptors located on postganglionic fibres are of the nicotinic type.

Autonomic ganglia

Figure 4.9 summarizes the differences between ganglionic nicAChR and those found on skeletal muscle at the NMJ.

Fig. 4.8 Somatic and autonomic nervous systems: organization and neurotransmitters. (ACh, acetylcholine; CNS, central nervous sytem; DA, dopamine; NA, noradrenaline.)

Fig. 4.9 Distinguishing features of the ganglionic nicotinic acetylcholine receptors and those found on skeletal muscle at the neuromuscular junction

	Skeletal muscle	Neurons
Structure	2α 1β 1γ or ε 1δ	2α 3β
Specific agonists	Suxamethonium	DMPP
Specific antagonists	Gallamine Tubocurarine α-bungarotoxin	Hexamethonium Mecamylamine κ-bungarotoxin
Function	End-plate region depolarization at NMJ	Neuronal depolarization in ganglia and CNS

DMPP, dimethylphenylpiperazinium

Ganglion-stimulating drugs

Nicotinic agonists

There are few agonists that act selectively on the nicAChR without affecting muscarinic receptors. Carbachol is the best example of a drug that shows preference for the nicotinic receptor, but still its action is not selective. Nicotine and lobeline both show preference for ganglionic nicotinic receptors (meaning slightly higher concentrations are needed when they stimulate the NMJ).

These drugs have no clinical use, since their range of effects is vast, affecting both sympathetic and parasympathetic transmission:

- Sympathetic effects include tachycardia and vasoconstriction leading to hypertension.
- Parasympathetic effects include increased gastrointestinal motility and glandular secretions.

Ganglion-blocking drugs

Autonomic ganglia can be blocked presynaptically by inhibiting ACh synthesis, vesicular packaging, or release (p. 77), or postsynaptically by blocking the nicotinic receptors.

Non-depolarizing ganglion blockers

A few of these drugs act solely as competitive antagonists, blocking receptors without depolarizing the ganglion. Most block the ion channel, as well as the associated receptor, and they produce their action through this former mechanism. For example:

- Some ganglion blockers, such as tubocurarine, are not antagonists at the ganglionic nicotinic receptor; they produce ganglion block through channel blockade.
- Tubocurarine also blocks transmission at the NMJ, but it does this through receptor antagonism.
- Hexamethonium was initially developed for use in treating hypertension, but it is no longer in clinical use.
- Trimetaphan, a ganglion blocker was used to reduce blood pressure during surgery since it had a short duration of action and could be administered intravenously. However, it has now been discontinued.

Ganglion-blocking drugs have a wide range of complex effects, although the sympathetic and parasympathetic systems tend to oppose one another. The effects of ganglion-blocking drugs include:

- Arteriolar vasodilatation leading to a marked reduction in blood pressure (block of sympathetic ganglia)
- Postural and postexercise hypotension (loss of cardiac reflexes)
- Slight reduction in cardiac output
- Inhibition of gastrointestinal secretions and motility, leading to constipation, urinary retention, impotence and failure of ejaculation.

Sympathetic nervous system

The fibres of the sympathetic nervous system leave the CNS from the thoracolumbar regions of the spinal cord (T1–L3). They synapse in ganglia located close to the spinal cord. These ganglia form a chain along each side of the spinal cord, which is known as sympathetic trunk.

The major transmitter released by postganglionic fibres at the junction with effector cells is noradrenaline (NA).

Sympathetic transmission is enhanced under conditions of stress, known as the 'fight-or-flight response'.

Adrenal medulla

Some postganglionic neurons in the sympathetic division do not have axons, but instead they release their transmitters directly into the bloodstream. These neurons are located in the adrenal medulla.

On stimulation by preganglionic fibres, the adrenal medulla acts as an endocrine gland, releasing its hormones/transmitters into the systemic circulation which consist of ~80% adrenaline, ~20% noradrenaline, as well as small amounts of dopamine, neuropeptides and ATP.

Adrenoceptors

In 1913 Henry Dale observed that adrenaline constricted some blood vessels but relaxed others, while in 1948 Ahlquist defined two receptor subtypes based on the rank order of potency of three agonists, namely isoprenaline, adrenaline and noradrenaline. The two receptor subtypes were α and β. Potency at:

- α receptors is noradrenaline > adrenaline > isoprenaline
- β receptors is isoprenaline > adrenaline > noradrenaline.

Effects mediated by α-adrenoreceptors

α_1-Receptors

α_1-Receptors are located postsynaptically. Their activation causes smooth muscle contraction (except for the non-sphincter part of the gastrointestinal tract, where activation causes relaxation), glycogenolysis in the liver, and potassium release from the liver and salivary glands. Transduction is via G-proteins and an increase in the second messengers inositol (1,4,5) triphosphate (IP_3) and diacylglycerol (DAG).

α_2-Receptors

α_2-Receptors are located mainly presynaptically, but also postsynaptically on liver cells, platelets and the smooth muscle of blood vessels. The activation of presynaptic α_2-receptors inhibits noradrenaline release and, therefore, provides a means of end-product negative feedback. Activation of postsynaptic α_2-receptors causes blood vessel constriction and platelet aggregation. Transduction is via G-proteins and a decrease in the second messenger cyclic adenosine monophosphate (cAMP).

Some drugs, such as phenoxybenzamine and phentolamine are non-selective α-adrenoceptor antagonists. Phenoxybenzamine is an irreversible antagonist as it forms covalent bonds with the receptor, while phentolamine binds reversibly and so has a much shorter duration of action. These drugs cause a fall in arterial blood pressure, due to block of α-receptor-mediated vasoconstriction.

Mrs Pharasha, a 26-year-old librarian, presents to her doctor with episodes of anxiety, sweating, tremor and palpitations. These attacks had been increasing in frequency and are now occurring almost daily. The only change Mrs Pharasha can think of is the increased stress at work, which she now feels she is not handling well. She is a non-smoker and seldom drinks alcohol. She is on no medication.

On examination, her heart rate is 106 beats per minute and her blood pressure is elevated. To treat her hypertension she is prescribed propranolol, a β-blocker, which causes her blood pressure to increase by 30 mmHg and her heart rate to reach 145 beats per minute. So her condition worsens markedly. She is rushed to accident and emergency where the doctor suspects phaeochromocytoma.

Resting plasma catecholamines and urinary metanephrines (catecholamine metabolites) are raised, supporting the diagnosis. Imaging reveals a tumour in the adrenal medulla, which is resectable. Intravenous phentolamine is given to safely reduce her blood pressure. Following stabilization of her blood pressure, she is put on phenoxybenzamine to achieve α-blockade, with propranolol added later to achieve β-blockade as well. She is maintained on this until complete α- and β-blockade is established and plasma volume has re-expanded. Surgery to remove the secreting tumour can then be performed, with an expert anaesthetist and surgeon, and readily available nitroprusside.

Effects mediated by β-adrenoceptors

β_1-Receptors

β_1-Receptors are mainly postsynaptic and located in the heart, platelets and non-sphincter part of the gastrointestinal tract. They can, however, be found presynaptically. Activation causes an increase in the rate and force of contraction of the heart, relaxation of the non-sphincter part of the gastrointestinal tract, aggregation of platelets, an increase in the release of noradrenaline, lipolysis in fat, and amylase

73

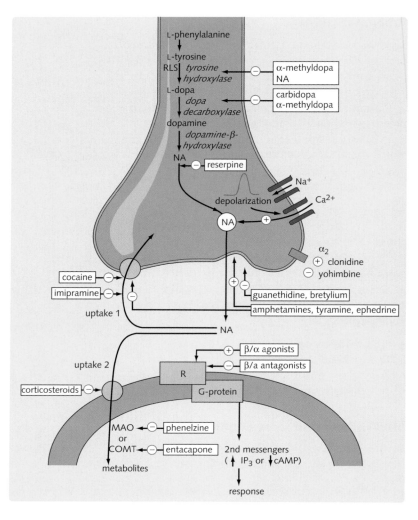

Fig. 4.10 Drugs affecting adrenergic transmission. (cAMP, cyclic adenosine monophosphate; COMT, catechol-O-methyltransferase; IP$_3$, inositol triphosphate; MAO, monoamine oxidase; NA, noradrenaline; RLS, rate-limiting step.)

secretion from the salivary glands. Presynaptically, their activation causes an increase in noradrenaline release. Transduction is via G-proteins and an increase in the second messenger cAMP.

β$_2$-Receptors

β$_2$-Receptors are located postsynaptically. Their activation causes smooth muscle relaxation, glycogenolysis in the liver, inhibition of histamine release from mast cells, and tremor in skeletal muscle. Transduction is via G-proteins and an increase in the second messenger cAMP.

Drugs acting on the sympathetic system

Figure 4.10 summarizes the drugs acting on the sympathetic system.

Presynaptic agents

Noradrenaline synthesis: The precursor to noradrenaline is L-tyrosine, which is taken up by adrenergic neurons.

Drugs decreasing noradrenaline synthesis: The rate-limiting step (RLS) is the conversion of tyrosine to dihydroxyphenylalanine (dopa), which is catalysed by tyrosine hydroxylase and inhibited by metyrosine. Noradrenaline provides a negative feedback upon this step. Carbidopa inhibits dopa decarboxylase and is used in Parkinson's disease to increase dopamine levels. Because this is not the RLS, drugs that inhibit dopa decarboxylase do not greatly affect noradrenaline synthesis. Administering α-methyldopa (used in hypertension) results in the formation of a false transmitter, α-methylnoradrenaline.

Fig. 4.11 Adrenoceptor agonists and their clinical uses

Drug	Receptor	Uses	Side effects	Phamacokinetics
Nordarenaline	α/β	No use clinically	Hypertension, tachycardia, ventricular arrhythmias	Poor oral absorption, metabolized by MAO and COMT, $t_{1/2} \sim 2$ min
Adrenaline	α/β	Anaphylactic shock Cardiac resuscitation with local anaesthetics	Hypertension, tachycardia, ventricular arrhythmias	Poor oral absorption, metabolized by MAO and COMT, $t_{1/2} \sim 2$ min given intravenously or intramuscularly
Oxymetazoline	α	Nasal decongestant	Rebound congestion	Given intranasally
Phenylephrine	α_1	Hypotension Nasal decongestant	Hypertension Reflex bradycardia	Metabolized by MAO $t_{1/2} <1$ min, given intramuscularly or intranasally
Clonidine	α_2	Hypertension Migraine	Drowsiness, hypotension	Good oral absorption, $t_{1/2} \sim 12$ h
Isoprenaline	β	Asthma Cardiac resuscitation	Arrhythmias, tachycardia	Metabolized by COMT, given sublingually or as aerosol $t_{1/2} \sim 2$ h
Dobutamine	β_1	Heart failure	Tachycardia	
Salbutamol	β_2	Asthma Premature labour	Arrhythmias, tachycardia, vasodilatation	Given by aerosol $t_{1/2} \sim 4$ h

COMT, catechol-O-methyltransferase; MAO, monoamine oxidase

Drugs increasing noradrenaline synthesis: Levodopa (L-dopa) administration bypasses the RLS and is used in Parkinson's disease. Noradrenaline is stored in vesicles as a complex with ATP and a protein called chromogranin A.

Drugs inhibiting noradrenaline storage: Reserpine is a drug used in the treatment of hypertension and schizophrenia. It reduces stores of noradrenaline by preventing the accumulation of noradrenaline in vesicles. Its action is effectively irreversible since it has a very high affinity for the noradrenaline storage site. The displaced noradrenaline is immediately broken down by monoamine oxygenase (MAO) and is therefore unable to exert sympathetic effects.

Drugs inhibiting the breakdown of leaked noradrenaline stores: These include monoamine oxidase inhibitors (MAOIs) and catechol-O-methyltransferase (COMT) inhibitors. They prevent the breakdown of leaked catecholamines so that noradrenaline that leaves the vesicles is protected and eventually leaks out from the nerve ending.

Drugs inhibiting noradrenaline release: These include guanethidine and bretylium. These are adrenergic neuron-blocking drugs that prevent the exocytosis of noradrenaline from nerve terminals; they are used as hypotensive drugs. They are taken up by uptake 1 and concentrated in nerve terminals where they have a local anaesthetic effect on impulse conduction. The tricyclic antidepressants, which inhibit uptake 1, prevent these drugs from exerting their effects. Clonidine is an α_2-receptor agonist and, therefore, inhibits noradrenaline release.

Drugs promoting noradrenaline release: These include: amphetamines, tyramine and ephedrine, which are sympathomimetic drugs that act indirectly. They are taken up by uptake 1 and displace noradrenaline from the vesicles. Because they also inhibit MAO, the displaced noradrenaline is not broken down, and it is able to exert sympathetic effects. These drugs act in part through a direct agonist effect on adrenoceptors. Yohimbine is an α_2-receptor antagonist and it, therefore, prevents noradrenaline from exerting a negative feedback effect on noradrenaline release.

Postsynaptic agents
Adrenoceptor agonists: These are termed 'sympathomimetics'. They activate postsynaptic receptors, eliciting a response (Fig. 4.11).

Fig. 4.12 Adrenoceptor antagonists and their clinical uses

Drug	Receptor	Uses	Side effects	Pharmacokinetics
Labetalol	α/β	Hypertension	Postural hypotension	Oral absorption $t_{1/2} \sim 4$ h
Phentolamine	α	No clinical use	Hypotension Tachycardia Nasal congestion	Metabolized by the liver, given intravenously $t_{1/2} \sim 4$ h
Prazosin	α_1	Hypertension	Hypotension Tachycardia Nasal congestion Drowsiness	Oral absorption, metabolized by the liver $t_{1/2} \sim 2$ h
Yohimbine	α_2	No clinical use	Hypertension Excitement	Oral absorption, metabolized by the liver $t_{1/2} \sim 4$ h
Propanolol	β	Hypertension Angina Arrhythmias	Bronchoconstriction Heart failure	Oral absorption, first-pass metabolism, 90% plasma-protein bound $t_{1/2} \sim 4$ h
Practolol	β_1	Hypertension Angina Arrhythmias	Bronchoconstriction Heart failure	Oral absorption $t_{1/2} \sim 4$ h
Butoxamine	β_2	No clinical use		

Adrenoceptor antagonists: These are termed 'sympatholytics'. They block postsynaptic receptors (Fig. 4.12).

Inactivation

Uptake 1: This is located on neuronal terminals, and it is the main mechanism for noradrenaline inactivation. Uptake 1 has a high affinity for the uptake of noradrenaline (K = 0.3 mmol/L in the rat) but the maximum rate of uptake is low (V_{max} = 1.2 nmol/g per minute in the rat). It has a specificity rank of noradrenaline > adrenaline > isoprenaline; it is blocked by cocaine, amphetamines and tricyclic antidepressants (e.g. imipramine), which therefore potentiate the actions of noradrenaline.

Uptake 2: This is located outside neurons (e.g. in smooth muscle, cardiac muscle and endothelium), and it is the main mechanism for the removal of circulating adrenaline from the bloodstream. It has a low affinity for the uptake of noradrenaline (K = 250 mmol/L in the rat) but a high maximum rate of uptake (V_{max} = 100 nmol/g per minute in the rat). Uptake 2 has a specificity rank of adrenaline > noradrenaline > isoprenaline, and it is blocked by corticosteroids.

Many of the adrenoceptor agonists and antagonists are not entirely specific for just the α- or the β-adrenoceptors, so side-effects are common, and they should be remembered.

Metabolism of catecholamines by the enzyme monoamine oxidase: MAO is found on the surface of mitochondria, principally within adrenergic nerve terminals but also in other cells, such as those of the liver and intestines. MAO metabolizes catecholamines into their corresponding aldehydes. It comprises two major forms: MAO_A and MAO_B. Noradrenaline is mainly broken down by MAO_A in nerve terminals. Inhibitors of MAO increase the releasable store of noradrenaline, but they do not greatly potentiate sympathetic transmission, since catecholamines are mainly inactivated by reuptake. MAOIs include the antidepressant drugs phenelzine and tranylcypromine.

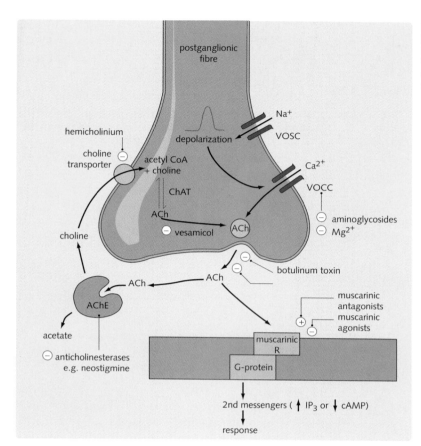

Fig. 4.13 Drugs acting on the parasympathetic nerve transmission. (VOSC, voltage-operated sodium channel; VOCC, voltage-operated calcium channel; AChE, acetylcholinesterase; ChAT, choline acetyl transferase.)

Metabolism of catecholamines by COMT: COMT is found in all tissues and breaks down most catecholamines and the byproducts of the actions of MAO. COMT metabolizes catecholamines to give a methoxy derivative. Entacapone, a COMT inhibitor, is a drug used clinically for parkinsonism.

Parasympathetic nervous system

The fibres of the parasympathetic nervous system leave the CNS from the sacral region (S3 and S4) of the spinal cord and via cranial nerves III, VII, IX and X. The fibres synapse in ganglia, which, unlike the sympathetic system, are located within the innervated organs themselves.

The major transmitter released by the postganglionic fibres at the junction with effector cells is ACh (Fig 4.13).

Parasympathetic receptors

The ACh released by postganglionic nerve fibres acts on muscarinic (M) receptors, of which between three and five subtypes exist.

'Neuroparietal' M_1 receptors

M_1 'neuroparietal' receptors are principally found in the CNS, peripheral neurons, and gastric parietal cells. Their effects tend to be excitatory, depolarizing membranes through a decrease in potassium conductance. Activation causes central excitation and gastric acid secretion, while transduction is via G-proteins and an increase in the second messengers IP_3 and DAG through stimulation of phospholipase C.

'Neurocardiac' M_2 receptors

M_2 'neurocardiac' receptors are found in the heart and on peripheral neurons. Their effects are inhibitory, increasing potassium conductance and inhibiting calcium channels. In the heart, their activation causes a decrease in the rate (via potassium) and force of contraction (via calcium). Transduction is via G-proteins and a decrease in the second messenger cAMP through inhibition of adenylyl cyclase.

'Smooth muscle-glandular' M_3 receptors

M_3 'smooth muscle-glandular' receptors are found in smooth muscle and glands. Their effects tend to be excitatory, increasing sodium conductance. Activation causes glandular secretions such as saliva and sweat, and smooth muscle contraction. Transduction is via G-proteins and an increase in the second messengers IP_3 and DAG. M_3 receptors are also located on vascular endothelium, activation of which causes vasodilatation, through the release of endothelium-derived relaxing factor (EDRF).

'Eye' M_4 receptors

M_4 'eye' receptors are believed to be exclusive to the eye. Their activation causes constriction of the pupil and accommodation for near vision. Transduction is via G-proteins and a decrease in the second messenger cAMP through inhibition of adenylyl cyclase.

Drugs acting on the parasympathetic system

Figure 4.13 summarizes the drugs that act on the parasympathetic system.

Presynaptic agents

For information regarding presynaptic agents, see p. 68.

Anticholinesterases

For information regarding anticholinesterases, see p. 70.

Postsynaptic agents

Muscarinic-receptor agonists: These are termed 'parasympathomimetic', they activate postsynaptic receptors (Fig. 4.14).

Muscarinic-receptor antagonists: These are termed 'parasympatholytic' and block postsynaptic receptors (Fig. 4.15).

Non-selective antagonists can be used in anaesthesia to prevent bronchial secretions and vagal slowing of heart rate.

Fig. 4.14 Muscarinic agonists and their clinical uses

Drug	Muscarinic receptors	Nicotinic receptors	Uses
Carbachol	++	+	Gut and bladder stimulation postoperatively
Methacholine	+++	+	
Bethanechol	+++	—	Gut and bladder stimulation postoperatively
Muscarine	+++	—	
Pilocarpine	++	—	To decrease intraocular pressure in glaucoma

Fig. 4.15 Muscarinic antagonists and their clinical uses

Drug	Muscarinic receptor	Specific uses
Atropine	Non-selective	Reduces gastrointestinal motility Cardiac arrest
Hyoscine	Non-selective	Motion sickness
Ipratropium	Non-selective	Bronchodilator
Cyclopentolate	M_4	Dilation of pupil
Tropicamide	M_4	Dilation of pupil
Pirenzepine	M_1	Reduces gastric acid secretion
Trihexyphenidyl (benzhexol)	M_1	Parkinson's disease

Fig. 4.16 Summary table of the opposing effects of sympathetic and parasympathetic nerve stimulation on body tissues

Target tissue	Sympathetic		Parasympathetic		Overall effect
Nerve terminals	α_2	Decreased release	M_2	Decreased release	Decreased transmission
Smooth muscle					
Blood vessels	$\alpha_{1/2}$	Contraction			Vasocontriction
	β_2	Relaxation	M_3	Relaxation (via EDRF)	Vasodilatation
Bronchi	β_2	Relaxation			Bronchodilation
	α_1	Contraction	M_3	Contraction	Bronchoconstriction
			M_3	Secretion	Bronchosecretion
Gastrointestinal tract:					Increased/decreased
non-sphincter	β_1/α_1	Relaxation	M_3	Contraction	motility and tone
sphincter	α_1	Contraction	M_3	Relaxation	GI secretions
secretions			M_3	Secretion	
Parietal cells			M_1	Contraction	Gastric acid secretion
Pancreas			M_3	Contraction	Increased secretions
Uterus	α_1	Contraction	M_3		
	β_2	Relaxation	M_3		
Bladder: detrusor	β_2	Relaxation	M_3	Contraction	Micturition
sphincter	α_1	Contraction	M_3	Relaxation	Urine retention
Seminal tract	α_1	Contraction			Ejaculation
	β_2	Relaxation			
Vas deferens	α_1	Contraction			Ejaculation
Penis venous sphincter			M_3	Vasodilatation	Erection
Radial muscle (iris)	α_1	Contraction	M_4	Relaxation	Pupil relaxation/constriction
Ciliary muscle	β_2	Relaxation	M_4	Contraction	Accommodation
Lacrimal gland			M_4	Contraction	Tear secretion
Heart	β_1	Increased rate and force	M_2	Decreased rate and force	
Liver	α_1/β_2	Glygenolysis			
Fat	β_1	Lipolysis			
Salivary glands	α_1/β_1	Secretion of thick saliva	M_3	Abundant secretion of watery saliva	
Platelets	α_2	Platelet aggregation			
Mast cells	β_2	Inhibition of histamine release			

Different tissues respond differently to muscarinic antagonists (Fig. 4.16). Salivary, sweat and bronchial glands are the most sensitive and can be blocked by very low doses of atropine. In contrast, the parietal cells are the most resistant, and the block of gastric acid secretion requires high doses of atropine.

The side-effects of muscarinic antagonists include:

- Dry mouth and skin, and increased body temperature (inhibition of salivary and sweat glands)
- Blurred vision and pupil no longer responsive to light (dilatation of pupil)
- Paralysis of accommodation: cycloplegia (relaxation of ciliary muscle)
- Urinary retention

- Central excitation: irritability and hyperactivity
- Sedation (hyoscine).

NITRERGIC NERVOUS SYSTEM

Nitric oxide is now well recognized as a neurotransmitter in the CNS, and more recently it has been attributed to have numerous roles to play in the peripheral nervous system too.

Nitric oxide is generated by the action of the enzyme nitric oxide synthase (NOS), of which constitutive and inducible isoforms exist. L-arginine is the amino acid precursor of nitric oxide synthesis.

Nitric oxide activates the guanylyl cyclase enzyme, which is responsible for generating cyclic guanosine monophosphate (cGMP). The synthesis of cGMP in turn activates a protein kinase, which phosphorylates ion channels in the plasma membrane, and causes hyperpolarization of the smooth muscle cell. Intracellular calcium ions are consequently sequestered into the endoplasmic reticulum, and further calcium influx into the cell inhibited by the closure of calcium channels. The overall effect of a fall in intracellular calcium is a relaxation of the smooth muscle.

The smooth muscle effects of nitric oxide in the peripheral nervous system are now recognized to be important in the gastrointestinal system, and in sexual arousal in both sexes, particularly in the male.

Therapeutic manipulation of the nitrergic nervous system is confined to the male reproductive system at present, and the agents currently used in the management of erectile dysfunction (e.g. sildenafil [Viagra®]) are discussed in Chapter 6.

Central nervous system

Objectives

After reading this chapter, you will:

- Understand the functions of the central nervous system and the diseases that can occur
- Know the drug classes used to treat these conditions, their mechanisms of action and adverse effects.

BASIC CONCEPTS

The central nervous system consists of the brain and the spinal cord, which are continuous with one another. The brain is composed of the cerebrum (which consists of the frontal, temporal, parietal and occipital lobes), the diencephalon (which includes the thalamus and hypothalamus), the brainstem (which consists of the midbrain, pons and medulla oblongata) and the cerebellum. The brain functions to interpret sensory information obtained about the internal and external environments and send messages to effector organs in response to a situation. Many different parts of the brain are associated with specific functions (Fig. 5.1). However, the brain is a complex organ and is not yet completely understood.

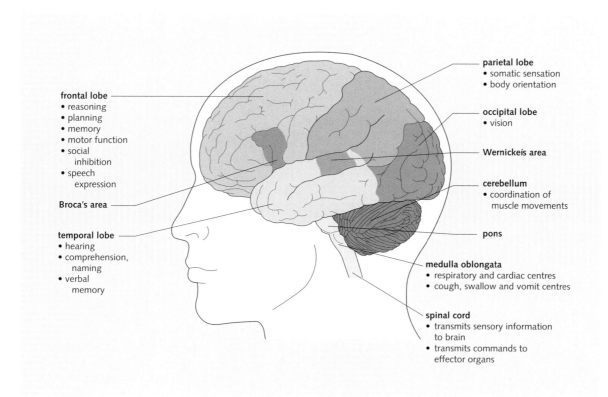

frontal lobe
- reasoning
- planning
- memory
- motor function
- social inhibition
- speech expression

Broca's area

temporal lobe
- hearing
- comprehension, naming
- verbal memory

parietal lobe
- somatic sensation
- body orientation

occipital lobe
- vision

Wernicke's area

cerebellum
- coordination of muscle movements

pons

medulla oblongata
- respiratory and cardiac centres
- cough, swallow and vomit centres

spinal cord
- transmits sensory information to brain
- transmits commands to effector organs

Fig. 5.1 Parts of the brain and their known functions.

PARKINSON'S DISEASE AND PARKINSONISM

Parkinsonism is characterized by a resting tremor, slow initiation of movements (bradykinesia), and muscle rigidity known collectively as the 'parkinsonian triad'. A patient with parkinsonism will present with characteristic signs including:

- A shuffling gait
- A blank 'mask-like' facial expression
- Speech impairment
- An inability to perform skilled tasks.

Parkinsonism is most commonly caused by Parkinson's disease, though numerous other causes do exist.

Parkinson's disease is a progressive neurological disorder of the basal ganglia that occurs most commonly in elderly people.

Aetiology

The cause of Parkinson's disease is unknown in most cases (idiopathic) although both endogenous and environmental neurotoxins are known to be responsible for causing parkinsonism.

Parkinson's disease is progressive, with continued loss of dopaminergic neurons in the substantia nigra correlating well with worsening of clinical symptoms. The possibility of a neurotoxic cause has been strengthened by the finding that 1-methyl-4-phenyl-1,2,3,6-tetrahydropyridine (MPTP), a chemical contaminant of heroin, causes irreversible damage to the nigrostriatal dopaminergic pathway. Thus, this damage can lead to the development of symptoms similar to those of idiopathic Parkinson's disease; it has been seen in drug users in California and has been experimentally induced in primates.

Drugs that block dopamine receptors can also induce parkinsonism. Neuroleptic drugs (pp. 96–100) used in the treatment of schizophrenia can produce parkinsonian symptoms as an adverse effect. Rare causes of parkinsonism are cerebral ischaemia (progressive atherosclerosis or stroke), viral encephalitis or other pathological damage.

Figure 5.2 summarizes the causes of parkinsonism.

RATS in the parking lot! Symptoms of parkinsonism include *Rigidity, Akinesia, Tremor* and *Shuffling gait.*

Fig. 5.2 Aetiological mechanisms in the development of parkinsonism

- Mostly unknown (idiopathic Parkinson's disease)
- Toxin induced: MPTP; carbon monoxide, manganese
- Drug induced: neuroleptics (dopamine antagonists)
- Rare causes: cerebral ischaemia; viral encephalitis and others?

MPTP, methyl-4-phenyl-1,2,3,6-tetrahydropyridine

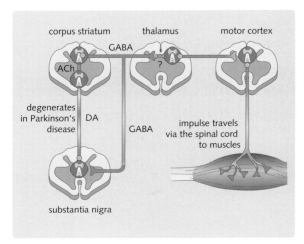

Fig. 5.3 Basal ganglia systems involved in Parkinson's disease. (ACh, acetylcholine; DA, dopamine; GABA, γ-aminobutyric acid.) (Redrawn from Page et al. 2002.)

Pathogenesis

Post-mortem analysis of brains of parkinsonian patients shows a substantially reduced concentration of dopamine (less than 10% of normal) in the basal ganglia. The basal ganglia exert an extrapyramidal neural influence that normally maintains smooth voluntary movement.

The main pathology in Parkinson's disease is a progressive degeneration of the dopaminergic neurons of the substantia nigra, which project via the nigrostriatal pathway to the corpus striatum (Fig. 5.3). The inhibitory dopaminergic activity of the nigrostriatal pathway is, therefore, considerably reduced (by 20–40%) in people with Parkinson's disease.

The reduction in the inhibitory dopaminergic activity of the nigrostriatal pathway results in unopposed cholinergic neuron hyperactivity from the corpus striatum, which contributes to the pathological features of parkinsonism. Frank symptoms of

Fig. 5.4 Drugs used to treat parkinsonism and their site of action. (ACh, acetylcholine; L-dopa, levodopa; MAO$_B$, monoamine oxidase B; COMT, catechol-O-methyl transferase; DA, dopamine.)

parkinsonism appear only when more than 80% of the dopaminergic neurons of the substantia nigra have degenerated.

Untreated Parkinson's eventually results in dementia and death.

Treatment of parkinsonism

The treatment of parkinsonism is based on correcting the imbalance between the dopaminergic and cholinergic systems at the basal ganglia (Fig. 5.4). Two major groups of drugs are used: drugs that increase dopaminergic activity between the substantia nigra and the corpus striatum, and anticholinergic drugs that inhibit striatal cholinergic activity.

Drugs that increase dopaminergic activity

Dopamine precursors

An example of a dopamine precursor is levodopa (L-dopa).

Mechanism of action: L-dopa is the immediate precursor of dopamine and is able to penetrate the blood–brain barrier to replenish the dopamine content of the corpus striatum. L-dopa is decarboxylated to dopamine in the brain by dopa decarboxylase, and it has beneficial effects produced through the actions of dopamine on D$_2$ receptors (see Fig. 5.4). Dopamine itself is not used, owing to its inability to cross the blood–brain barrier.

Route of administration: L-dopa is administered orally. It reaches peak plasma concentrations after 1–2 hours and only 1% reaches the brain, owing to peripheral metabolism.

Indications: L-dopa is used in the treatment of parkinsonism (excluding drug-induced extrapyramidal symptoms).

Contraindications: Closed-angle glaucoma.

Adverse effects: The extensive peripheral metabolism of L-dopa means that large doses have to be given to produce therapeutic effects in the brain. Large doses are more likely to produce adverse effects. These include:

- Nausea and vomiting
- Psychiatric side-effects (schizophrenia-like symptoms)
- Cardiovascular effects (hypotension)
- Dyskinesias.

Nausea and vomiting are caused by stimulation of dopamine receptors in the chemoreceptor trigger zone in the area postrema (p. 158), which lies outside the blood–brain barrier.

Psychiatric side-effects are common limiting factors in L-dopa treatment; these include vivid dreams, confusion and psychotic symptoms more commonly seen in schizophrenia. These effects are probably a result of increased dopaminergic activity in the mesolimbic area of the brain, possibly similar to that found pathologically in schizophrenia (dopaminergic overactivity is implicated in schizophrenia, p. 96).

Hypotension is common but usually asymptomatic. Cardiac arrhythmias are due to increased catecholamine stimulation following the excessive peripheral metabolism of L-dopa.

Dyskinesias can often develop and tend to involve the face and limbs. They usually reflect overtreatment and respond to simple dose reduction.

Three strategies have been developed to optimize L-dopa treatment, to maximize the central effects of L-dopa within the brain, and minimize its unwanted peripheral effects. These strategies involve co-administration of:

- Carbidopa (given with L-dopa as co-careldopa) or benserazide (given with L-dopa as co-beneldopa), inhibitors of dopa decarboxylase in the periphery, that cannot penetrate the blood–brain barrier. Hence, extracerebral conversion of L-dopa to dopamine is inhibited.

- Domperidone, a dopamine antagonist, that does not penetrate the blood–brain barrier and can, therefore, block the stimulation of dopamine receptors in the periphery.
- Selegiline and entacapone, monoamine oxidase $(MAO)_B$ and catechol-O-methyltransferase (COMT) inhibitors, respectively, which inhibit dopamine degradation in the central nervous system (CNS).

Therapeutic notes: Initially, treatment with L-dopa is effective in 80% of patients with possible restoration of near-normal motor function. Although L-dopa restores dopamine levels in the short term, therapy has no effect on the underlying degenerative disease process.

As progressive neuronal degeneration continues, the capacity of the corpus striatum to convert L-dopa to dopamine diminishes. This affects the majority of patients within 5 years and manifests itself as 'end of dose deterioration' (a shortening of duration of each dose of L-dopa), and the 'on-off effect' (rapid fluctuations in clinical state, varying from increased mobility and a general improvement to increased rigidity and hypokinesia). The latter effect occurs suddenly and for short periods from a few minutes to a few hours, tending to worsen with length of treatment.

Dopamine agonists

Examples of dopamine agonists include bromocriptine, ropinirole, cabergoline (longer acting), pergolide, pramipexole, lisuride and apomorphine.

Mechanism of action: Bromocriptine, ropinirole, cabergoline (longer acting), pergolide, pramipexole, lisuride and apomorphine are dopamine agonists selective for the D_2 receptor (see Fig. 5.4). Apomorphine also has agonist action at D_1 receptors. Pramipexole has a particularly high affinity for D_3 receptors.

Route of administration: Oral. Apomorphine is given by the subcutaneous route.

Indications: Dopamine agonists are used in combination with L-dopa in an attempt to reduce the late adverse effects of L-dopa therapy ('end of dose deterioration' and 'on-off effect') or when L-dopa alone does not adequately control the symptoms.

Adverse effects: The adverse effects of dopamine agonists are essentially similar to those of L-dopa (i.e. nausea, postural hypotension, psychiatric symptoms), but they tend to be more common and more severe. Apomorphine produces profound nausea and vomiting. Ergot-derived dopamine agonists (bromocriptine, cabergoline, lisuride and pergolide) can cause fibrosis.

Therapeutic notes: Currently bromocriptine is the most used of the dopamine agonists in the treatment of Parkinson's disease.

Drugs stimulating release of dopamine
Amantadine is an example of a drug that stimulates the release of dopamine (see Fig. 5.4).

Mechanism of action: Facilitation of neuronal dopamine release and inhibition of its reuptake into nerves, and additional muscarinic blocking actions.

Route of administration: Oral.

Indications: Amantadine has a synergistic effect when used in conjunction with L-dopa therapy in Parkinson's disease.

Adverse effects: Anorexia, nausea, hallucinations.

Therapeutic notes: Amantadine has modest antiparkinsonian effects, but it is only of short-term benefit, since most of its effectiveness is lost within 6 months of initiating treatment.

MAO$_B$ inhibitors
Selegiline is an example of a MAO$_B$ inhibitor.

Mechanism of action: Selegiline selectively inhibits the MAO$_B$ enzyme in the brain that is normally responsible for the degradation of dopamine (see Fig. 5.4). By reducing the catabolism of dopamine, the actions of L-dopa are potentiated, thus allowing the dose to be reduced by up to a third. There is evidence to suggest that selegiline may slow the progression of the underlying neuronal degeneration in Parkinson's disease.

Route of administration: Oral.

Indications: MAO$_B$ inhibitors can be used on their own in mild cases of parkinsonism or in conjunction with L-dopa to reduce 'end-of-dose' deterioration in severe parkinsonism.

Adverse effects: The adverse effects of MAO$_B$ inhibitors are those that might be expected by potentiation of L-dopa.

Note that with the possible exception of selegiline, none of the drugs used in Parkinson's disease affect the inevitable progressive degeneration of nigrostriatal dopaminergic neurons. The disease process is unaffected, just compensated for by drug therapy.

Mrs Patches, a 62-year-old barrister, presents to her GP complaining of shaking arms, the right arm more prominently so than the left. She notes that alcohol does not help to steady the shaking and that people at work have started complaining about her handwriting becoming too small to read. She also mentions her body muscles have been feeling rather stiff.

She is referred to a neurologist, who observes her face to be expressionless, a resting tremor and increased muscle tone. Her power, reflexes, coordination and sensation are found to be normal. Examination of her gait shows she is slow getting started and has difficulty stopping and starting.

A diagnosis of Parkinson's disease is made and the implications discussed with Mrs Patches. She returns 3 months later and says she now wishes to commence treatment; she has the same symptoms as before, however, they are interfering more with her daily life. She is given co-beneldopa and this helps to control her symptoms.

COMT inhibitors
Entacapone and tolcapone are examples of COMT inhibitors.

Mechanism of action: Dopamine is broken down by a second pathway, in addition to that of MAO$_B$. The enzyme COMT is responsible for the degradation of dopamine to inactive methylated metabolites. COMT inhibitors specifically inhibit this enzyme.

Route of administration: Oral.

Indications: As an adjunct to L-dopa preparations when 'end-of-dose' is problematic.

Contraindications: Phaeochromocytoma.

Adverse effects: Nausea, vomiting, abdominal pain, diarrhoea.

Therapeutic notes: Due to hepatotoxicity, tolcapone should only be prescribed under specialist supervision.

Drugs that inhibit striatal cholinergic activity

Anticholinergic agents

Benzatropine, procyclidine and orphenadrine are examples of anticholinergic (antimuscarinic) agents.

Mechanism of action: Benzatropine, procyclidine and orphenadrine are antagonists at the muscarinic receptors that mediate striatal cholinergic excitation (see Fig. 5.4). Their major action in the treatment of Parkinson's disease is to reduce the excessive striatal cholinergic activity that characterizes the disease.

Route of administration: Oral.

Adverse effects: Typical peripheral anticholinergic effects, such as a dry mouth and blurred vision, are less common. More often, patients experience a variety of CNS effects, ranging from mild memory loss to acute confusional states.

Therapeutic notes: Termination of anticholinergic treatment should be gradual, as parkinsonism can worsen when these drugs are withdrawn. Anticholinergic drugs are most effective in controlling tremor rather than other symptoms of Parkinson's disease.

Transplantation

The transplantation of cells from the substantia nigra of human fetuses into the putamen of patients with Parkinson's disease has shown some success in controlling parkinsonian symptoms.

Transplantation in the treatment of Parkinson's disease is still experimental, and its role is highly controversial.

DEMENTIA

Alzheimer's disease is a specific process that results in dementia, and is unrelated to the dementias associated with stroke, brain trauma and alcohol. Alzheimer's disease is very common in elderly people, and its prevalence increases markedly with age.

Alzheimer's disease is progressive, and it is associated with shrinkage of the brain substance, loss of neuronal tissue and deposition of so-called amyloid plaques. The clinical features include deterioration in cognitive function, disorientation and generalized confusion.

Neuropharmacological studies have shown that despite widespread shrinkage of the brain, loss of neurons in the forebrain is most marked, and a relative selective loss of cholinergic neurons most likely accounts for the features of this dementia. The obvious therapeutic target is, therefore, restoration of cholinergic function.

Certain cholinesterase inhibitors appear to improve cognitive functioning in as many as 50% of patients, and delay subsequent deterioration in mental capacity.

Cholinesterase inhibitors

Donepezil, galantamine and rivastigmine are cholinesterase inhibitors, licensed for use in dementia in the UK.

Mechanism of action: The cholinesterase inhibitors prevent the breakdown of acetylcholine within the synaptic cleft, and they enhance endogenous cholinogenic activity within the CNS and peripheral tissues.

Route of administration: Oral.

Indications: Mild to moderate dementia in Alzheimer's disease.

Contraindications: Pregnancy, breastfeeding, hepatic and renal impairment.

Adverse effects: Nausea, vomiting, diarrhoea, anorexia, agitation.

ANXIETY AND SLEEP DISORDERS

Anxiety and anxiolytics

Anxiety is a state characterized by psychological symptoms such as a diffuse, unpleasant and vague feeling of apprehension, often accompanied by physical symptoms of autonomic arousal such as palpitations, light-headedness, perspiration, 'butterflies' and, in some people, restlessness.

While occasional anxiety is perfectly normal, it is a common and disabling symptom in a variety of mental illnesses including phobias, panic disorders and obsessive compulsive disorders. Drugs used to treat such anxiety disorders are called anxiolytics.

Sleep disorders and hypnotics

Insomnia is a common and non-specific disorder that may be reported by 40–50% of people at any given time.

Causes of insomnia include medical illness, alcohol or drugs, periodic limb movement disorder, sleep apnoea and psychiatric illness. Without an obvious underlying cause, it is known as primary or psycho-physiological.

Hypnotics are drugs used to treat psycho-physiological (primary) insomnia. The distinction between the treatment of anxiety and that of sleep disorders is not clear-cut, particularly if anxiety is the main impediment to sleep.

γ-Aminobutyric acid receptor

The γ-aminobutyric acid (GABA) receptors of the $GABA_A$ type are involved in the actions of some classes of hypnotic/anxiolytic drugs, notably:

- The benzodiazepines, which are currently the most commonly used clinically
- Newer non-benzodiazepine hypnotics, e.g. zopiclone
- The now obsolete barbiturates.

The $GABA_A$ receptor belongs to the superfamily of ligand-gated ion channels. It consists of several subunits – α, β, γ and δ – which form the GABA/Cl⁻ channel complex, as well as containing benzodiazepine and barbiturate modulatory receptor sites. The GABA binding site appears to be located on the α and β subunits whereas the benzodiazepine modulatory site is distinct and located on the γ subunit.

GABA released from nerve terminals binds to postsynaptic $GABA_A$ receptors, the activation of which increases the Cl^- conductance of the neuron. Occupation of the benzodiazepine sites by benzodiazepine receptor agonists enhances the actions of GABA on the Cl^- conductance of the neuronal membrane. The barbiturates similarly enhance the action of GABA, but by occupying a distinct modulatory site (Fig. 5.5).

Anxiolytic and hypnotic drugs

The pharmacotherapy of anxiety and sleep disorders involves several different classes of drug, as shown in Figure 5.6, and non-pharmacological management relying on cognitive and behaviour psychotherapy.

Benzodiazepines

Benzodiazepines are drugs with anxiolytic, hypnotic, muscle relaxation and anticonvulsant actions that are used in the treatment of both anxiety states and insomnia.

Benzodiazepines are marketed as either hypnotics or anxiolytics. It is mainly the duration of action that determines the choice of drug (see below).

Mechanism of action: Benzodiazepines potentiate the action of GABA, the primary inhibitory neurotransmitter in the CNS. They do this by binding to a site on $GABA_A$ receptors, increasing their affinity for GABA. This results in an increased opening frequency of these ligand-gated Cl^- channels, thus potentiating the effect of GABA release in terms of inhibitory effects on the postsynaptic cell (Fig. 5.5).

Indications: Benzodiazepines are used clinically in the short-term relief of severe anxiety and severe insomnia, preoperative sedation, status epilepticus and acute alcohol withdrawal.

Route of administration: Oral is the usual route. Intravenous, intramuscular and rectal preparations are available.

Contraindications: Benzodiazepines should not be given to people with bronchopulmonary disease, and they have additive or synergistic effects with other central depressants such as alcohol, barbiturates and antihistamines.

Adverse effects: Benzodiazepines have several adverse effects:

- Drowsiness, ataxia and reduced psychomotor performance are common; therefore, care is necessary when driving or operating machinery.
- Dependence becomes apparent after 4–6 weeks, and is both physical and psychological. The withdrawal syndrome (in 30% of patients) comprises rebound anxiety and insomnia, tremulousness and twitching.

Although in overdose benzodiazepines alone are relatively safe when compared with other sedatives, such as barbiturates, if benzodiazepines are taken in combination with alcohol the CNS-depressant effects are potentiated and fatal respiratory depression can result. Treatment is with the benzodiazepine antagonist flumazenil.

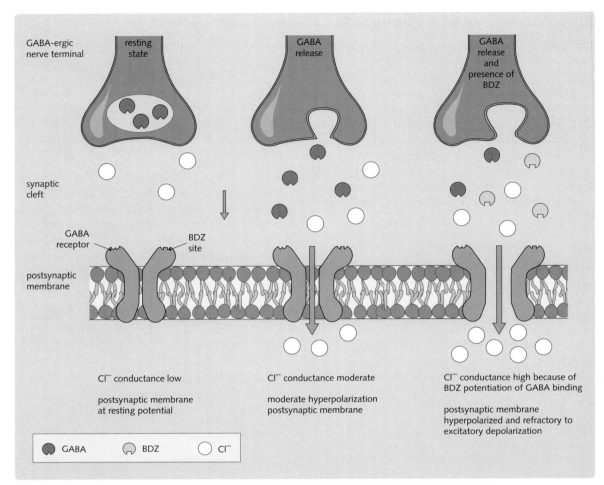

Fig. 5.5 Diagrammatic representation of the GABA$_A$ receptor and how its activity is enhanced by benzodiazepines and similarly by barbiturates. (BDZ, benzodiazepine; GABA, γ-aminobutyric acid; Cl⁻, chloride ion.) (Redrawn from Page et al. 2002.)

Fig. 5.6 Drugs used to treat anxiety and sleep disorders	
Anxiolytics	**Hypnotics**
Benzodiazepines (act on GABA$_A$ receptors) e.g. diazepam, lorazepam	Benzodiazepines (act on GABA$_A$ receptors) e.g. triazolam, temazepam, lormetazepam, nitrazepam
Acting on serotonergic receptors (act on 5-HT$_{1A}$ or 5-HT$_3$ receptors) e.g. buspirone	Non-benzodiazepine hypnotics (act on GABA$_A$ receptors) e.g. zopiclone, zolpidem and zaleplon
Other drugs e.g. proparnolol antidepressants	Other drugs e.g. chloral hydrate clomethiazole barbiturates (obsolete) sedative antidepressants sedative antihistamines

GABA, γ-aminobutyric acid; 5-HT, 5-hydroxytryptamine

Therapeutic notes: Benzodiazepines are active orally, and they differ mainly in respect of their duration of action (Fig. 5.7). Short-acting agents (e.g. lorazepam and temazepam) are metabolized to inactive compounds, and these are used mainly as sleeping pills because of the relative lack of 'hangover' effects in the morning. Some long-acting agents (e.g. diazepam) are converted to long-lasting active metabolites with a half-life longer than the administered parent drug. With others (e.g. nitrazepam) it is the parent drug itself that is metabolized slowly. Such drugs are more suitable for an anxiolytic effect maintained all day long, or when early morning waking is the problem.

Non-benzodiazepine hypnotics

Zopiclone, zolpidem and zaleplon are the newer-generation hypnotics that have a short duration of

Fig. 5.7 Approximate elimination half-lives of the benzodiazepines

Benzodiazepine	Approximate half-life (hours)
Midazolam	2 – 4
Temazepam	8 – 12
Lormetazepam	10
Lorazepam	12
Nitrazepam	24
Diazepam	32 (one metabolite is active for up to 200 hours)

action with little or no hangover effect. Although these drugs are not benzodiazepines, they act in a comparable manner to benzodiazepines on the GABA$_A$ receptor, although not at exactly the same sites.

Anxiolytic drugs acting at serotonergic receptors

The serotonergic theory of anxiety suggests that serotonergic transmission is involved in anxiety as, in general, stimulation of this system causes anxiety whereas a reduction in serotonergic neuronal activity reduces anxiety.

The serotonergic theory prompted the development of anxiolytic drugs that act to moderate serotonergic neurotransmission while not causing sedation and incoordination.

5-HT$_{1A}$ agonists

Buspirone is a serotonergic (5-HT$_{1A}$) agonist.

Mechanism of action: In the raphe nucleus the dendrites of serotonergic neurons possess inhibitory presynaptic autoreceptors of the 5-HT$_{1A}$ subtype that, when stimulated, decrease the firing of 5-HT neurons. This class of anxiolytic agents called the azapirones are thought to reduce 5-HT transmission by acting as partial agonists at these 5-HT$_{1A}$ receptors. Buspirone is the first of this new class of anxiolytics.

Route of administration: Oral.

Indications: Buspirone is indicated for the short-term relief of generalized anxiety disorder.

Contraindications: 5-HT$_{1A}$ agonists should not be used in people with epilepsy.

Adverse effects: The adverse effects of 5-HT$_{1A}$ agonists include nervousness, dizziness, headache and light-headedness.

In contrast to benzodiazepines, buspirone does not cause significant sedation or cognitive impairment, and it carries only a minimal risk of dependence and withdrawal. It does not potentiate the effects of alcohol.

Therapeutic notes: The anxiolytic effect of buspirone gradually evolves over 1–3 weeks.

5-hydroxytryptamine 3 antagonists

Ondansetron is a 5-HT$_3$ receptor antagonist that is well established for use as an antiemetic drug.

Ondansetron also has anxiolytic properties by virtue of its antagonism at the excitatory postsynaptic 5-HT$_3$ receptor.

β-Adrenoreceptor blockers

β-Adrenoreceptor blockers or β-blockers, e.g. propranolol, can be very effective in alleviating the somatic manifestations of anxiety caused by marked sympathetic arousal, such as palpitations, tremor, sweating and diarrhoea.

Mechanism of action: β-Blockers act by antagonism at β-adrenoreceptors so that excessive catecholamine release does not produce the sympathetic responses of tachycardia, sweating, etc. β-Blockers are also used in cardiovascular disease (p. 35).

Route of administration: Oral.

Indications: β-Blockers are indicated in patients with predominantly somatic symptoms; this, in turn, may prevent the onset of worry and fear. Patients with predominantly psychological symptoms may obtain no benefit. β-Blockers can be useful in social phobias and to reduce performance anxiety in musicians, for whom fine motor control may be critical.

Contraindications: β-Blockers should not be used in people with asthma or heart failure.

Adverse effects: β-Blockers can cause bradycardia, heart failure, bronchospasm and peripheral vasoconstriction.

Barbiturates

Barbiturates are non-selective CNS depressants that produce effects ranging from sedation and reduction of anxiety to unconsciousness and death from respiratory and cardiovascular failure. Barbiturates increase GABA-mediated inhibition by acting on the same receptor as benzodiazepines (the $GABA_A$ receptor), though at a different site.

At low doses, barbiturates prolong the duration of individual Cl^- channel openings triggered by a given GABA stimulus (benzodiazepines increase the frequency of Cl^- channel openings). At high doses, they are far more depressant than benzodiazepines because they start to increase Cl^- conductance directly, thus decreasing the sensitivity of the postsynaptic membrane to excitatory transmitters.

Although very popular until the 1960s as sedative/hypnotic agents, they are now obsolete since they readily lead to psychological and physical dependence, and a relatively small overdose can be fatal. Conversely, benzodiazepines, which have largely replaced barbiturates as sedative/hypnotics, have been taken in huge overdoses without serious long-term effects.

Barbiturates, however, still have a place in anaesthesia (p. 104) and to a lesser extent in the treatment of epilepsy (p. 104).

An understanding of the $GABA_A$/Cl^- channel complex is central to the mechanism of action of several classes of hypnotic/anxiolytic drugs. You should be aware what these are.

Miscellaneous agents

A number of miscellaneous hypnotic agents have been used historically and are still prescribed under certain circumstances.

Chloral hydrate and derivatives

Chloral hydrate is metabolized to trichloroethanol, which is an effective hypnotic. It is cheap, but causes gastric irritation and there is no convincing evidence that it has any advantage over the newer benzodiazepines.

Chloral hydrate and its derivatives were previously popular hypnotics for children. Current thinking does not justify the use of hypnotics in children, and these drugs now have very limited uses.

Clomethiazole (chlormethiazole)

Clomethiazole may be a useful hypnotic in elderly people because of the relative freedom from hangover effects. It has no advantage over benzodiazepines in younger adults.

Clomethiazole was once indicated to attenuate the symptoms of acute alcohol withdrawal, though it has been largely replaced by the benzodiazepine, chlordiazepoxide.

Antidepressants

If the underlying cause of insomnia is associated with depression, or particularly in depressed patients exhibiting anxiety and agitation, then tricyclic antidepressants (TCAs) with sedative actions (p. 91), e.g. amitriptyline, may be useful, as they act as hypnotics when given at bedtime. Alternatively, selective serotonin reuptake inhibitors (SSRIs, p. 92) may correct the mood disorder and lessen the symptoms of anxiety or insomnia.

Sedative antihistamines

The older antihistamine drugs, e.g. diphenhydramine, have antimuscarinic actions and pass the blood–brain barrier, commonly causing drowsiness and psychomotor impairment.

Proprietary brands of diphenhydramine are on sale to the public to relieve temporary sleep disturbances, as these drugs are relatively safe.

AFFECTIVE DISORDERS

Affective disorders involve a disturbance of mood (cognitive/emotional symptoms) associated with changes in behaviour, energy, appetite and sleep (biological symptoms). Affective disorders can be thought of as pathological extremes of the normal continuum of human moods, from extreme excitement and elation (mania) to severe depressive states.

There are two types of affective disorder: unipolar affective disorders and bipolar affective disorders.

Unipolar affective disorders

A common unipolar affective disorder is depression, which is characterized by misery, malaise, despair, guilt, apathy, indecisiveness, low energy and fatigue, changes in sleeping pattern, loss of appetite and suicidal thoughts. Attempts have been made to classify types of depression as either 'reactive' or 'endogenous' in origin.

Reactive depression is where there is a clear psychological cause, e.g. bereavement. It involves less-severe symptoms and less likelihood of biological disturbance. It affects 3–10% of the population, with the incidence increasing with age, and it is more common in females.

Endogenous depression is where there is no clear cause and more severe symptoms, e.g. suicidal thoughts, and a greater likelihood of biological disturbance, e.g. insomnia, anorexia. It affects 1% of the population, usually starting in early adulthood, and affecting both sexes equally.

The distinction between reactive and endogenous depression is of importance since there is some evidence that depressions with endogenous features tend to respond better to drug therapy.

Bipolar affective disorders

Bipolar affective disorder presents with mood and behaviour oscillating between depression and mania, and it is, therefore, also known as manic-depressive disorder.

Bipolar affective disorder develops earlier in life than unipolar depressive disorders, and it tends to be inherited. It affects 1% of the population, and it can have associated elements of psychotic phenomena.

Mania hardly ever exists in isolation from depression, which is why it is referred to as bipolar affective disorder, as it has two faces.

Monoamine theory of depression

The aetiology of major depressive disorders is not clear. Genetic, environmental and neurochemical influences have all been examined as possible aetiological factors.

The most widely accepted neurochemical explanation of endogenous depression involves the monoamines (noradrenaline; serotonin [5-HT]; dopamine). The original hypothesis of depression, 'the monoamine theory', stated that depression resulted from a functional deficit of these transmitter amines, whereas conversely mania was caused by an excess.

The monoamine theory explains why:

- Drugs that deplete monoamines are depressant, e.g. reserpine and methyldopa.

- A wide range of drugs that increase the functional availability of monoamine neurotransmitters improve mood in depressed patients, e.g. tricyclic antidepressants (TCAs) and MAO inhibitors.
- The concentration of monoamines and their metabolites is reduced in the cerebrospinal fluid (CSF) of depressed patients.
- In some post-mortem studies the most consistent finding is an elevation in cortical $5\text{-}HT_2$ binding.

The monoamine theory cannot explain why:

- A number of compounds that increase the functional availability of monoamines, e.g. amphetamines, cocaine and L-dopa, have no effect on the mood of depressed patients.
- Some older, atypical antidepressants e.g. iprindole, worked without manipulating monoaminergic systems.
- There is a 'therapeutic delay' of 2 weeks between the full neurochemical effects of antidepressants and the start of their therapeutic effect.

It is unlikely, therefore, that monoamine mechanisms alone are responsible for the symptoms of depression. Other systems that may be involved in depression include:

- The GABA system
- The neuropeptide systems, particularly vasopressin and the endogenous opiates
- Secondary-messenger systems also appear to have a crucial role in some treatments.

Treatment of unipolar depressive disorders

The major classes of drug that are used to treat depression, and their mechanisms of action, are summarized in Figure 5.8.

Although almost certainly flawed and incomplete, the monoamine theory is probably the best way to rationalize your thinking about affective disorders, and to understand the mechanism of action of the drugs used in their treatment.

TCAs and related drugs

Examples of TCAs and related drugs include amitriptyline, imipramine, dosulepin (dothiepin) and lofepramine.

Fig. 5.8 Major classes of antidepressant drugs and their mechanisms of action

Class of anti-depressant drug	Examples	Mode of action
Tricyclic antidepressants (TCAs)	Amitriptyline Imipramine Lofepramine	Non-specific blockers of monoamine uptake
Selective serotonin reuptake inhibitors (SSRIs)	Fluoxetine Paroxetine Sertraline	Selective blockers of 5-HT reuptake
Serotonin–noradrenaline reuptake inhibitors (SNRIs)	Venlafaxine	Selective blockers of 5-HT and noradrenalline uptake
Monoamine oxidase inhibitors (MAOIs)	Phenelzine Tranylcrpromine	Non-competitive, non-selective irreversible blockers of MAO_A and MAO_B
Reversible inhibitors of MAO_A (RIMAs)	Moclobemide	Reversibly inhibit MAO_A selectively
Atypical	Reboxetine Mirtazapine	Act by various mechanisms that are poorly understood

5-HT, 5-hydroxytryptamine; MAO, monoamine oxidase

Mechanism of action: TCAs act by blocking 5-HT and noradrenaline uptake into the presynaptic terminal from the synaptic cleft (Fig. 5.9). They also have a certain affinity for H_1 and muscarinic receptors, and for α_1- and α_2-receptors.

Contraindications: TCAs and related drugs should not be used in:

- Recent myocardial infarction or arrhythmias (especially heart block) since TCAs increase the risk of conduction abnormalities
- Manic phase
- Severe liver disease
- Epilepsy, where TCAs lower the seizure threshold
- Patients taking other anticholinergic drugs, alcohol and adrenaline as TCAs potentiate the effects of these.

Lidocaine is contraindicated in combination with TCAs, owing to a potentially fatal drug interaction.

Adverse effects: Although TCAs are an effective therapy for depression, their adverse effects can reduce patient compliance and acceptability. Side-effects include:

- Muscarinic blocking effects such as a dry mouth, blurred vision, constipation
- α-Adrenergic blocking effects causing postural hypotension
- Noradrenaline uptake block in the heart, increasing the risk of arrhythmias
- Histamine-blocking effects leading to sedation
- Weight gain.

TCAs are relatively dangerous in overdose. Patients present with confusion, mania, and potentially fatal arrhythmias due to the cardiotoxic nature of the drug.

Therapeutic notes: No individual TCA has superior antidepressant activity, and the choice of drug is usually determined by the most acceptable or desired side-effects. For example, drugs with sedative actions, such as amitriptyline or trimipramine, are the TCAs of choice for patients in agitated or anxious states. The most recent TCA is lofepramine, which causes fewer antimuscarinic side-effects, and is less dangerous if taken in overdose.

Therapeutic effects take 2–3 weeks to develop. TCA-related antidepressants should be withdrawn slowly.

Selective serotonin reuptake inhibitors (SSRIs)

SSRIs are the most recently introduced class of anti-depressant agent. Fluoxetine (Prozac®) is an SSRI. Other examples include citalopram, fluvoxamine, paroxetine and sertraline.

Mechanism of action: SSRIs act with a high specificity for potent inhibition of serotonin reuptake into nerve terminals from the synaptic cleft, while having only minimal effects on noradrenaline uptake (see Fig. 5.9). They block serotonin transporters, which belong to a class of Na^+/Cl^--coupled transporters.

Contraindications: Contraindications with SSRIs are few. They should not be used with MAO inhibitors as the combination can cause a potentially fatal serotonergic syndrome of hyperthermia and cardiovascular collapse.

Adverse effects: The side-effect profile of SSRIs is much better than that of TCAs and MAO inhibitors as there are no amine interactions, anticholinergic actions, adrenergic blockade or toxic effects in overdose. Adverse effects, however, caused by their effect on serotonergic nerves throughout the body, include nausea, diarrhoea, insomnia, anxiety and

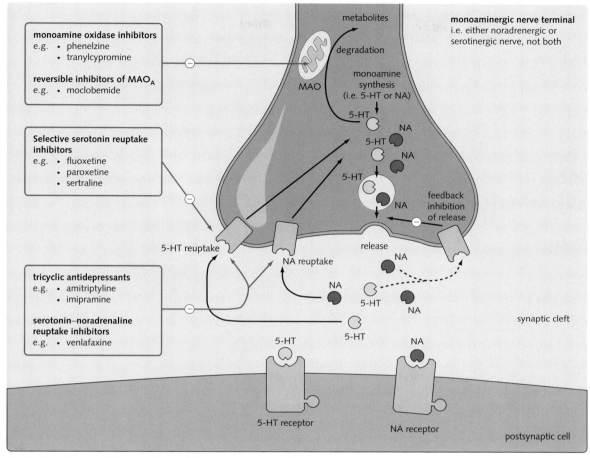

Fig. 5.9 Site of action of the major classes of drug used to treat unipolar depression. (5-HT, 5-hydroxytryptamine (serotonin); MAO, monoamine oxidase; NA, noradrenaline.)

agitation. Sexual dysfunction is sometimes a problem.

Therapeutic notes: SSRIs have a similar efficacy to that of TCAs. It is their clinical advantages and lack of side-effects that have led to their popularity. These include no anticholinergic effects, no toxicity in overdose and no cardiotoxic effects. SSRIs are now the most widely prescribed antidepressants.

Serotonin-noradrenaline reuptake inhibitors

Venlafaxine was the first and is the most commonly used serotonin-noradrenaline reuptake inhibitor (SNRI)-type antidepressant.

Mechanism of action: SNRIs cause potentiation of neurotransmitter activity in the CNS, by blocking the norepinephrine and serotonin reuptake transporter (see Fig. 5.9).

Contraindications: The drug interactions of SNRIs are much like those of SSRIs; however, extra care must be taken with hypertensive patients as venlafaxine raises blood pressure.

Adverse effects: The adverse effects of SNRIs are similar to those of SSRIs, but they occur with lower frequency.

Therapeutic notes: The pharmacological effects of venlafaxine are similar to those of the TCAs, but adverse effects are reduced because it has little affinity for cholinergic and histaminergic receptors or α-adrenoreceptors.

MAO inhibitors

Examples of irreversible MAO inhibitors include phenelzine, tranylcypromine and isocarboxazid, and an example of reversible inhibitors of MAO_A (RIMAs) is moclobemide.

Mechanism of action: MAO inhibitors block the action of MAO_A and MAO_B, which are neuron enzymes that metabolize (degrade) the monoamines (noradrenaline, 5-HT and dopamine) (see Fig. 5.9). MAO has two main isoforms, MAO_A and MAO_B, which differ in terms of substrate preference; inhibition of the MAO_A form correlates best with antidepressant efficacy. Both non-selective irreversible blockers of MAO_A and MAO_B, and drugs that reversibly inhibit MAO_A are available.

Adverse effects: Dietary interactions may occur, such as the 'cheese reaction'. MAO in the gut wall and liver normally breaks down ingested tyramine. When the enzyme is inhibited, tyramine reaches the circulation and this causes the release of noradrenaline from sympathetic nerve terminals; this can lead to a severe and potentially fatal rise in blood pressure. Patients on MAO inhibitors must, therefore, avoid foods rich in tyramine, which include cheese, game and alcoholic drinks. Preparations containing sympathomimetic amines (e.g. cough mixtures and nasal decongestants) should also be avoided. MAO inhibitors are not specific, and they reduce the metabolism of barbiturates, opioids and alcohol. Side-effects include CNS stimulation causing excitement and tremor, sympathetic blockade causing postural hypotension, and muscarinic blockade causing a dry mouth and blurred vision. Phenelzine can be hepatotoxic.

Therapeutic notes: Response to treatment with MAO inhibitors may be delayed for 3 weeks or more. Phobic and depressed patients with atypical, hypochondriacal or hysterical features are said to respond best to MAO inhibitors. Because of the dietary and drug restrictions outlined above, MAO inhibitors are largely reserved for depression refractory to other antidepressants and treatment.

Atypical antidepressants

Examples of atypical antidepressants include reboxetine, mirtazapine and tryptophan.

Mechanism of action: Reboxetine is a selective inhibitor of noradrenaline reuptake, increasing the concentration of this mediator in the synaptic cleft. Mirtazapine has α_2-adrenoreceptor-blocking activity, which, by acting on inhibitory α_2-autoreceptors on central noradrenergic nerve endings, may increase the amount of noradrenaline in the synaptic cleft. Tryptophan is an amino acid precursor for serotonin.

Contraindications: The contraindications for atypical antidepressants are similar to those for TCAs.

Adverse effects: Atypical antidepressants generally cause less autonomic side-effects and are less dangerous in overdose, owing to their lower cardiotoxicity compared with TCAs. Mirtazapine may cause agranulocytosis. Tryptophan is associated with eosinophil-myalgia syndrome.

Therapeutic notes: Mirtazapine is sedative, and it is, therefore, used in depression when a degree of sedation is desirable. Neither reboxetine nor mirtazapine are currently first-line drugs for the treatment of depression. Tryptophan requires specialist supervision due to the stated adverse affect.

Treatment of bipolar affective disorders

Bipolar affective disorder is treated with a combination of mood stabilizers and antidepressants, and sometimes antipsychotics (p. 96). Mood stabilizers include lithium and carbamazepine.

Lithium

Lithium is administered as lithium carbonate, and it is the most widely used mood stabilizer, with antimanic and antidepressant activity.

Mechanism of action: The mechanism of action of lithium is unclear, but it probably involves modulation of secondary-messenger pathways of cAMP and inositol triphosphate (IP_3). It is known that lithium inhibits the pathway for recapturing inositol for the resynthesis of polyphosphoinositides. It may exert its effect by reducing the concentrations of lipids important in secondary signal transduction in the brain.

Indications: Lithium salts are mainly used in the prophylaxis and treatment of bipolar affective disorder, but also in the prophylaxis and treatment of acute mania and in the prophylaxis of resistant recurrent depression.

Contraindications: Some drugs may interact, causing a rise in plasma lithium concentration and so should be avoided. Such drugs include antipsychotics, non-steroidal anti-inflammatory drugs (NSAIDs), diuretics and cardioactive drugs. Lithium is excreted via the kidney, and caution should be employed in patients with renal impairment.

Adverse effects: Lithium has a long plasma half-life and a narrow therapeutic window; therefore, side-effects are common and plasma concentration monitoring is essential. Early side-effects include thirst, nausea, diarrhoea, tremor and polyuria; late side-effects include weight gain, oedema, acne, nephrogenic diabetes insipidus and hypothyroidism. Toxicity/overdose (serum level >2–3 mmol/L) effects include vomiting, diarrhoea, tremor, ataxia, confusion and coma.

Therapeutic notes: The decision to give prophylactic lithium requires specialist advice, and careful monitoring after initiation of treatment is essential.

Carbamazepine

Carbamazepine is as effective as lithium in the prophylaxis of bipolar affective disorder and acute mania, particularly in rapidly alternating bipolar affective disorder.

Mechanism of action: Carbamazepine is a GABA agonist, and this may be the basis of its antimanic properties. The relevance of its effect in stabilizing neuronal sodium, and on calcium channels, is unclear.

Adverse effects: Drowsiness, diplopia, nausea, ataxia, rashes and headache; blood disorders such as agranulocytosis and leucopenia; and drug interactions with lithium, antipsychotics, TCAs and MAO inhibitors. Many other drugs can be affected by the effect of carbamazepine on inducing hepatic enzymes. Diplopia, ataxia, clonus, tremor and sedation are associated with acute carbamazepine toxicity.

Therapeutic notes: At the start of treatment with carbamazepine, plasma concentrations should be monitored to establish a maintenance dose.

PSYCHOTIC DISORDERS

Psychotic disorders are characterized by a mental state that is out of touch with reality, involving a variety of abnormalities of perception, thought and ideas.
Psychotic illnesses include:

- Schizophrenia
- Schizoaffective disorder
- Delusional disorders
- Some depressive and manic illnesses.

Schizophrenia is the most important of these psychotic illnesses, because of its prevalence, young age of onset, and chronic and disabling nature.

Neuroleptics, or antipsychotics, are drugs used in the treatment of psychotic disorders.

Schizophrenia

Epidemiology

Schizophrenia characteristically develops in people aged 15–45 years; it has a relatively stable cross-cultural incidence affecting 1% of the population; with a greater proportion being male.

Symptoms and signs

Schizophrenia is a psychotic illness characterized by multiple symptoms affecting thought, perceptions, emotion and volition.

Symptoms fall into two groups (positive and negative) that may have different underlying causes. Positive symptoms include:

- Delusions – false personal beliefs held with absolute conviction.
- Hallucinations – false perceptions in the absence of a real external stimulus; most commonly, these are auditory (hearing voices) and occur in 60–70% of schizophrenics, but they can be visual, tactile or olfactory.
- Thought alienation and disordered thought – belief that one's thoughts are under the control of an outside agency (e.g. aliens, MI5). This type of belief is common, and thought processes are often incomprehensible.

Negative symptoms include:

- Poverty of speech – restriction in the amount of spontaneous speech.
- Flattening of affect – loss of normal experience and expression of emotion.
- Social withdrawal.
- Anhedonia – inability to experience pleasure.
- Apathy – reduced drive, energy, and interest.
- Attention deficit – inattentiveness at work or on interview.

The distinction between the positive and negative symptoms found in schizophrenia is of importance as neuroleptic drugs tend to have most effect on positive symptoms, whereas negative symptoms are fairly refractory to treatment and carry a worse prognosis.

Theories of schizophrenia

The cause of schizophrenia remains mysterious. Any theory of the cause of schizophrenia must take into account the strong, though not invariable, hereditary tendency (50% concurrence in monozygotic twins), as well as the environmental factors known to predispose towards its development.

Many hypotheses have been suggested to explain the manifestations of schizophrenia at the level of neurotransmitters in the brain. The potential role of excessive dopaminergic activity, in particular, has attracted considerable attention. Evidence for this theory includes the following:

- Most antipsychotic drugs block dopamine receptors, the clinical dose being proportional to the ability to block D_2 receptors.
- Single photon emission computed tomography (SPECT) ligand scans show that there are increased D_2 receptors in the nucleus accumbens of schizophrenic patients.
- Psychotic symptoms can be induced by drugs that increase dopaminergic activity, such as some of the antiparkinsonian agents.

However, there is much evidence that the dopaminergic theory fails to explain. Current research indicates a likely role for other neurotransmitters in schizophrenia, including 5-HT, GABA and glutamate. Although the dopamine theory cannot explain many of the features and findings in schizophrenia, most current pharmacological treatment (typical neuroleptics) is aimed at dopaminergic transmission (Fig. 5.10).

> Mr Sarhan is a 28-year-old postman who was found at 5 am standing on the edge of Tower Bridge and shouting 'Freedom is through flying'. He was previously seen erratically throwing his mailbag into the River Thames. The police manage to grab him just before he jumped and took him to accident and emergency. The on-call psychiatrist sees him. Mr Sarhan is very agitated and shouting 'They gave me powers to fly! Let me prove it! I can prove it! Don't try to steal my powers, go away!'. A mental state examination supports a diagnosis of schizophrenia. A collateral history is obtained from his parents, who say that he has been acting more and more bizarrely over the past year but they just thought it was due to stress. Shortly after admission, he began shouting abuse and pushing past staff with the intention of leaving despite their discouragement. He was, thus, rapidly tranquillized using haloperidol and sectioned under section 2 of the Mental Health Act.

Neuroleptic drugs

The treatment of schizophrenia and all other psychotic illnesses involves the use of antipsychotic medication, the neuroleptic drugs. Neuroleptic drugs produce a general improvement in all the acute positive symptoms of schizophrenia, but it is less clear how effective they are in the treatment of chronic schizophrenia and negative symptoms.

Mechanism of action: Antipsychotic drugs have a variety of structures and fall into various classes (Fig. 5.11). There is a strong correlation between clinical potency and affinity for D_2 receptors among the typical neuroleptics.

Neuroleptics take days or weeks to work, suggesting that secondary effects (e.g. increase in number of D_2 receptors in limbic structure) may be more important than a direct effect of D_2 receptor block. It was once thought, therefore, that neuroleptics exerted their antipsychotic effect by interfering with dopamine

Fig. 5.10 Classes of dopamine receptor		
Type	2nd messenger + cellular effects	Location in CNS and postulated function
D_1	cAMP increase	• Mainly postsynaptic inhibition • Functions unclear
D_2	cAMP decrease K^+ conductance up Ca^{2+} conductance down	• Mainly presynaptic inhibition of dopamine synthesis/release in nigrostriatal, mesolimbic and tuberoinfundibular systems • Affinity of neuroleptics for D_2 receptors correlates with antipsychotic potency
D_3	Unknown	• Localized mainly in limbic and cortical structures concerned with cognitive functions and emotional behaviour • Not clear whether antipsychotic effects of neuroleptics are mediated by the D_3 type
D_4	Unknown	• Similar to D_3 type; clozapine has particular affinity for D_4 receptors

CNS, central nervous system

Fig. 5.11 Classes of neuroleptic drugs

Class	Chemical classification	Examples
Typical anti-psychotics	Phenothiazines: • propylamine side chains • piperidine side chains • piperazine side chains Butyrophenones Thioxanthines	Chlorpromazine Thioridazine Fluphenazine Haloperidol Flupentixol
Atypical anti-psychotics	Dibenzodiazepines Dopamine/5-HT blockers: • diphenylbutylpiperidines • substituted benzamides • benzixasoles	Clozapine, olanzapine Pimozide Sulpiride Risperidone

5-HT, 5-hydroxytryptamine

transmission at D_2 receptors in the mesocortical and mesolimbic systems. The development of newer atypical neuroleptics that are not very active at the D_2 receptor but which are still clinically effective has challenged this hypothesis.

Most neuroleptics also block other monoamine receptors, and this is often the cause of some of the side-effects of these drugs.

The distinction between typical and atypical groups is not clearly defined, but it rests partly on the incidence of extrapyramidal motor side-effects and partly on receptor specificity. Atypical neuroleptics are less prone to producing motor disorders than other drugs, and they tend to have different pharmacological profiles with respect to dopamine and other receptor specificity.

Route of administration: All the neuroleptic drugs can be given orally, though some of the typical drugs can be given by the intramuscular route, which prolongs their release and aids drug compliance.

Typical neuroleptics

Phenothiazines
This class of compounds is subdivided into three groups by the type of side chain attached to the mother structure (phenothiazine ring) (Fig. 5.11). Side-effect patterns vary with the different side chains:

- Propylamine side chains – e.g. in chlorpromazine, produce strong sedation, a moderate muscarinic block, and moderate motor disturbance. Indicated for violent patients, owing to their sedative effect.

- Piperidine side chains – e.g. in thioridazine, produce moderate sedation, strong muscarinic block and low motor disturbance. Favoured for use in elderly patients.
- Piperazine side chains – e.g. in fluphenazine, produce low sedation, low muscarinic block and strong motor disturbance. Contraindicated for use in elderly patients, owing to the motor effects.

Butyrophenones and thioxanthenes
The butyrophenone and thioxanthene groups of compounds have the same profile of low sedation, low muscarinic block and high incidence of motor disturbance.

An example of a butyrophenone compound is haloperidol; flupentixol is an example of the thioxanthenes.

Atypical neuroleptics

Dibenzodiazepines
Dibenzodiazepines such as clozapine and olanzapine have a low affinity for the D_2 receptor and a higher affinity for D_1 and D_4 receptors.

Indications: In the UK and US, atypical neuroleptics are indicated only in chronic cases refractory to other drugs, or with severe motor disturbance. This is because of a 1% risk of potentially fatal neutropenia in those patients on these agents.

Adverse effects: Clozapine has a low incidence of adverse motor effects because of its low affinity for the D_2 receptor. Side-effects of dibenzodiazepines include hypersalivation, sedation, weight gain, tachycardia and hypotension.

Therapeutic notes: Olanzapine is similar to clozapine, though carries less risk of agranulocytosis.

Dopamine/5-HT blockers
Examples of dopamine/5-HT blockers include the diphenylbutylpiperidines and the benzixasoles. Examples of the former include pimozide and substituted benzamides (e.g. sulpiride); examples of the latter include risperidone.

Sulpiride, and the newer agent pimozide, show high selectivity for D_2 receptors compared with D_1 or other neurotransmitter receptors. Both drugs are effective in treating schizophrenia but, sulpiride is claimed to have less tendency to cause adverse motor effects. Pimozide appears to be similar to conventional neuroleptic agents, but it has a longer duration of action, allowing once-daily medication.

Fig. 5.12 Adverse effects of the neuroleptics

- Acute neurological effects: acute dystonia, akathisia, parkinsonism
- Chronic neurological effects: tardive dyskinesia, tardive dystonia
- Neuroendocrine effects: amenorrhoea, galactorrhoea, infertility
- Idiosyncratic: neuroleptic malignant syndrome
- Anticholinergic: dry mouth, blurred vision, constipation, urinary retention, ejaculatory failure
- Antihistaminergic: sedation
- Antiadrenergic: hypotension, arrhythmia
- Miscellaneous: photosensitivity, heat sensitivity, cholestatic jaundice, retinal pigmentation

Redrawn from Page et al. 2002

Benzixasoles such as risperidone show a high affinity for 5-HT receptors and a lower affinity for D_2 receptors. With this class of drugs, extrapyramidal motor side-effects occur with less frequency than with 'classic' neuroleptics.

Quetiapine fumarate is a dibenzothiazepine derivative and acts an as antagonist at the D_1, D_2, 5-HT_{1A} and 5-HT_2 receptors.

Aripiprazole appears to mediate its antipsychotic effects primarily by *partial agonism* at the D_2 receptor. It is also a partial agonist at the 5-HT_{1A} receptor, and like the other atypical antipsychotics, aripiprazole displays an antagonist profile at the 5-HT_{2A} receptor, as well as moderate affinity for histamine and α-adrenergic receptors.

Zotepine has good efficacy against negative symptoms of schizophrenia. This is thought to be due to its noradrenaline reuptake inhibition. It also has a high affinity for the *dopamine* D_1 and D_2 receptors. It also affects the 5-HT_{2A}, 5-HT_{2C}, 5-HT_6 and 5-HT_7 receptors.

Adverse effects of neuroleptics

Neuroleptic drugs cause a variety of adverse effects (Fig. 5.12). The majority of the unwanted effects of neuroleptics can be inferred from their pharmacological actions, such as the disruption of dopaminergic pathways (the major action of most neuroleptics) and the blockade of monoamine and other receptors, including muscarinic receptors, α-adrenoreceptors and histamine receptors.

In addition, individual drugs may cause immunological reactions or have their own characteristic side-effect profile.

Adverse effects on the dopaminergic pathways

There are three main dopaminergic pathways in the brain (Fig. 5.13):

- Mesolimbic and/or mesocortical dopamine pathways running from groups of cells in the midbrain to the nucleus accumbens and amygdala. This pathway affects thoughts and motivation.
- Nigrostriatal dopamine pathways running from the midbrain to the caudate nuclei. This pathway is important in smooth motor control.
- Tuberoinfundibular neurons running from the hypothalamus to the pituitary gland, the secretions of which they regulate.

Antagonism of dopamine receptors leads to interference with the normal functioning of these pathways, bringing about unwanted side-effects as well as the desired antipsychotic effect. This antagonism is the cause of the most serious side-effects associated with neuroleptic use, which include:

- Psychological effects – due to D_2 receptor blockade of the mesolimbic/mesocortical pathway.
- Movement disorders – due to D_2 receptor blockade of the nigrostriatal pathways.
- Neuroendocrine disorders – due to D_2 receptor blockade of the tuberoinfundibular pathway.

It is by dopaminergic antagonism of the mesolimbic mesocortical pathway that it is thought that typical neuroleptics exert their antipsychotic effects. However, as a side-effect of mesolimbic and mesocortical dopaminergic inhibition, sedation and impaired performance are common.

Blocking of dopamine receptors in the basal ganglia (corpus striatum) frequently results in distressing and disabling movement disorders. Two main types of movement disorder occur. Acute reversible parkinsonian-like symptoms (tremor, rigidity and akinesia) are treated by dose reduction, anticholinergic drugs or switching to an atypical neuroleptic. Slowly developing tardive dyskinesia, often irreversible, and manifesting as involuntary movements of the face, trunk and limbs, appears months or years after the start of neuroleptic treatment. It may be a result of proliferation or sensitization of dopamine receptors. Incidence is

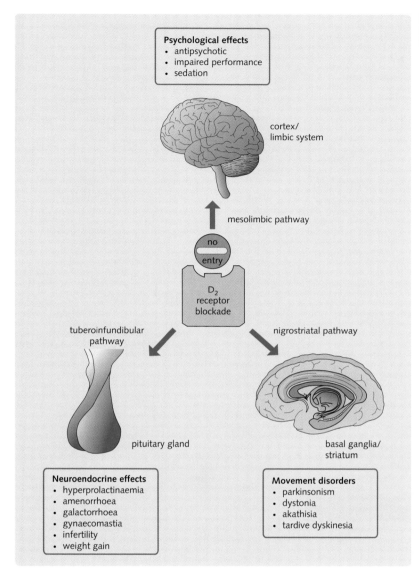

Fig. 5.13 Effect of D$_2$ dopamine receptor blockade on the dopaminergic pathways in the brain.

unpredictable, and it affects approximately 20% of long-term users of neuroleptics. Treatment is generally unsuccessful. The newer atypical neuroleptics may be less likely to induce tardive dyskinesia.

By reducing the negative feedback on the anterior pituitary, over-secretion of prolactin can result (hyperprolactinaemia). This can lead to gynaecomastia, galactorrhoea, menstrual irregularities, impotence and weight gain in some patients (Fig. 5.13).

Adverse effects from non-selective receptor blockade

The adverse effects of neuroleptics from non-selective receptor blockade include:

- Anticholinergic effects due to muscarinic-receptor blockade, such as dry mouth, urinary retention, constipation, blurred vision, etc.
- Adverse effects due to α-adrenoreceptor blockade. Many neuroleptics have the capacity to block α-adrenoreceptors and cause postural hypotension.

- Adverse effects due to histamine-receptor blockade. Antagonism of central histamine H_1 receptors may contribute to sedation.

Adverse effects due to individual drugs or immune reactions

The neuroleptic drug clozapine can cause neutropenia due to toxic bone marrow suppression, while pimozide can cause sudden death secondary to cardiac arrhythmia.

Immune reactions to neuroleptic drugs can include dermatitis, rashes, photosensitivity and urticaria. Such reactions are more common with the phenothiazines, which can also cause deposits in the cornea and lens.

Neuroleptic malignant syndrome: This is the most lethal adverse effect of neuroleptic use. It is an idiosyncratic reaction of unknown pathophysiology. Symptoms include fever, extrapyramidal motor disturbance, muscle rigidity and coma. Urgent treatment is indicated.

Neuroleptics have many side-effects, some related to their principal mechanism of action (dopamine receptor antagonism) and some unrelated to this. Learn these well as they are a popular examination topic.

NAUSEA AND VERTIGO

Nausea and vertigo are common clinical problems, and they may represent a whole array of pathologies. The use of antiemetic drugs can be very effective at alleviating these symptoms, though caution must be taken to ensure the underlying mechanism for the symptoms is investigated.

Antiemetic drugs are discussed in Chapter 8, page 158.

EPILEPSY

Epilepsy is a chronic disease, in which seizures result from the abnormal discharge of cerebral neurons.

A seizure is a particular behaviour produced by an abnormal high-frequency discharge of a group of neurons, starting focally and spreading to a varying extent to affect other parts of the brain. According to

Fig. 5.14 Classification of common epileptic syndromes

Partial (local, focal) seizures	Generalized seizures
• Psychomotor (temporal lobe) epilepsy • Partial motor epilepsy	• Tonic–clonic seizure or grand-mal epilepsy • Absence seizure or petit-mal epilepsy

the focus and spread of discharges, seizures may be classified as:

- Partial (focal) – which originate at a specific focus and do not spread to involve other cortical areas.
- Generalized – which usually have a focus (often in the temporal lobe) and then spread to other areas.

Different epileptic syndromes can be classified on the basis of seizure type and pattern, with other clinical features (such as age of onset), anatomical location of focus, and aetiology taken into account.

Common types of epileptic syndrome

Epileptic syndromes result from either generalized seizures or focal seizures (Fig. 5.14).

Generalized seizure involves loss of consciousness, and it may be convulsive or non-convulsive:

- Tonic-clonic or grand-mal epilepsy – convulsive generalized seizure characterized by periods of tonic muscle rigidity followed later by massive jerking of the body (clonus).
- Absence or petit-mal seizures – generalized seizures characterized by changes in consciousness lasting less than 10 seconds. They occur most commonly in children, where they can be confused with day-dreaming.

The effect on the body of focal seizures depends on the location of the abnormal signal focus: e.g. involvement of the motor cortex will produce convulsions whereas involvement of the brainstem can produce unconsciousness. Psychomotor or temporal lobe epilepsy results from a partial seizure with cortical activity localized to the temporal lobe. Such seizures are characterized by features including impaired consciousness or confusion, amnesia, emotional instability, atypical behaviour and outbursts.

Partial motor seizures have their focus in cortical motor regions and they present with convulsive or tonic activity corresponding to the neurons involved, e.g. the left arm.

Another type of epileptic syndrome is status epilepticus. This is a state in which fits follow each other without consciousness being regained. Status epilepticus constitutes a medical emergency because of possible exhaustion of vital centres.

Causes of epilepsy

The aetiology of epilepsy is unknown in 60–70% of cases, but heredity is an important factor. Damage to the brain – for example, by tumours, head injury, infections or cerebrovascular accident – may subsequently cause epilepsy.

The neurochemical basis of the abnormal discharges in epilepsy are not known, but it may involve altered GABA metabolism.

Treatment of epilepsy

Remember that epilepsy is simply aberrant electrical activity spreading throughout an area of, or the whole of, the brain. Antiepileptic medications limit the propagation of this spread and inhibit development of symptoms.

Drugs used to treat epilepsy are termed antiepileptics; the term anticonvulsant is also used.

The aim of pharmacological treatment of epilepsy is to minimize seizure activity/frequency, without producing adverse drug effects.

Mechanisms of action of antiepileptics

Antiepileptic drugs act generically to inhibit the rapid, repetitive neuronal firing that characterizes seizures. There are three established mechanisms of action by which the antiepileptic drugs achieve this (Fig. 5.15).

1. Inhibition of ionic channels involved in neuronal excitability

Drugs such as phenytoin, carbamazepine and valproate inhibit the 'fast' sodium current. These drugs bind preferentially to inactivated (closed) sodium channels, preventing them from opening. The high-frequency repetitive depolarization of neurons during a seizure increases the proportion of sodium channels in the inactivated state susceptible to blockade. Eventually, sufficient sodium channels become blocked so that the 'fast' neuronal sodium current is insufficient to cause a depolarization. Note that neuronal transmission at normal frequencies is relatively unaffected because a much smaller proportion of the sodium channels are in the inactivated state.

Ethosuximide inhibits 'T-type' low-threshold, fast-inactivating calcium. Absence seizures involve oscillatory neuronal activity between the thalamus and the cerebral cortex. The oscillation involves 'T-type' calcium channels, which produce low-threshold spikes, thus allowing groups of cells to fire in bursts. It appears that the anti-absence drug ethosuximide reduces this fast-inactivating calcium current, dampening the thalamocortical oscillations that are critical in the generation of such absence seizures.

2. Inhibition of excitatory transmission

Drugs that block excitatory amino acid receptors (*N*-methyl-D-aspartate [NMDA] antagonists) have been shown to be antiepileptic in animal models. Such drugs may prove useful in the clinical treatment of epilepsy in the future. Lamotrigine, one of the newer antiepileptic agents, inhibits the release of glutamate as one of its actions, and this may contribute to its antiepileptic activity.

3. Enhancement of GABA-mediated inhibition

This can take any of the following forms:

- Enhancement by direct GABA agonist properties, e.g. by gabapentin, another of the newer antiepileptics, agent which has been designed to mimic GABA in the CNS.
- Potentiation of chloride currents through the $GABA_A/Cl^-$ channel complex, e.g. by benzodiazepines and barbiturates. The increased postsynaptic inhibitory chloride current at $GABA_A$ receptors, hyperpolarizes neurons and makes them refractory to excitation (see Fig. 5.5).
- Inhibition of GABA degradation in the CNS, e.g. by vigabatrin, which is an irreversible inhibitor of GABA transaminase ($GABA_T$), the enzyme normally responsible for metabolism of GABA

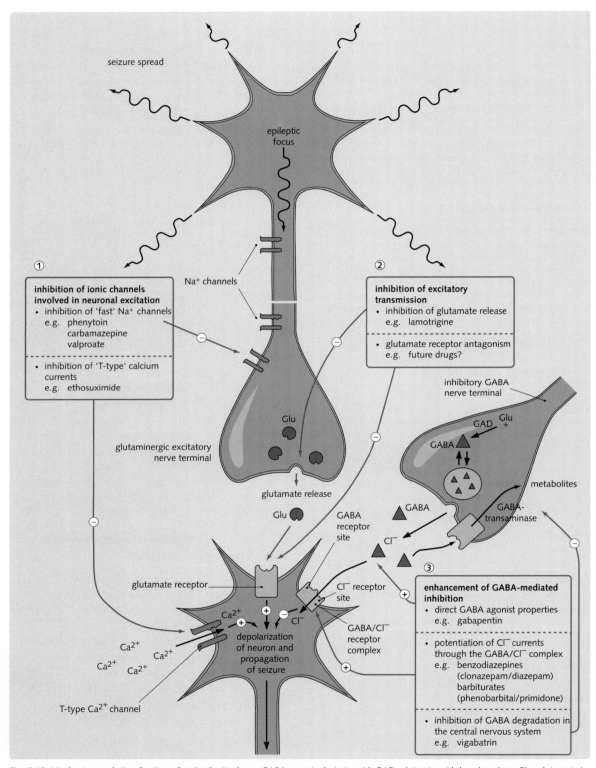

Fig. 5.15 Mechanism and site of action of antiepileptic drugs. GABA, γ-aminobutyric acid; GAD, glutamic acid decarboxylase; Glu, glutamate.)

Fig. 5.16 Drugs used for epilepsy classified by clinical use

Seizure type	Primary drugs	Secondary drugs
Partial and/or generalized tonic–clonic seizures	• Sodium valproate • Carbamazepine	• Phenytoin • Vigabatrin • Gabapentin • Lamotrigine • Phenobarbital
Absence seizures	• Ethosuximide • Sodium valproate	• Phenobarbital • Lamotrigine
Status epilepticus	• Lorazepam	• Diazepam • Clonazepam

in the neuron. Inhibition of $GABA_T$, therefore, leads to an increase in synaptic levels of GABA and so enhances GABA-mediated inhibition.

Antiepileptic drugs (anticonvulsants)

Antiepileptic drugs can be classified according to their mechanism of action (Fig. 5.15), but in clinical practice it is useful to think of the drugs according to their use (Fig. 5.16).

Phenytoin

Mechanism of action: This involves use-dependent block of voltage-gated sodium channels. Phenytoin reduces the spread of a seizure. Electroencephalographic (EEG) recordings show that phenytoin does not stop the 'spiking' at a focus (i.e. it does not prevent the ignition of an epileptic discharge), but it does stop it spreading and causing overt clinical symptoms.

Route of administration: Oral, intravenous.

Indications: Phenytoin is indicated in all forms of epilepsy except absence seizures; neuralgic pain (p. 173).

Contraindications: Phenytoin has many contraindications, mainly because it induces the hepatic cytochrome P_{450} oxidase system, increasing the metabolism of oral contraceptives, anticoagulants, dexamethasone and pethidine.

Adverse effects: The adverse effects of phenytoin may be dosage- or non-dosage-related. The dosage-related effects of phenytoin affect the cerebellovestibular system, leading to ataxia, blurred vision and hyperactivity. Acute toxicity causes sedation and confusion. The non-dosage-related

effects include collagen effects such as gum hypertrophy and coarsening of facial features; allergic reactions, e.g. rash, hepatitis and lymphadenopathy; haematological effects, e.g. megaloblastic anaemia; endocrine effects, e.g. hirsutism (hair growth); and teratogenic effects (it may cause congenital malformations).

Therapeutic notes: The use of phenytoin is complicated by its zero-order pharmacokinetics, characteristic toxicities, and necessity for long-term administration. Phenytoin has a narrow therapeutic index, and the relationship between dose and plasma concentration is non-linear. This is because phenytoin is metabolized by a hepatic enzyme system that is saturated at therapeutic levels. Small dosage increases may, therefore, produce large rises in plasma concentrations with acute side-effects. Monitoring of plasma concentration greatly assists dosage adjustment. Because of its adverse effects and narrow therapeutic window, phenytoin is no longer a first-line treatment for any of the seizure syndromes.

Sodium valproate

Mechanism of action: Sodium valproate has two mechanisms of action: like phenytoin, it causes use-dependent block of voltage-gated sodium channels; it also increases the GABA content of the brain when given over a prolonged period.

Route of administration: Oral, intravenous.

Indications: Sodium valproate is useful in all forms of epilepsy.

Contraindications: Sodium valproate should not be given to people with acute liver disease or a history of hepatic dysfunction.

Adverse effects: Sodium valproate has many fewer side-effects than other antiepileptics; the main problems are gastrointestinal upset and, more importantly, liver failure. Hepatic toxicity appears to be more common when sodium valproate is used in combination with other antiepileptics.

Therapeutic notes: Sodium valproate is well absorbed orally and has a half-life of 10–15 hours. Sodium valproate is now the first-line drug for most types of seizure syndromes.

Carbamazepine

Mechanism of action: Like phenytoin, carbamazepine causes use-dependent block of voltage-gated sodium channels. Oxcarbazepine, another antiepileptic, is structurally a derivative of carbamazepine. It has an extra oxygen atom on the dibenzazepine ring, which helps reduce the impact on the liver of metabolizing the drug, and also prevents the serious forms of anaemia occasionally associated with carbamazepine. It is thought to have the same mechanism of action as carbamazepine.

Route of administration: Oral, rectal.

Indications: Carbamazepine can be used in all forms of epilepsy except absence seizures; neuralgic pain (p. 173).

Contraindications: Like phenytoin, carbamazepine is a strong enzyme inducer and so causes similar drug interactions.

Adverse effects: The adverse effects of carbamazepine are really limited to the nervous system – ataxia, nystagmus, dysarthria, vertigo, sedation.

Therapeutic notes: Carbamazepine is well absorbed orally with a long half-life (25–60 hours) when first given. Enzyme induction subsequently reduces this half-life.

Ethosuximide

Mechanism of action: Ethosuximide exerts its effects by inhibition of low-threshold calcium currents (T-currents).

Route of administration: Oral.

Indications: Ethosuximide is the drug of choice in simple absence seizures and is particularly well tolerated in children.

Contraindications: Ethosuximide may make tonic-clonic attacks worse.

Adverse effects: The adverse effects of ethosuximide include gastrointestinal upset, drowsiness, mood swings and skin rashes. Rarely, it causes serious bone marrow depression.

Vigabatrin

Mechanism of action: Vigabatrin exerts its effects by irreversible inhibition of GABA transaminase.

Route of administration: Oral.

Indications: Vigabatrin is indicated in epilepsy not satisfactorily controlled by other drugs.

Contraindications: Vigabatrin should not be used in people with a history of psychosis because of the side-effect of hallucinations.

Adverse effects: Drowsiness, dizziness, depression, visual hallucinations.

Therapeutic notes: Vigabatrin is a new drug, used as an adjunct to other therapies.

Lamotrigine

Mechanism of action: Lamotrigine appears to act via an effect on sodium channels, and inhibiting the release of excitatory amino acids.

Route of administration: Oral.

Indications: Monotherapy and adjunctive treatment of partial seizures and generalized tonic-clonic seizures; neuralgic pain (p. 173).

Contraindications: Hepatic impairment.

Adverse effects: Rashes, fever, malaise, drowsiness and, rarely, hepatic dysfunction.

Gabapentin

Mechanism of action: Gabapentin is a lipophilic drug that was designed to act like GABA in the CNS (agonist), though it does not appear to have GABA-mimetic actions. Its mechanism of action remains elusive, but its antiepileptic action almost certainly involves voltage-gated calcium-channel blockade.

Route of administration: Oral.

Indications: As an adjunct to therapy in partial epilepsy with or without secondary generalization.

Contraindications: Caution to avoid sudden withdrawal, in elderly patients and in those with renal impairment.

Adverse effects: Somnolence, dizziness, ataxia, fatigue and, rarely, cerebellar signs.

Barbiturates

Examples of barbiturates include phenobarbital and primidone (which itself, is largely converted to phenobarbital).

Mechanism of action: Barbiturates cause potentiation of chloride currents through the $GABA_A/Cl^-$ channel complex.

Route of administration: Oral, intravenous.

Indications: Barbiturates are used in all forms of epilepsy, including status epilepticus.

Contraindications: Barbiturates should not be used in children, elderly people, and people with respiratory depression.

Adverse effects: The main side-effect of barbiturates is sedation, which limits their use clinically, along with the danger of potentially fatal CNS depression in overdose. Phenobarbital is a good inducer of cytochrome P_{450}, and so it can be involved in drug interactions.

Therapeutic notes: Only the long-acting barbiturates are antiepileptic. Phenobarbital has a plasma half-life of 10 hours. The strong sedating nature of these drugs now limits their use in the management of epilepsy.

Benzodiazepines
Examples of benzodiazepines include clonazepam and clobazam.

Mechanism of action: Benzodiazepines cause potentiation of chloride currents through the $GABA_A/Cl^-$ channel complex (see Fig. 5.5).

Route of administration: Oral, intravenously.

Indications: Clonazepam is occasionally used for tonic-clonic and partial seizures. Lorazepam and diazepam are effective in the management of status epilepticus.

Contraindications: Benzodiazepines should not be used in people with respiratory depression.

Adverse effects: The most common adverse effect of the benzodiazepines is sedation. Intravenous lorazepam and diazepam can depress respiration.

Therapeutic notes: The repeated seizures of status epilepticus can damage the brain and be potentially life-threatening, so they should be controlled by administration of intravenous diazepam. Lorazepam has a longer half-life than diazepam.

Other anticonvulsants
Other agents used as antiepileptics include levetiracetam, tiagabine, topiramate, acetazolamide and piracetam. Their indications and side-effect profiles can be obtained from the *British National Formulary* (*BNF*).

Emmett Hezz, a 19-year-old student car mechanic is brought to accident and emergency following a collapse while waiting for a taxi. His fiancée was with him at the time and tells staff that he fell to the ground all of a sudden and that his breathing appeared to stop for about 30 seconds. He then developed jerking movements of his arms and legs and by this time his face had turned blue. He was incontinent of urine and on regaining consciousness was drowsy, confused and complaining of aching muscles. In hospital he was able to explain that 8 months ago, he experienced a similar episode when in a park, but was too embarrassed to tell anybody.

On examination, his pulse is 76 beats per minute and regular. No abnormalities are found, other than a bleeding tongue. The history is very indicative of a tonic-clonic (grand mal) seizure. He is admitted for 24 hours and sent for blood investigations, ECG, head CT and EEG. EEG reveals generalized spike-and-wave activity, but no other abnormality. He is warned not to drive or operate heavy machinery until he has been seizure-free for a year. Emmett agrees to start taking the anticonvulsant sodium valproate and return for a follow-up appointment.

Status epilepticus

Intravenous benzodiazepines (lorazepam or diazepam) are first-line drugs in status epilepticus. If these fail to bring an end to seizure activity, intravenous sodium valproate or phenytoin, or carbamazepine via a nasogastric tube should be attempted, ideally in an intensive care setting. Alternatively intravenous fosphenytoin, a prodrug of phenytoin, can be given more rapidly but requires ECG monitoring. Thiopental (p. 178) can be used as a final option.

DRUG MISUSE

Concepts of drug misuse

Historically there has been a long relationship between humans and the non-therapeutic use of drugs that act on the mind and body. Drugs have been used for non-therapeutic purposes in virtually all cultures: for instance, the Incas used psychoactive fungi and the ancient Egyptians (and many other cultures since) used alcohol.

It is important to realize that the misuse of drugs is a socially defined concept that has as much to do with the legal, religious, moral and cultural framework of a society as the pharmacological properties of the drug itself. Drugs now banned in the UK, e.g. opium, were once popular and legal in nineteenth century England, while attitudes to alcohol vary both historically and geographically from total prohibition to deep entrenchment in the culture.

Humans show great ingenuity in creating, harvesting, obtaining and taking drugs for non-therapeutic reasons, and they go to great lengths to do so. The sheer prevalence and associated co-morbidity makes drug misuse an important medical subject.

Definitions

Drug misuse

Drug misuse is defined as the use of drugs that causes actual physical or mental harm to an individual or to society, or that is illegal. Therefore, drug misuse includes alcohol, nicotine, and the damaging overprescription of tranquillizers, as well as the more obvious illicit drugs such as ecstasy or amphetamines.

Drug dependence

Drug dependence is defined as the compulsion to take a drug repeatedly, with distress being caused if this is prevented. Drugs of dependence all have rewarding effects (this is why they are taken), but they also have unpleasant (aversive) effects, often as the drug is metabolized and excreted.

Dependence involves psychological factors as well as physical aspects. These are not exclusive and there is a mixture of both in most people who are dependent on drugs. Psychological dependence is when the rewarding effects (positive reinforcement) predominate to cause a compulsion to continue taking the drug. Physical dependence is when the distress on stopping the drug (negative reinforcement) is the main reason for continuing to take it, i.e. avoidance of the 'withdrawal syndrome'.

Drug tolerance

Drug tolerance is the necessity to increase the dose of an administered drug progressively to maintain the effect that was produced by the (smaller) original doses. Drug tolerance is a phenomenon that develops with chronic administration of a drug.

Many different mechanisms can give rise to drug tolerance, though they are rather poorly understood. They include:

- Down-regulation of receptors
- Changes in receptors
- Exhaustion of biological mediators or transmitters
- Increased metabolic degradation (enzyme induction)
- Physiological adaptation.

Withdrawal

Withdrawal is the term used to describe the syndrome of effects caused by stopping administration of a drug. It results from the change of (neuro)physiological equilibrium induced by the presence of the drug (Fig. 5.17).

Legal aspects of drug misuse (UK)

Misuse of Drugs Act 1971

The Misuse of Drugs Act 1971 prohibits certain activities in relation to 'controlled drugs', in particular their manufacture, supply and possession. The Act is primarily a legal document for use by the police and judiciary. The penalties applicable to offences involving the different drugs are graded broadly according to the harmfulness attributable to a drug when it is misused, and for this purpose the drugs are categorized into three classes (Fig. 5.18).

Misuse of Drugs Regulations 1985

The Misuse of Drugs Regulations 1985 are a set of working regulations that define the classes of persons who are authorized to supply and possess controlled drugs while acting in their professional capacities, and lay down the conditions under which these activities may be carried out.

In these regulations, drugs of addiction or high misuse potential are divided into five schedules, each specifying the requirements governing such aspects as import, export, production, supply, possession, prescription and record keeping that apply to them (Fig. 5.19).

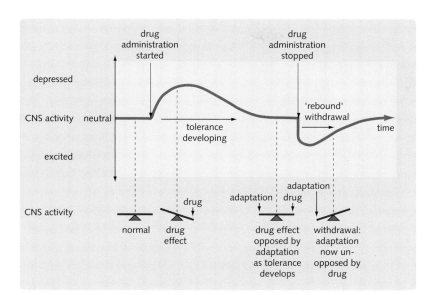

Fig. 5.17 Tolerance to, and withdrawal from central nervous system (CNS) depressant drugs, e.g. alcohol. The graph for tolerance of and withdrawal from CNS stimulant drugs, e.g. cocaine, would be a mirror image in the x-axis of what is shown.

Fig. 5.18 Classes of controlled drugs		
Class A drugs	**Class B drugs**	**Class C drugs**
Cocaine	Amphetamines	Benzodiazepines
MDMA ('ecstasy')	Barbiturates	Cannabis
Diamorphine (heroin) and other strong opioids	Some weak opioids	Androgenic and anabolic steroids
	Others	Human chorionic gonadotrophin
Lysergic acid diethylamide (LSD) class B substance when prepared for injection		Others
Others		

MDMA, methylenedioxymethamfetamine

These regulations are more relevant than the 1971 Act to the clinical practice of health professionals (Fig. 5.19).

Notification and Supply to Addicts Regulations 1973

The Notification and Supply to Addicts Regulations 1973 require that any doctor who attends to a person who he or she suspects is addicted to a notifiable drug is legally required to furnish details, in writing, of that person's particulars to the Chief Medical Officer. The idea of this is to maintain a confidential 'index of addicts' that can be checked, to safeguard against addicts obtaining supplies simultaneously from two or more doctors.

Drugs of misuse

Drugs with a high potential for misuse fall into many distinct pharmacological categories. They may or may not be used therapeutically, and they may be illegal or legal (Fig. 5.20).

Central stimulants

Try to use the correct chemical name when describing drugs of misuse, rather than a street name or personal favourite, i.e. amphetamines rather than Whizz or Speed, as it tends to go down better with examiners!

Amphetamines
Street names: Speed, Whizz, Billy, Base.

Mechanism of action: Amphetamines cause the release of monoamines and the inhibition of monoamine reuptake, especially of dopamine and noradrenaline in neurons.

Route of administration: Amphetamines are administered orally, or 'snorted' as a powder nasally; sometimes used intravenously.

Effects: The effects of amphetamines include the following: increased motor activity; euphoria and

Fig. 5.19 Misuse of drugs regulations 1985

Classification and example	Controlled drug requirements
Schedule 1 • drugs that have no medicinal use e.g. cannabis, LSD	Possession and supply prohibited without Home Office authority (given e.g. for research)
Schedule 2 • medicinal drugs with high misuse potential e.g. heroin, morphine, pethidine, cocaine	Drugs subject to full controlled drug requirements, e.g. special prescription requirements, safe custody, register keeping
Schedule 3 • medicinal drugs of lesser misuse potential e.g. minor stimulants, barbiturates, some analgesics	Drugs subject to some controlled drug requirements, e.g. special prescription requirements, but not safe custody or register keeping
Schedule 4 • mainly benzodiazepines with abuse potential e.g. benzodiazepines, anabolic steroids	Minimal requirements
Schedule 5 • high-strength preparations of non-controlled drugs	Virtually no controlled drug requirements other than the retention of invoices for 2 years

LSD, lysergic acid diethylamide

Fig. 5.20 Drugs with high potential for misuse

Drug class	Examples
Central stimulants	Cocaine Amphetamines MDMA (ecstasy) Nicotine
Central depressants	Alcohol Benzodiazepines Barbiturates
Opioid analgesics	Morphine Heroin (diamorphine) Methadone
Cannabinoids	Cannabis Tetrahydrocannabinoids (THCs)
Hallucinogens	LSD Mescaline Psilocybin
Dissociative anaesthetics	Ketamine Phencyclidine

LSD, lysergic acid diethylamide; MDMA, methylenedioxymethamfetamine

excitement; anorexia and insomnia; peripheral sympathomimetic effects, such as hypertension and inhibition of gut motility; and stereotyped behaviour and psychosis, which develop with prolonged usage.

Clinical uses: The (very few) clinical uses of amphetamines are for narcolepsy and for hyperkinesis in children. They are no longer recommended as appetite suppressants, owing to their adverse effects.

Tolerance, dependence and withdrawal: Tolerance to the peripheral sympathomimetic stimulant effects of amphetamines develops rapidly, but it develops much more slowly to other effects such as locomotor stimulation. Amphetamines cause strong psychological dependence but no real physical dependence. After stopping chronic use, the individual will usually enter a deep, long sleep ('REM rebound') and awake feeling tired, depressed and hungry. This state may reflect the depletion of the normal monoamine stores.

Adverse effects: Acute amphetamine toxicity causes cardiac arrhythmias, hypertension and stroke.

Chronic toxicity causes paranoid psychosis, vasocon-striction, tissue anoxia at sites of injection or snorting, and damage to the fetal brain *in utero*.

Cocaine
Street names: Coke, Charlie, Snow, Crack (free base).

Mechanism of action: Cocaine strongly inhibits the reuptake of catecholamines at noradrenergic neurons, and thus strongly enhances sympathetic activity.

Route of administration: Cocaine hydrochloride is usually snorted nasally. 'Crack' is the free base, which is more volatile and which does not decompose on heating. It can, therefore, be smoked, producing a brief intense 'rush'.

Effects: The behavioural effects produced by cocaine are similar to those produced by amphetamines, such as euphoria. The euphoric effects may be greater, and there is less of a tendency for stereotypical behaviour and paranoid delusions.

The effects of cocaine hydrochloride (lasting about an hour) are not as long lasting as those of amfetamine, while those obtained from crack are brief (minutes).

Clinical uses: Cocaine is occasionally used as a topical anaesthetic by ear, nose and throat specialists.

Tolerance, dependence and withdrawal: Cocaine causes strong psychological dependence but no real physical dependence. Withdrawal causes a marked deterioration in motor performance, which is restorable on provision of the drug.

Adverse effects: Acute cocaine toxicity causes toxic psychosis, cardiac arrhythmias, hypertension and stroke. Chronic toxicity causes paranoid psychosis, vasoconstriction, tissue anoxia at sites of injection or snorting and damage to the fetal brain.

Methylenedioxymethamfetamine (MDMA)
Street names: Ecstasy, E, Disco Biscuits, Pills.

Mechanism of action: MDMA is an amphetamine derivative that has a mechanism of action similar to that of amphetamines (release of monoamines, inhibition of monoamine reuptake). MDMA especially has actions on serotonergic neurons, potentiating 5-HT.

Route of administration: MDMA is usually taken as a pill containing other psychoactive drugs, such as amfetamine or ketamine.

Effects: MDMA has mixed stimulant and hallucinogenic properties, especially in its pure form. Euphoria, arousal and perceptual disturbances are common. Uniquely, MDMA has the effect of creating a feeling of euphoric empathy, so that social barriers are reduced.

Clinical uses: MDMA has no clinical use. Trials have been licensed in the USA for its evaluation as a treatment for people with social avoidant personality disorders.

Tolerance, dependence and withdrawal: It is not currently known to what extent tolerance and dependence occur with MDMA. The withdrawal syndrome is similar to that with amphetamines.

Adverse effects: The most serious acute consequences of acute MDMA toxicity appear to be hyperthermia, exhaustion and dehydration caused indirectly by the repetitive locomotor behaviour induced (dancing!). Rarely this results in fatality. Chronic MDMA toxicity causes neurodegeneration of serotonergic nerves in the brains of experimental primates. The correlation to humans is not known.

Nicotine
Nicotine is found in cigarettes, cigars, pipes and chewing tobacco. Various therapeutic products are available which contain nicotine as part of nicotine replacement therapy for those wishing to withdraw from their nicotine addiction. These are discussed on page 112.

Mechanism of action: Nicotine exerts its effects by causing nicotinic acetylcholine receptor (nicAChR) excitation leading to neurotransmitter release and nicAChR desensitization.

Route of administration: Nicotine is usually inhaled, although it can be chewed.

Effects: Nicotine has both stimulant and relaxant properties. Physiologically, nicotine increases alertness, decreases irritability and relaxes skeletal muscle tone. Peripheral effects due to ganglionic stimulation include tachycardia, increased blood pressure and decreased gastrointestinal motility.

Clinical uses: Nicotine has no clinical use.

Tolerance, dependence, and withdrawal: Tolerance to nicotine occurs rapidly, first to peripheral effects but later to central effects.

Nicotine is highly addictive, causing both physical and psychological dependence. Withdrawal from tobacco often leads to a syndrome of craving, irritability, anxiety and increased appetite for approximately 2–3 weeks.

Adverse effects: Acute nicotine toxicity causes nausea and vomiting. Chronic toxicity caused by smoking leads to more morbidity in the UK than all other drugs combined, predisposing to all of the following diseases, often greatly so:

- Cardiovascular diseases, including atherosclerosis, hypertension and coronary heart disease
- Cancer of the lung, bladder and mouth
- Respiratory diseases such as bronchitis, emphysema and asthma
- Fetal growth retardation.

Central depressants

Ethanol
Mechanism of action: Ethanol, or alcohol, acts in a similar way to volatile anaesthetic agents, as a general CNS depressant. The cellular mechanisms involved may include inhibition of calcium entry, hence reduction in transmitter release, as well as potentiation of inhibitory GABA transmission.

Route of administration: Ethanol is administered orally.

Effects: The familiar effects of ethanol intoxication range from increased self-confidence and motor incoordination through to unconsciousness and coma. Peripheral effects include a self-limiting diuresis and vasodilatation.

Clinical uses: Ethanol is used as an antidote to methanol poisoning.

Tolerance, dependence and withdrawal: Tolerance, and physical and psychological dependence all occur with ethanol, such that 15 000 people a year are admitted to psychiatric hospital for alcohol dependence and psychosis, and up to 20% of males on a medical ward have alcohol-related disabilities.

The alcohol withdrawal syndrome is a rebound of the nervous system after adaptation to the depression caused by alcohol. This syndrome occurs in two stages:

- Early stage ('hangover') – which is common and starts 6–8 hours after cessation of drinking. It involves tremulousness, nausea, retching and sweating.
- Late stage (delirium tremens) – which is much less common and starts 48–72 hours after cessation of drinking. It involves delirium, tremor, hallucinations and confusion.

Management of these late withdrawal symptoms involves sedation with clomethiazole or benzodiazepines; clonidine may be useful.

Adverse effects: Acute ethanol toxicity causes ataxia, nystagmus, coma, respiratory depression and death. Chronic ethanol toxicity causes neurodegeneration (potentiated by vitamin deficiency), dementia, liver damage, pancreatitis, etc., and accompanying psychiatric illness-depression/psychosis is common.

Benzodiazepines
Mechanism of action: Benzodiazepines exert their effects by potentiation of inhibitory GABA transmission (p. 87).

Route of administration: Benzodiazepines are administered orally.

Effects: The effects of benzodiazepines include sedation, agitation and ataxia.

Clinical uses: Benzodiazepines are heavily prescribed as anxiolytics and hypnotics.

Tolerance, dependence and withdrawal: Benzodiazepines have a potential for misuse – tolerance and dependence are common.

A physical withdrawal syndrome can occur in patients given benzodiazepines, even for short periods. Symptoms include rebound anxiety and insomnia with depression, nausea and perceptual changes that may last from weeks to months.

Adverse effects: The adverse effects of acute benzodiazepine toxicity include hypotension and confusion. Cognitive impairment occurs in chronic benzodiazepine toxicity.

Mr Alrum is a 45-year-old banker who lives by himself. He presents to accident and emergency following a fall in the road. The examining doctor sees some minor cuts and bruises on his right arm and leg but also notices the patient smells strongly of alcohol. On talking to the patient, the doctor discovers Mr Alrum has recently lost his job due to poor performance, elicits some feelings of low mood, hopelessness and helplessness and that at the time of the fall he was on his way to buy some bottles of rum since he had run out. The AUDIT questionnaire is used and supports a diagnosis of alcohol dependence. Mr Alrum is admitted for assistance. Blood tests are done and show a macrocytic anaemia, elevated γ-glutamyl transferase and alanine aminotransferase (liver transaminases). A couple of hours after the blood was taken, he is found at the wrong end of the ward, disorientated, sweating and trembling. He is given chlordiazepoxide, the dose of which is gradually reduced over 10 days to help manage his withdrawal symptoms.

Opioid analgesics

Heroin addicts are able to tolerate 300–600-mg doses several times per day. This is 30–60 times the normal dose needed to produce an analgesic effect. A non-addict given this would die of respiratory depression.

Diamorphine (heroin) and other opioids

Street names: Smack, H, Gear, Junk, Jack, Brown.

Mechanism of action: Opioids, e.g. diamorphine, show agonist action at opioid receptors (p. 169).

Note that the sense of euphoria and well-being produced by strong opioids undoubtedly contributes to their analgesic activity by helping to reduce the anxiety and stress associated with pain. This effect also accounts for the illicit use of these drugs by addicts.

Route of administration: Opioids are generally taken intravenously by misusers as this produces the most intense sense of euphoria ('rush').

Effects: Opioids produce feelings of euphoria and well-being. Other effects are mentioned on p. 171.

Clinical uses: Opioids are used in analgesia for moderate to severe pain.

Tolerance, dependence and withdrawal: Tolerance to opioid analgesics develops quickly in addicts and results in larger and larger doses of the drug being needed to achieve the same effect.

Dependence involves both psychological factors and physical factors. Psychological dependence is based on the positive reinforcement provided by euphoria.

There is a definite physical withdrawal syndrome in addicts following cessation of drug treatment with opioids. This syndrome comprises a complex mixture of irritable and sometimes aggressive behaviour, combined with extremely unpleasant autonomic symptoms such as fever, sweating, yawning, pupillary dilatation, and piloerection that gives the state its colloquial name of 'cold turkey'. Patients are extremely distressed and restless and strongly crave the drug. Symptoms are maximal at 2 days and largely disappear in 7–10 days.

Treatment of withdrawal: Methadone is a long-acting opiate, active orally, that is used to wean addicts from their addiction. The withdrawal symptoms from this longer-acting compound are more prolonged, but less intense than, for example, those of heroin. Treatment usually involves substitution of methadone followed by a slow reduction in dose over time.

Clonidine, an α_2-adrenoreceptor agonist, inhibits firing of locus ceruleus neurons, and it is effective in suppressing some components of the opioid withdrawal syndrome, especially the nausea, vomiting and diarrhoea.

Adverse effects: Acute opioid toxicity causes the following:

- Confusion, drowsiness and sedation. Initial excitement is followed by sedation and finally coma on overdose.
- Shallow and slow respiration – due to reduction of sensitivity of the respiratory centre to CO_2.
- Vomiting – due to stimulation of the chemoreceptor trigger zone.
- Autonomic effects such as tremor and pupillary constriction.
- Bronchospasm, flushing and arteriolar dilatation due to histamine release.

Acute toxicity may be countered by use of an opioid antagonist such as naloxone. The adverse effects of direct chronic toxicity are minor (p. 171).

Cannabinoids

Cannabis

There are two forms of cannabis: marijuana is the dried leaves and flowers of the cannabis plant, and hashish is the extracted resin of the cannabis plant.

Street names: Hashish, Weed, Skunk, Pot, Dope, Gear, Grass, Ganja, Blow.

Mechanism of action: How cannabis exerts its effects is not clearly defined, but it includes both depressant, stimulant and psychomimetic effects. The active constituent of cannabis is D^9-tetrahydrocannabinol (THC), though metabolites that also have activity may be important.

Route of administration: Cannabis is usually smoked, although it may be eaten.

Effects: Cannabis has several effects:

- Subjectively, users feel relaxed and mildly euphoric.
- Perception is altered, with apparent sharpening of sensory experience.
- Appetite is enhanced.
- Peripheral actions include vasodilatation and bronchodilatation, and a reduction in intraocular pressure.

Clinical uses: Cannabis is not currently licensed for use in the UK. It is being evaluated for palliative or symptomatic relief use in certain conditions in the USA, e.g. for the antiemetic effect of THC, and a possible role in treatment of multiple sclerosis and glaucoma.

Tolerance, dependence and withdrawal: Tolerance to cannabis occurs to a minor degree. It is not dangerously addictive, with only moderate physical and psychological withdrawal effects noted, such as mild anxiety/dysphoria and sleep disturbances.

Adverse effects: Acute cannabis toxicity causes confusion and hallucinations. Chronic toxicity may cause flashbacks, memory loss and 'de-motivational syndrome'. There is a clear correlation between cannabis use and schizophrenia. One study showed the chance of developing schizophrenia later in life was six times higher in cannabis users than the group not using it.

Psychotomimetic drugs or hallucinogens

Examples of psychotomimetic drugs include LSD, mescaline and psilocybin.

Street names: Acid, Trips, Magic mushrooms.

Mechanism of action: How LSD, mescaline and psilocybin produce changes in perception is not well understood, but it seems to involve serotonin. LSD appears to affect serotonergic systems by acting on 5-HT_2 inhibitory autoreceptors on serotonergic neurons to reduce their firing. Whether LSD is an agonist, an antagonist or both is not clear.

Route of administration: Psychotomimetic drugs are administered orally as a liquid, pills or paper stamps.

Effects: Psychotomimetic drugs cause a dramatically altered state of perception-vivid and unusual sensory experiences combined with euphoric sensations. Hallucinations, delusions and panic can occur; this is known as a 'bad trip' and it can be terrifying.

Clinical uses: Psychotomimetic drugs have no clinical uses.

Tolerance, dependence and withdrawal: Tolerance to, dependence on, and withdrawal from psychotomimetic drugs are not significant.

Adverse effects: Acute toxicity from psychotomimetic drugs causes frightening delusions or hallucinations that can lead to accidents or violence. In chronic toxicity, 'flashbacks' (a recurrence of hallucination) may occur long after the 'trip'. Other psychotic symptoms may also occur.

Smoking cessation

The most successful smoking cures combine psychological and pharmacological treatments.

Pharmacological options largely rely on nicotine replacement, once the patient has stopped smoking, with gradual reduction in nicotine. The latest drug to be used to help cigarette smokers is bupropion (Zyban®), which is derived from an antidepressant.

Nicotine products

Mechanism of action: Measured doses of nicotine are used to replace nicotine derived from cigarettes once the patient has stopped smoking, meeting the physical nicotine needs. The dose of nicotine is gradually reduced over 10–12 weeks.

112

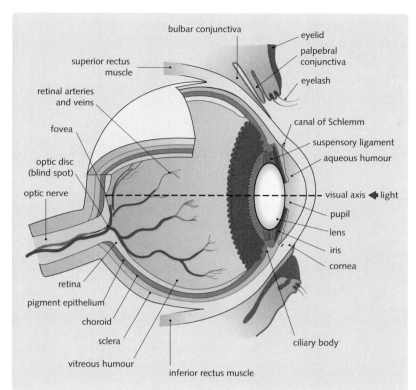

superior rectus muscle
bulbar conjunctiva
eyelid
palpebral conjunctiva
eyelash
retinal arteries and veins
fovea
canal of Schlemm
suspensory ligament
aqueous humour
optic disc (blind spot)
optic nerve
visual axis ◀ light
pupil
lens
iris
cornea
retina
pigment epithelium
choroid
sclera
vitreous humour
inferior rectus muscle
ciliary body

Fig. 5.21 Anatomy of the eye. (Redrawn from Page et al. 2002.)

Route of administration: Oral (chewing gum, sublingual tablets), transdermal (patches), nasal (spray), inhalation.

Indications: Adjunct to smoking cessation.

Contraindications: Severe cardiovascular disease, recent cerebrovascular accident, pregnancy, breast-feeding.

Adverse effects: Nausea, dizziness, headache and cold, influenza-like symptoms, palpitations.

Therapeutic notes: Nicotine products are available over the counter or GPs can prescribe them for patients intending to stop smoking.

Bupropion (Zyban®)

Mechanism of action: Bupropion is a selective inhibitor of the neuronal uptake of noradrenaline and dopamine. This is believed to reduce nicotine craving and withdrawal symptoms.

Route of administration: Oral.

Indications: Adjunct to smoking cessation.

Contraindications: History of epilepsy and eating disorders, pregnancy, breastfeeding.

Adverse effects: Dry mouth, gastrointestinal disturbances, insomnia, tremor, impaired concentration.

Therapeutic notes: Bupropion is available on the NHS.

THE EYE

The eyeball is a 25 mm sphere made up of two fluid-filled compartments (the aqueous humour and the vitreous humour) separated by an translucent lens, all encased within four layers of supporting tissue (Fig. 5.21). These four layers consist of:

- The cornea and sclera
- The uveal tract, comprising the iris, ciliary body and choroid
- The pigment epithelium
- The retina (neural tissue containing photoreceptors).

Fig. 5.22 Mechanisms involved in controlling pupil size. (Redrawn from Page et al. 2002.)

Light entering the eye is focused by the lens onto the retina, and the signal reaches the brain via the optic nerve.

Control of pupil size

Light

Light levels affect the pupil in two ways (Fig. 5.22):

- High light levels cause pupil constriction, termed miosis
- Low light levels cause pupil dilation, termed mydriasis.

Autonomic control

The pupils are innervated by the autonomic nervous system, such that:

- Parasympathetic stimulation causes miosis
- Sympathetic stimulation causes mydriasis.

The dilator pupillae (radial smooth muscle of the iris) is innervated by the sympathetic system, which causes contraction when noradrenaline activates α_1-adrenoceptors. The constrictor pupillae (sphincter smooth muscle of the iris) is innervated by the parasympathetic system, which causes contraction when acetylcholine activates M_3 receptors.

Accommodation

Accommodation is the ability of the eye to change its refractive power. This is determined by the curvature of the lens.

Suspensory ligaments connect the lens to the ciliary muscle. When the ciliary muscle contracts (parasympathetic M_3 receptor activation), the suspensory ligaments relax, resulting in the lens becoming more spherical so that it is able to focus near objects. When the ciliary muscle relaxes, the suspensory ligaments tighten, and the lens becomes elongated and thin, allowing far objects to be focused on the retina.

An Argyll Robertson pupil is one which constricts upon convergence but not in response to light. This is due to a lesion in the brainstem and is almost diagnostic of neurosyphilis.

Production of aqueous humour

Aqueous humour fills the anterior chamber of the eyeball. It is continuously produced at a rate of 3 mL/day by a special vascular tissue associated with the ciliary body (Fig. 5.23). The ciliary epithelial cells contain carbonic anhydrase and an ATPase, which transport bicarbonate and sodium.

The aqueous humour flows through the pupil and into the anterior aqueous chamber. Draining fluid leaves the aqueous chamber via the trabecular meshwork and the canal of Schlemm within the surface of the sclera before entering the episcleral veins.

Glaucoma

Glaucoma describes a group of disorders characterised by a loss in visual field associated with cupping of the optic disc and optic nerve damage.

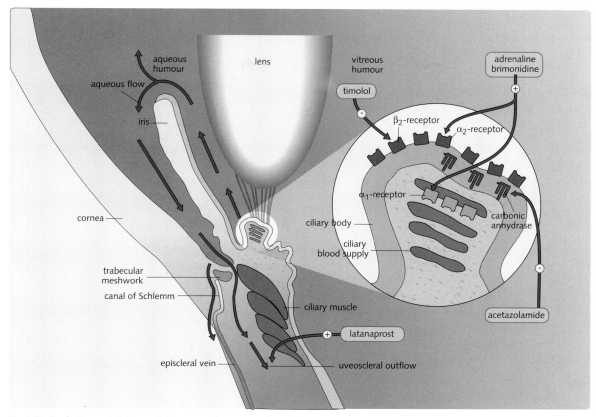

Fig. 5.23 Production and drainage of the aqueous humour. (Redrawn from Page et al. 2002.)

The glaucomas are the second commonest cause of blindness in the world and the commonest cause of irreversible blindness. Glaucoma is generally associated with raised intraocular pressure (IOP), but can occur when the IOP is within normal limits.

There are two types of glaucoma: open-angle and closed-angle.

Open-angle glaucoma is the most common type of glaucoma and it may be congenital. It is caused by pathology of the trabecular meshwork that reduces the drainage of the aqueous humour into the canal of Schlemm. Treatment involves either reducing the amount of aqueous humour produced or increasing its drainage.

In closed-angle glaucoma, the angle between the iris and the cornea is very small, and this results in forward ballooning of the iris against the back of the cornea.

It is important to differentiate between acute closed-angle glaucoma and chronic open-angle glaucoma because chronic open-angle glaucoma is of insidious onset and often picked up at routine check up, whereas acute closed-angle glaucoma symptoms include painful, red eyes and blurred vision. Acute closed-angle glaucoma is a medical emergency and requires admission to save sight. It is difficult for patient to notice gradual loss of visual fields associated with chronic open-angle glaucoma and so regular check ups are vital for at-risk groups, such as elderly people.

Treatment of open-angle glaucoma

The most effective way of preventing this damage to the eye is by lowering the IOP. Most drugs used to treat eye disease can be given topically in the form of drops and ointments. To enable these drugs to penetrate the cornea, they must be lipophilic or uncharged.

Drugs used to inhibit aqueous production

β-Adrenoceptor antagonists and prostaglandin analogues are the current choice for first-line treatment.

β-Adrenoceptor antagonists

Timolol and betaxolol are examples of β-adrenoceptor antagonists used in glaucoma.

Mechanism of action: α-Adrenoceptor antagonists block β_2-receptors on the ciliary body, and they may also block β-receptors on ciliary blood vessels, resulting in vasoconstriction (they are almost universally referred to as 'β-blockers' in clinical practice) (Fig. 5.23) and reduced aqueous production.

Route of administration: Topical.

Indications: Open-angle glaucoma. β-Adrenoceptor antagonists are also used in cardiovascular disease (Ch. 2).

Contraindications: β-Adrenoceptor antagonists should not be given to patients with asthma, bradycardia, heart block or heart failure.

Adverse effects: Systemic side-effects include bronchospasm in asthmatic patients, and potentially bradycardia owing to their non-selective action on β-receptors. Other side-effects include transitory dry eyes and allergic blepharoconjunctivitis.

Prostaglandin analogues

Examples include latanoprost and travoprost.

Mechanism of action: Promote outflow of aqueous from the anterior chamber via an alternative drainage route, called the uveoscleral pathway.

Indications: Open angle glaucoma, ocular hypertension.

Contraindication: Pregnancy.

Adverse effects: Brown pigmentation of the iris may occur.

Sympathomimetics (adrenoceptor agonists)

Adrenaline, dipivefrine and brimonidine are commonly used sympathomimetics.

Mechanism of action: Agonism at α-adrenoceptors is thought to be the principal means by which these agents reduce aqueous production from the ciliary body. Adrenaline may also increase drainage of aqueous via the trabecular meshwork (see Fig. 5.23).

Route of administration: Topical.

Indications: Open-angle glaucoma. Sympathomimetics are also used in the management of cardiac (Ch. 2) and anaphylactic emergencies and in reversible airways disease (Ch. 3).

Contraindications: Closed-angle glaucoma, hypertension, heart disease.

Adverse effects: Pain and redness of the eye.

Therapeutic notes: Adrenaline is not very lipophilic and, therefore, it does not penetrate the cornea effectively. This can be overcome by administering dipivefrine hydrochloride, a prodrug that crosses the cornea and that is metabolized to adrenaline once inside the eye.

Carbonic anhydrase inhibitors (CAIs)

Acetazolamide and dorzolamide are CAIs.

Mechanism of action: CAIs inhibit the enzyme carbonic anhydrase, which catalyses the conversion of carbon dioxide and water to carbonic acid, which dissociates into bicarbonate and H^+. Bicarbonate is required by the cells of the ciliary body, and underproduction of bicarbonate limits aqueous secretion (Fig. 5.23). CAIs given systemically have a weak diuretic effect (Ch. 7).

Route of administration: Oral, topical, intravenous.

Indications: Open-angle glaucoma.

Contraindications: Hypokalaemia, hyponatraemia, renal impairment. These effects can be reduced if the drug is given in a slow-release form.

Adverse effects: Irritation of the eye, nausea, vomiting, diarrhoea, diuresis.

Drugs used to increase the drainage of aqueous humour

Miotics–muscarinic agonists.

Pilocarpine is a muscarinic agonist.

Mechanism of action: Pilocarpine causes contraction of the constrictor pupillae muscles of the iris, constricting the pupil, and allowing aqueous to drain from the anterior chamber into the trabecular meshwork (Fig. 5.23).

Route of administration: Topical.

Indications: Open-angle glaucoma.

Contraindications: Acute iritis, anterior uveitis.

Adverse effects: Eye irritation, headache and brow ache, blurred vision, hypersalivation. May exacerbate asthma.

Treatment of closed-angle glaucoma

Drugs to treat closed-angle glaucoma are used in emergencies as a temporary measure to lower IOP.

Pilocarpine and a carbonic anhydrase inhibitor are often first-line treatments, with mannitol and glycerol being administered systemically, and reduce IOP for resistant or more serious cases.

YAG (yttrium-aluminium-garnet) laser surgery provides a permanent cure for closed-angle glaucoma. A hole is made in the iris (iridectomy) to allow increased flow of aqueous humour.

Stimuli that cause the pupils to dilate, such as sitting awake in a dark room, increase the tightness of the angle between the iris and the cornea and can thus precipitate an attack of acute closed-angle glaucoma.

Examining the eye

Mydriatic drugs dilate the pupil, i.e. cause mydriasis, while cycloplegic drugs cause paralysis of the ciliary muscle, i.e. cycloplegia. Mydriatic and cycloplegic drugs are used in ophthalmoscopy to allow a better view of the interior of the eye.

Mydriasis and cycloplegia reduce the drainage of the aqueous humour, and they should, therefore, be avoided in patients with closed-angle glaucoma.

Fig. 5.24 Mydriatic and cycloplegic effects of the commonly used muscarinic antagonists

Drug	Duration (h)	Mydriatic effect	Cycloplegic effect
Tropicamide	1 – 3	++	+
Cyclopentolate	12 – 24	+++	+++
Atropine	168 – 240	+++	+++

Muscarinic antagonists

The most effective mydriatics are the muscarinic antagonists. These block the parasympathetic control of the iris sphincter muscle.

The type of muscarinic antagonist chosen will depend on the length of the procedure and on whether or not cycloplegia is required.

The most commonly used muscarinic antagonists, their duration of action, and their mydriatic and cycloplegic effects are summarized in Fig. 5.24.

α-Adrenoceptor agonists

α-Adrenoceptor agonists can cause mydriasis by stimulating the sympathetic control of the iris dilator muscle. The sympathetic system does not control the ciliary muscle, however, and, therefore, these drugs do not produce cycloplegia. The α-agonist most commonly used to produce mydriasis is phenylephrine.

Muscarinic agonists and α-antagonists

A muscarinic agonist such as pilocarpine, or an α-antagonist such as moxisylyte may be used to reverse mydriasis at the end of an ophthalmic examination. This is not usually necessary.

Endocrine and reproductive systems

Objectives

After reading this chapter, you will:

- Understand the main functions of the endocrine and reproductive systems
- Know which drugs affect the functioning of these systems and how
- Be aware of indications, contraindications and adverse drug reactions

THE THYROID GLAND

Basic concepts

Production of thyroid hormones

The thyroid gland secretes three hormones, tri-iodothyronine (T_3), thyroxine (T_4) and calcitonin, although T_3 and T_4 are regarded as the 'true' thyroid hormones and reference to thyroid hormones will relate to these. Calcitonin is discussed in the last section of this chapter.

The principal effects of the thyroid hormones are: determination of basal metabolic rate and influence of growth through stimulation of growth hormone synthesis and action. Other effects are summarized in Figure 6.1.

The follicular cells of the thyroid gland synthesize and glycosylate thyroglobulin before secreting it into their lumen. Iodination of the tyrosine residues on this molecule is catalysed by thyroid peroxidase and results in the formation of monoiodotyrosine (MIT) or diiodotyrosine (DIT), according to the position on the ring at which this occurs. The coupling

---

Fig. 6.1 Physiological effects of thyroid hormones

- Fetal development (physical and cognitive)
- Metabolic rate
- Body temperature
- Cardiac rate and contractility
- Peripheral vasodilatation
- Red cell mass and circulatory volume
- Respiratory drive
- Peripheral nerves (reflexes)
- Hepatic metabolic enzymes
- Bone turnover
- Skin and soft tissue effects

From Page et al. 2002

---

of MIT with DIT produces T_3, and the coupling of two DIT molecules produces T_4. Coupling is also catalysed by thyroid peroxidase.

Thyroglobulin, now known as colloid, is endocytosed into the follicular cells, where it is broken down to release T_3, T_4, MIT and DIT. T_3 and T_4 are secreted into the plasma; MIT and DIT are metabolized within the cells and their iodide is recycled (Fig. 6.2).

The iodine required for the synthesis of T_3 and T_4 comes mainly from the diet in the form of iodide. Through the action of a thyrotrophin-dependent pump, iodide is concentrated in the follicular cells, where it is converted into iodine by thyroid peroxidase.

Control of thyroid hormone secretion

The production of thyroid hormones is slow but constant, and control of their plasma levels is determined by varying their rate of secretion (Fig. 6.3).

The hypothalamus contains thyroid-hormone receptors that are able to detect and respond to decreased levels of T_3 and T_4 by causing the release of thyrotrophin-releasing hormone (TRH). TRH reaches the anterior pituitary via the portal circulation and stimulates TRH receptors on thyrotroph cells which in turn secrete thyroid-stimulating hormone (TSH).

TSH reaches the thyroid gland through the systemic circulation where it stimulates thyroid hormone secretion. Both T_3 and T_4 bind to proteins in the plasma (mostly thyroxine-binding globulin), and less than 1% of total thyroid hormones are free. It is the free thyroid hormones which exert the physiological effects. T_3 is about five times more biologically active than T_4, and T_4 is converted to T_3 in some peripheral tissues.

Fig. 6.2 Synthesis of thyroid hormones and the site of action of some antithyroid drugs. (DIT, diiodotyrosine; MIT, monoiodotyrosine; PTU, propylthiouracil; T_3, triiodothyronine; T_4, thyroxine; TSH, thyroid-stimulating hormone.) (Redrawn from Page et al. 2002.)

T_3 and T_4 exert negative feedback on the hypothalamus and pituitary.

Most modern laboratory thyroid function tests measure just TSH, although levels of free and total T_3 and T_4 can be measured as well as thyroxine-binding globulin.

Thyroid dysfunction

Hypothyroidism

Hypothyroidism, thyroid insufficiency, is relatively common in adults and associated with tiredness and lethargy, weight gain, intolerance to cold, dry skin, bradycardia and mental impairment. Children with hypothyroidism manifest delayed bone growth, whereas a deficiency in utero also results in mental retardation – this condition is known as cretinism.

Hashimoto's thyroiditis is an autoimmune disease resulting in fibrosis of the thyroid gland. It is the most common cause of hypothyroidism and, like most autoimmune diseases, is more prevalent in women. Myxoedema is also immunological in origin, and represents the most severe form of hypothyroidism, sometimes causing coma.

Thyroid-hormone resistance and reduced TSH secretion will also produce the symptoms of hypothyroidism.

The causes of hypothyroidism are summarized in Figure 6.4.

Hyperthyroidism

Hyperthyroidism, thyroid excess, results either from the overproduction of endogenous hormone or exposure to excess exogenous hormone. Symptoms include increased basal metabolic rate (BMR) with consequent weight loss, increased appetite, increased body temperature, and sweating, as well as nervousness, tremor, tachycardia and classic ophthalmic signs.

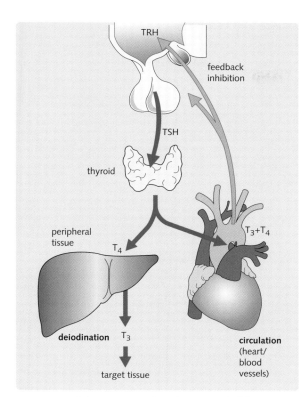

Fig. 6.3 Hypothalamic–pituitary–thyroid axis: control of thyroid hormone synthesis. (T_3, triiodothyronine; T_4, thyroxine; TSH, thyroid-stimulating hormone; TRH, thyrotrophin-releasing hormone.) (Redrawn from Page et al. 2002.)

Fig. 6.5 Causes of hyperthyroidism

- Excess exogenous thyroid hormone
- Diffuse toxic goitre (Graves' disease)
- Hyperfunctioning adenoma (toxic nodule)
- Toxic multinodular goitre
- Painless thyroiditis
- Subacute thyroiditis
- Thyroid-stimulating hormone (TSH)-secreting adenoma
- Human chorionic gonadotropin (hCG)-secreting tumours

From Page et al. 2002

Graves' disease (diffuse toxic goitre) is the most common cause of hyperthyroidism. It is an autoimmune disease caused by the activation of TSH receptors by antibodies. This results in an enlargement of the gland and therefore excess hormone production.

Toxic nodular goitre is the second most common cause of hyperthyroidism. It is due to either a single adenoma (hyperfunctioning adenoma) or multiple adenomas (multinodular goitre).

The causes of hyperthyroidism are summarized in Figure 6.5.

Mrs Akasuki, 41 years old, presents to her GP with tremor and weight loss of 6.5 kg (1 stone) over 4 weeks, despite increased appetite. She admits to feeling hot and sweaty both day and night, which has affected her sleep. On examination a diffuse goitre is seen. Her pulse is rapid and she has noticeable exophthalmos. A pregnancy test is negative. A blood sample is taken and reveals an elevated serum T_3 and T_4 with suppressed TSH levels. Mrs Akasuki is diagnosed as having hyperthyroidism. She is given propanolol for her symptoms and is started on carbimazole to suppress her thyroid. After 4 weeks she is reviewed and checked for neutropenia, a possible dangerous side-effect of carbimazole treatment.

Management of thyroid dysfunction

Hyperthyroidism and antithyroid drugs

Thioureylenes

The thioureylenes are the first-line drugs for treatment of hyperthyroidism. Carbimazole, thiamazole,

---

Fig. 6.4 Causes of hypothyroidism

Primary	Chronic lymphocytic thyroiditis (Hashimoto's disease)
	Subacute thyroiditis
	Painless thyroiditis (postpartum thyroiditis)
	Radioactive iodine ingestion
	Post thyroidectomy
	Iodine deficiency or excess
	Inborn errors of thyroid hormone synthesis
Secondary	Pituitary disease
Target tissues	Thyroid hormone resistance

From Page et al. 2002

and propylthiouracil (PTU) are examples of thioureylenes.

In the body, carbimazole is rapidly converted to active compound thiamazole.

Mechanism of action: The thioureylenes cause inhibition of thyroid peroxidase with a consequent reduction in thyroid hormone synthesis and storage (see Fig. 6.2). The effects of PTU may take several weeks to manifest as the body has stores of T_3 and T_4. PTU also inhibits the peripheral deiodination of T_4 to T_3.

Route of administration: Oral.

Indications: Thioureylenes are used for hyperthyroidism. Patients sensitive to carbimazole are given PTU.

Contraindications: Thioureylenes should not be given to people with a large goitre. PTU should be given at a reduced dose in patients with renal impairment.

Adverse effects: Nausea and headache; allergic reactions, including rashes; hypothyroidism; and, rarely hepatotoxicity, bone marrow suppression, alopecia.

Therapeutic regimen: Carbimazole is given at 20–60 mg daily until the patient is euthyroid (4–11 weeks later), then the dose is progressively reduced to a maintenance level of 5–15 mg daily. Treatment is usually given for 18 months. PTU is given at 300–600 mg daily until the patient is euthyroid, then the dose is progressively reduced to a maintenance level of 50–150 mg daily.

Anion inhibitors

Iodine, iodide and potassium perchlorate are examples of anion inhibitors.

Potassium perchlorate inhibits the uptake of iodine by the thyroid (Fig. 6.2), but is no longer used owing to the risk of aplastic anaemia.

Iodide is the most rapidly acting treatment against thyrotoxicosis and is given in thyrotoxic crisis (thyroid storm).

Mechanism of action: Iodine and iodide cause inhibition of conversion of T_4 to T_3, of organification, and of hormone secretion. They also reduce the size and vascularity of the gland, which is evident after 10–14 days.

Route of administration: Oral.

Indications: Thyrotoxicosis; preoperatively.

Contraindications: Iodine and iodide should not be given to breastfeeding women as they cause goitre in infants.

Adverse effects: Iodine and iodide can cause hypersensitivity reactions including rashes, headache, lacrimation, conjunctivitis, laryngitis and bronchitis. With long-term treatment, depression, insomnia and impotence can occur.

Therapeutic regimen: Iodine and iodide are given 10–14 days before partial thyroidectomy, with either carbimazole or PTU. They should not be given long term as iodine becomes less effective.

β-Adrenoceptor antagonists

Propranolol and atenolol are examples of β-adrenoceptor antagonists. They are used to attenuate the symptoms of increased thyroid hormone levels, and the effect of increased numbers of adrenoceptors caused by thyroid hormone.

Mechanism of action: β-Adrenoceptor antagonists reduce tachycardia, the basal metabolic rate, nervousness and tremor.

Route of administration: Oral.

Indications: Thyrotoxic crisis; preoperatively.

Contraindications: β-Adrenoceptor antagonists should not be given to people with asthma.

Adverse effects: The side-effects of β-Adrenoceptor antagonists are given in Chapter 2.

Radioiodine

The use of radioactive iodine to treat hyperthyroidism is not classically considered pharmacology, although readers should be aware of its place in the management of thyroid disorders, and are advised to consult a general medical textbook.

Hypothyroidism and thyroid replacement therapy

Levothyroxine

Thyroxine is given as levothyroxine sodium in maintenance therapy. It has a half-life of 6 days and a peak onset of 9 days.

Mechanism of action: Levothyroxine is converted to T_3 in vivo.

Route of administration: Oral.

Indications: Hypothyroidism.

Contraindications: Levothyroxine should not be given to people with thyrotoxicosis, and should be used with caution in those who have cardiovascular disease.

Adverse effects: Arrhythmias, tachycardia, anginal pain, cramps, headache, restlessness, sweating, weight loss.

Therapeutic regimen: The starting dose of levothyroxine sodium should be no greater than 100 µg daily (reduce in elderly or those with cardiovascular disease) and increased by 25–50 µg every 4 weeks until a dose of 100–200 µg is reached.

Liothyronine sodium (L-triiodothyronine sodium)

As liothyronine is bound only slightly by thyroid binding globulin, it has a more rapid onset of effects and a shorter duration of action than levothyroxine.

Mechanism of action: Liothyronine is rapidly metabolized in vivo to T_3. It has a half-life of 2–5 days and a peak onset of 1–2 days.

Route of administration: Oral, intravenous.

Indications: Liothyronine is given for severe hypothyroidism where a rapid effect is needed.

Contraindications: Liothyronine should not be given to people with cardiovascular disorders.

Adverse effects: Arrhythmias, tachycardia, anginal pain, cramps, headache, restlessness, sweating, weight loss.

Therapeutic regimen: The dosage of liothyronine sodium should be gradually increased as with levothyroxine sodium (20 µg liothyronine sodium is equivalent to 100 µg levothyroxine sodium). Intravenous liothyronine is the drug of choice in the emergency treatment of myxoedema (hypothyroid) coma.

THE ENDOCRINE PANCREAS AND DIABETES MELLITUS

Control of plasma glucose

Blood glucose levels are maintained at a concentration of about 5 mmol/L, and usually do not exceed 8 mmol/L. A plasma glucose concentration of 2.2 mmol/L or less may result in hypoglycaemic coma and death due to a lack of energy reaching the brain. A plasma glucose concentration of more than 10 mmol/L exceeds the renal threshold for glucose and means that glucose will be present in the urine. Osmotic diuresis then occurs.

The islets of Langerhans, located in the pancreas, contain glucose receptors and secrete the hormones glucagon and insulin. These hormones are short-term regulators of plasma glucose levels with opposite effects. In addition, their release can be influenced by gastrointestinal hormones and autonomic nerves.

Glucose receptors are also found in the ventro-medial nucleus and lateral areas of the hypothalamus. These are able to regulate appetite and feeding, and also indirectly stimulate the release of a variety of hormones, including adrenaline, growth hormone and cortisol, all of which affect glucose metabolism.

The hormones involved in blood glucose regulation target the liver, skeletal muscle and adipose tissue.

Insulin

Insulin is a 51 amino acid peptide made up of an α- and a β-chain linked by disulphide bonds. It has a half-life of 3–5 minutes and is metabolized to a large extent by the liver (40–50%), but also by the kidneys and muscles.

In response to high blood glucose levels (as occurs after a meal), as well as to glucosamine, amino acids, fatty acids, ketone bodies and sulphonylureas (see below), the β-cells of the endocrine pancreas secrete insulin along with a C-peptide.

Insulin release is mediated by ATP-dependent potassium channels, located in the membrane of the β-cells. These close in response to elevated cytoplasmic ATP and decreased cytoplasmic ADP levels, resulting in depolarization of the membrane. This triggers calcium entry into the cell through voltage-dependent calcium channels, and subsequent insulin release (Fig. 6.6).

Insulin release is inhibited by low blood glucose levels, growth hormone, glucagon, cortisol and sympathetic nervous system activation.

The insulin receptor consists of two α and two β subunits linked by disulphide bonds. Insulin binds to the extracellular α subunits, resulting in the internalization of the receptor and its subsequent breakdown. The β subunits display tyrosine kinase activity on the binding of insulin to the receptor. Autophosphorylation of the β subunits ensues, resulting in the phosphorylation of phospholipase

Fig. 6.6 Mechanism of insulin secretion from pancreatic β-cells.

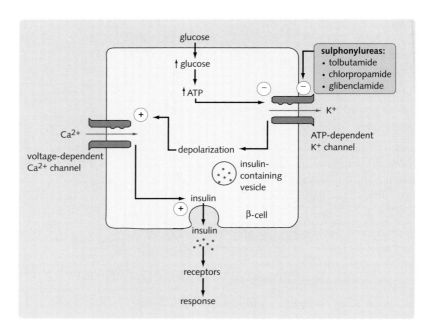

C with subsequent liberation of diacylglycerol (DAG) and inositol triphosphate (IP_3).

The effects of insulin are summarized in Figure 6.7.

Mrs Raye, 26 years, is 25 weeks into her first pregnancy. Her body mass index (BMI) is 30 and there is a family history of both diabetes and stroke. She is found to have glucose in her urine on routine testing. She has an oral glucose tolerance test. Her fasting plasma glucose is 4.7 mmol/L and her 2 hours post glucose load level is 12.1 mmol/L, indicative of diabetes. The test should be repeated to confirm the result, however, prompt action is also required to prevent harm to the fetus. There is a higher chance of congenital abnormalities with elevated plasma glucose concentrations. Fetal ultrasound is used to exclude this. Mrs Raye is told to try a diabetic diet with small and frequent meals. Since she is overweight, her diet should also be calorie-restricted. After 4 days it is noted this has not worked and insulin injections are started. Her insulin regimen is insulin aspart (rapid and short action), before meals and isophane insulin (delayed onset and intermediate length of action), at breakfast and bedtime. She is warned about symptoms of hypoglycaemia and told to eat if she recognizes them.

Fig. 6.7 Metabolic effects of insulin on fuel homeostasis

Carbohydrates	Increase glucose transport Increase glycogen synthesis Increase glycolysis Inhibit gluconeogenesis
Fats	Increase lipoprotein lipase activity Increase fat storage in adipocytes Inhibit lipolysis (hormone-sensitive lipase) Increase hepatic lipoprotein synthesis Inhibit fatty acid oxidation
Proteins	Increase protein synthesis Increase amino acid transport

From Page et al. 2002

Diabetes mellitus

Diabetes mellitus is characterized by an inability to regulate plasma glucose within the normal range. There is an absolute or relative insulin deficiency, leading to hyperglycaemia, glycosuria (glucose in the urine), polyuria (production of large volumes of dilute urine) associated with cellular potassium depletion and polydipsia (intense thirst).

There are two types of diabetes mellitus:

- Insulin-dependent
- Non-insulin-dependent.

Fig. 6.8 Features of type 1 and type 2 diabetes mellitus

Type 1 diabetes (IDDM)	Type 2 diabetes (NIDDM)
0.5% prevalence in adults	5% prevalence in adults
Juvenile onset (<30 years)	Maturity onset (> 30 years)
Absolute lack of insulin	Relative lack of, or excess, insulin
Not associated with obesity	Often associated with obesity
Insulin therapy	Oral agents (sulphonylureas) usually suffice
Ketoacidosis frequent	Ketoacidosis uncommon
Linked to the presence of islet cell antibody and genetic markers (HLA antigens)	No known autoimmune origin

The differences between the two types are summarized in Figure 6.8.

The long-term consequences of both types of diabetes are similar, and include increased risk of cardiovascular and cerebrovascular events, peripheral and autonomic neuropathy, nephropathy and retinopathy.

Type 1 diabetes

In type 1 diabetes (insulin-dependent diabetes mellitus [IDDM]), pancreatic β-cells are destroyed by an autoimmune T-cell attack. This leads to a complete inability to secrete insulin and ketoacidosis is a problem. Some untreated patients have a plasma glucose concentration of up to 100 mmol/L due to insulin deficiency. In this situation, lipolysis is increased, as is the production of ketone bodies from fatty acids. This leads to ketonuria and metabolic acidosis; body fluids become hypertonic, resulting in cellular dehydration, and eventually in hyperosmolar coma.

Type 1 diabetes is apparent at a young age.

Type 2 diabetes

In type 2 diabetes (non-insulin-dependent diabetes mellitus [NIDDM]), insulin is often secreted as on average 50% of the β-cells remain active, although there is also peripheral resistance to insulin. Unlike type 1 diabetes, this is relatively common in all populations enjoying an affluent life-style. The prevalence of type 2 diabetes increases with age and the degree of obesity.

Ketosis is not a feature of type 2 diabetes as ketone production is suppressed by the small amounts of insulin produced by the pancreas. Hyperosmolar non-ketotic coma is the type 2 diabetes equivalent to ketoacidosis, and can be fatal if untreated, although responds rapidly to fluids and insulin.

Secondary diabetes mellitus

Not to be confused with type 2 diabetes, secondary diabetes mellitus accounts for less than 2% of all new cases of diabetes, and is most commonly due to pancreatic disease (pancreatitis, carcinoma, cystic fibrosis), endocrine disease (Cushing's syndrome, acromegaly) or drug-induced (thiazide diuretics or corticosteroid therapy).

Management of diabetes mellitus

Insulin

The aim of exogenous insulin preparations is to mimic basal levels of endogenous insulin and meal-induced increases in insulin.

Nowadays the insulin preparation used is mostly the human (recombinant) insulin (however, insulin preparations of bovine origin are also available).

- Available as short-, intermediate-, and long-acting preparations (Figure 6.9).

Short-acting insulins are soluble. These preparations most resemble endogenous insulin, and can be given intravenously in hospital. The rapid-acting insulins aspart and lispro have a faster onset and shorter duration of action than the traditional short-acting insulin. Exubera® is the newest short-acting insulin, available to patients in the form of an inhaled powder. This new method of delivering insulin hopes to reduce the number of injections

Fig. 6.9 Insulin preparations

Insulin preparation	Action	Peak activity (h)	Duration (h)
Rapid-acting insulin	Very rapid	0–2	3–4
Short-acting insulin	Rapid	1–3	3–7
Isophane insulin	Intermediate	2–12	12–22
Insulin zinc suspension	Prolonged	4–24	24–28

some patients need to take and has increased the choices available for patients in their disease management. However, patients must have stopped smoking for 6 months prior to commencement of Exubera® and must not also have severe lung disease.

Intermediate- and long-acting insulins are not as soluble as the short-acting preparations. Their solubility is decreased by precipitating the insulin with zinc or protamine (a basic protein), which prolongs their release into the blood stream.

The intermediate- and long-acting preparations include:

- Isophane insulin
- Biphasic isophane insulin
- Insulin zinc suspension
- Protamine zinc insulin

Mechanism of action: Insulin preparations mimic endogenous insulin.

Route of administration: Insulin must always be given parenterally (intravenously, intramuscularly or subcutaneously), as it is a peptide and thus destroyed in the gastrointestinal tract. Short-acting insulin is given intravenously in emergencies, but administration of the insulin preparations in maintenance treatment is usually subcutaneous.

Indications: Type 1 diabetes; type 2 diabetes uncontrolled by other means.

Adverse effects: Local reactions and, in overdose, hypoglycaemia. Protamine can cause allergic reactions. Rarely, there may be immune resistance.

Therapeutic regimen: The following regimens are recommended according to the patient's needs:

- Short-acting insulin three times daily (before breakfast, lunch and dinner) and intermediate-acting insulin at bedtime.
- Short-acting insulin and intermediate-acting insulin mixture twice daily before meals.
- Short-acting insulin and intermediate-acting insulin mixture before breakfast, short-acting insulin before dinner, and intermediate-acting insulin before bedtime.
- Short-acting insulin and intermediate-acting insulin mixture before breakfast is adequate for some type 2 diabetes patients needing insulin.

Therapeutic notes: Preparations are now available which contain mixtures of short and intermediate- and long-acting insulins, allowing patients to inject themselves only once each time they administer their insulin.

Oral hypoglycaemics

Oral hypoglycaemics are administered orally, and like insulin act to lower plasma glucose. The sulphonylureas and the biguanides are the main drugs uses from this class, but newer drugs are also now available.

Sulphonylureas

Gliclazide, tolbutamide, chlorpropamide and glibenclamide are examples of sulphonylureas.

Mechanism of action: Sulphonylureas block ATP-dependent potassium channels in the membrane of the pancreatic β-cells, causing depolarization, calcium influx and insulin release.

Route of administration: Oral.

Indications: Sulphonylureas are given for diabetes mellitus, in patients with residual β-cell activity.

Contraindications: Breastfeeding women, or people with ketoacidosis. Long-acting sulphonylureas (chlorpropamide, glibenclamide) should be avoided in elderly people and in those with renal and hepatic insufficiency, as these drugs can induce hypoglycaemia.

Adverse effects: Weight gain; sensitivity reactions, including rashes; gastrointestinal disturbances; headache; hypoglycaemia.

Therapeutic regimen: Tolbutamide is given at 500 mg two or three times daily and lasts for 6 hours; chlorpropamide is given at 100–250 mg daily and lasts for 12 hours; and glibenclamide is given at 2.5–15 mg daily and lasts for 12 hours.

Biguanides

Metformin is the only drug in this class.

Mechanism of action: Metformin increases the peripheral utilization of glucose, by increasing uptake, and decreasing gluconeogenesis. To work, metformin requires the presence of endogenous insulin; thus, patients must have some functioning β-cells.

Route of administration: Oral.

Indications: Type 2 diabetes where dieting and sulphonylureas have proved ineffective.

Contraindications: Metformin should not be given to patients with hepatic or renal impairment (owing to the risk of lactic acidosis) or heart failure.

Adverse effects: Anorexia, headache, nausea and vomiting, lactic acidosis and decreased vitamin B_{12} absorption.

Therapeutic regimen: Metformin is given at 1 g two or three times daily. It can be used alone or with sulphonylureas. Metformin should be taken with or after food.

Other antidiabetics

α-Glucosidase inhibitors

Acarbose is the only available drug in this class.

Mechanism of action: Acarbose inhibits intestinal α-glucosidases, and delays the absorption of starch and sucrose.

Route of administration: Oral.

Indications: Diabetes mellitus inadequately controlled by diet alone or in combination with other oral hypoglycaemics.

Contraindications: Pregnancy, breastfeeding, bowel disease.

Adverse effects: Flatulence, diarrhoea.

Therapeutic notes: Like metformin, acarbose is particularly useful in the obese diabetic patient.

Thiazolidinediones

Rosiglitazone and pioglitazone belong to the thiazolidinediones.

Mechanism of action: These agents are believed to reduce peripheral insulin resistance, leading to a reduction in plasma glucose.

Route of administration: Oral.

Indications: Type 2 diabetes inadequately controlled by diet alone or in combination with other oral hypoglycaemics.

Contraindications: Hepatic impairment, history of heart failure.

Adverse effects: Gastrointestinal disturbance, weight gain. Potentially liver failure.

Therapeutic notes: The thiazolidinediones should only be prescribed by a physician experienced in treating type 2 diabetes, and are currently only licensed for use in combination with either a sulphonylurea or metformin.

Diet and fluid replacement

Dietary control

Dietary control is important for both type 1 and type 2 diabetes.

The diet should aim to derive its energy from the following constituents, in the following amounts:

- 50% carbohydrate (slowly absorbed forms)
- 35% fat
- 15% protein.

This regimen aims to reduce total fat intake, increase protein intake, and increase the intake of high fibre foods, which slow the rate of absorption from the gut.

Simple sugars, as found in sweet drinks and cakes, should be avoided. Meals should be small and regular, thus avoiding large swings in blood glucose levels.

Rehydration therapy

In the acute diabetic patient the fluid deficit can be as high as 7–8 L. Rehydration therapy is essential to regain fluid and electrolyte balance and takes precedence over the administration of insulin.

It is essential to know about the management of the acute diabetic patient. Not only is this a very common exam question, you will also encounter such patients on the wards.

Untreated diabetic patients have hyperkalaemia as potassium requires insulin to enter cells. As soon as insulin is administered, however, potassium follows glucose into cells, and hypokalaemia becomes the danger. The rehydration fluid should therefore contain potassium, but plasma K^+ should be measured hourly.

Diabetic patients are also at risk of metabolic acidosis due to excessive ketone production. If the acidosis is severe (pH <7.0), bicarbonate can be administered intravenously, although evidence to support this is weak.

Hypoglycaemia

Hypoglycaemia is an uncommon presentation in the untreated diabetic patient, although very common in those taking insulin, and sulphonylureas.

The symptoms of hypoglycaemia are driven by the sympathetic nervous system and include:

- Sweating
- Tremor
- Anxiety
- Altered consciousness.

The history may reveal the patient has not eaten as scheduled, exercised or taken too much insulin.

Management depends on the consciousness of the patient. If the patient is alert, glucose can be given orally as a syrup, or as simple sugar. If consciousness is altered, oral administration of glucose is dangerous, and there is a risk of the patient aspirating. In this situation, glucose should be administered intravenously or glucagon can be given by intramuscular or intravenous injection.

Glucose (dextrose monohydrate)
Glucose is administered parenterally as dextrose monohydrate.

Mechanism of action: Dextrose mimics endogenous glucose and is utilized by cells.

Route of administration: Intravenous.

Indications: Hypoglycaemia, as part of rehydration therapy.

Contraindications: Hyperglycaemia.

Adverse effects: Venous irritation, thrombophlebitis. Hypokalaemia may occur.

Therapeutic notes: Glucose is also available in numerous oral preparations, although the patient

must be alert and conscious before these are administered as aspiration can occur.

Glucagon
Glucagon is a polypeptide hormone, normally secreted by the pancreatic α-cells.

Mechanism of action: Glucagon acts on the liver to convert glycogen to glucose, and to synthesize glucose from non-carbohydrate precursors (gluconeogenesis). The overall effect is to raise plasma glucose levels.

Route of administration: Parenteral.

Indications: Insulin-induced hypoglycaemia.

Contraindications: Phaeochromocytoma.

Adverse effects: Nausea, vomiting, diarrhoea, hypokalaemia.

Therapeutic notes: Unlike intravenous glucose, glucagon can be administered easily by non-medical personnel, and can be carried by the patient as a prefilled syringe-pen.

> In an acute hyperglycaemic attack, it is essential that fluids and soluble insulin are given intravenously to rehydrate the patient rapidly and decrease blood sugar levels.

ADRENAL CORTICOSTEROIDS

Basic concepts

The adrenal cortex secretes several steroid hormones into the bloodstream. These are categorized by their actions into two main classes – mineralocorticoids and glucocorticoids.

Of the mineralocorticoids, aldosterone is the main endogenous hormone, synthesized in the zona glomerulosa. It affects water and electrolyte balance, and possesses salt-retaining activity.

Of the glucocorticoids, hydrocortisone (cortisol) and cortisone are the main endogenous hormones, synthesized in the zona fasciculata and zona reticularis. These affect carbohydrate, fat and protein metabolism, and suppress inflammatory and immune responses. Cortisol and cortisone also possess some mineralocorticoid activity.

Small quantities of some sex steroids, mainly androgens, are also produced by the adrenal cortex.

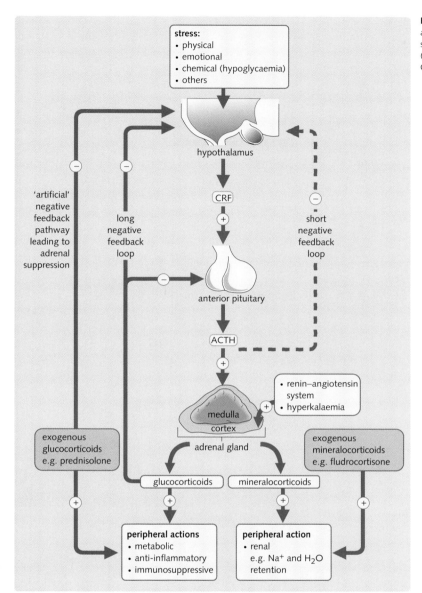

Fig. 6.10 Hypothalamic–pituitary–adrenal axis: control of adrenal corticosteroid synthesis and secretion.
(ACTH, adrenocorticotrophic hormone; CRF, corticotrophin-releasing factor.)

Synthesis and release

Adrenal corticosteroids are not pre-formed, but are synthesized when required from cholesterol (Fig. 6.10).

Glucocorticoids

The release of cortisol is controlled by negative feedback to the hypothalamic–pituitary–adrenal axis (Fig. 6.10). There is a diurnal pattern of activity with an early morning peak in cortisol release.

A variety of sensorineural inputs regulate the release of corticotrophin-releasing factor (CRF) in the hypothalamus; examples include physiological and psychological 'stress', injury and infection. CRF, a 41-amino-acid polypeptide, reaches the anterior pituitary in the hypothalamo-hypophysial portal system where it stimulates the release of adrenocorticotrophic hormone (ACTH). ACTH is formed from a larger molecule, pro-opiomelanocortin, and is released into the circulation where it stimulates the synthesis and release of cortisol from the adrenal cortex.

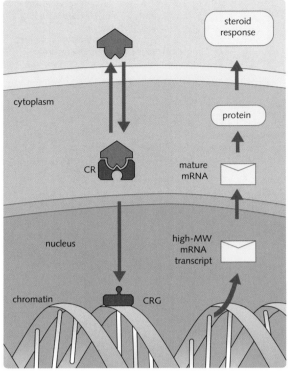

Fig. 6.11 Mechanism of action of corticosteroids at the cellular level. (CR, corticosteroid receptor; CRG, corticosteroid response gene; MW, molecular weight.) (Redrawn from Page et al. 2002.)

Natural and artificial glucocorticoids circulating in the blood exert a negative feedback effect on the production of both CRH and ACTH.

Mineralocorticoids

Aldosterone release is also partially controlled by ACTH, but other factors, especially the renin–angiotensin system (RAS), and plasma potassium levels, are more important.

Mechanism of action of corticosteroids

Endogenous and synthetic corticosteroids act in a similar way (Fig. 6.11). The hormone or drug circulates to peripheral tissues where it enters cells (steroids are lipid soluble) and binds to cytosolic corticosteroid receptors (CR). After hormone binding, these receptors are translocated to the nucleus where they interact with DNA and lead to the transcription of corticosteroid-responsive genes (CRG).

The products of these CRGs have diverse effects on the target tissues (Fig. 6.12). The actions of corticosteroids are divided into effects on inorganic metabolism (mineralocorticoid effects) and effects on organic metabolism (glucocorticoid effects).

Therapeutic use of corticosteroids

Corticosteroids have wide-ranging and powerful effects on human physiology. There are two main areas where these properties are taken advantage of in the therapeutic use of corticosteroids – physiological replacement therapy of corticosteroid deficiency, and anti-inflammatory therapy and immunosuppression (Chs 10 and 11).

Exogenous corticosteroids

Both naturally occurring, and a number of synthetic corticosteroids are available for clinical use. These vary in their potency, half-life and the balance between glucocorticoid versus mineralocorticoid activity (Fig. 6.13).

Mechanism of action: Exogenous corticosteroids imitate endogenous corticosteroids.

Indications: The therapeutic use of corticosteroids falls into the two main categories of physiological replacement therapy, and anti-inflammatory therapy and immunosuppression.

Corticosteroid replacement therapy is necessary when endogenous hormones are deficient, as happens in:

- Primary adrenocortical destruction (Addison's disease)
- Secondary adrenocortical failure due to deficient ACTH from the pituitary or post adrenalectomy
- Suppression of the hypothalamic–pituitary–adrenal axis due to prolonged glucocorticoid therapy.

As all the actions of natural corticosteroids are required, a glucocorticoid with mineralocorticoid activity (cortisol) or separate glucocorticoid and mineralocorticoid are given.

The anti-inflammatory and immunosuppressive effects of glucocorticoids are used to treat a wide variety of conditions (Fig. 6.14). In these cases, synthetic glucocorticoids with little mineralocorticoid activity are used (Ch 10).

Fig. 6.12 Major effects of corticosteroids

Glucocorticoids

Immunological	• decreased production of T and B lymphocytes and macrophages, involution of lymphoid tissue • decreased function of T and B lymphocytes, and reduced responsiveness to cytokines • inhibition of complement system
Antiinflammatory	• profound generalized inhibitory effects on inflammatory response • reduced production of acute inflammatory mediators, especially the eicosanoids (prostaglandins, leukotrienes, etc.), owing to production of lipocortin, an enzyme that inhibits phospholipase A_2, thus blocking the formation of arachidonic acid and its metabolites—see Chapter 10 • reduced numbers and activity of circulating immunocompetent cells, neutrophils, and macrophages • decreased activity of macrophages and fibroblasts involved in the chronic stages of inflammation, leading to decreased inflammation and decreased healing
Carbohydrate metabolism	• increased gluconeogenesis, decreased cellular uptake and utilization of glucose, increased storage of glycogen in the liver (hyperglycaemic actions)
Fat metabolism	• redistribution of lipid from steroid-sensitive stores (limbs) to steroid-resistant stores (face, neck, trunk)
Protein metabolism	• increased catabolism, decreased anabolism, leading to protein degradation
Cardiovascular	• increased sensitivity of vascular system to catecholamines, reduced capillary permeability leading to raised blood pressure
Central nervous system	• high levels can cause mood changes (euphoria/depression) or psychotic states, perhaps due to electrolyte changes
Anterior hypothalamus and pituitary	• negative feedback effect of CRF and ACTH with the result that endogenous secretion of glucocorticoids is reduced, and may remain so after prolonged glucocorticoid therapy ('adrenal suppression')

Mineralocorticoids

Kidney	• increased permeability of the apical membrane of cells in the distal renal tubule to sodium • stimulation of the Na^+/K^+ ATPase pump leading to reabsorption of Na^+ and loss of K^+ in the urine • water is passively reabsorbed owing to sodium retention; thus extracellular fluid and blood volume are increased (raising blood pressure)

Fig. 6.13 Examples of therapeutically used corticosteroids

Glucocorticoids		Mineralocorticoids
'Natural hormones'	Synthetic	Synthetic
Hydrocortisone (cortisol)	Prednisolone Betamethasone Dexamethasone Beclometasone Triamcinolone	Fludrocortisone Deoxycortone

Contraindications: Exogenous corticosteroids should not be given to people with systemic infection, unless specific antimicrobial therapy is being given.

Route of administration: Replacement therapy is given orally twice a day at physiological doses to try to mimic as closely as possible the level and rhythm of natural corticosteroid secretion.

When used to suppress inflammatory and immune responses, corticosteroids may be given orally or intravenously, but, depending on the condition, the

131

Fig. 6.14 Examples of conditions in which corticosteroids are used for their anti-inflammatory and immunosuppressive effects

Systemic uses	Topical uses	
Acute inflammatory conditions 　e.g. anaphylaxis, status asthmaticus, 　fibrosing alveolitis, angioneurotic oedema	Asthma	Aerosol
Chronic inflammatory conditions 　e.g. rheumatoid arthritis, inflammatory 　bowel disease, systemic lupus 　erythematosus, glomerulonephritis	Allergic rhinitis	Nasal spray
Neoplastic disease 　myelomas, lymphomas, lymphatic 　leukaemias	Eczema	Ointment or cream
Miscellaneous 　organ transplantation	Inflammatory bowel disease	Foam enema

topical administration of glucocorticoids is preferred, if feasible, as it can deliver high concentrations to the target site while minimizing systemic absorption and adverse effects (Fig. 6.14).

At high doses, even topically administered glucocorticoids can achieve systemic penetration.

Adverse effects: Overdosage or prolonged use of corticosteroids may exaggerate some of their normal physiological actions (see earlier), leading to mineralocorticoid and glucocorticoid side-effects. Many of these effects are similar to those seen in Cushing's syndrome, a condition caused by excess secretion of endogenous corticosteroids (Fig. 6.15).

The metabolic side-effects of glucocorticoids include:

- Central obesity and a 'moon' face, as fat is redistributed
- Hyperglycaemia, which may lead to clinical diabetes mellitus, due to disturbed carbohydrate metabolism
- Osteoporosis, due to catabolism of protein matrix in bone
- Loss of skin structure, with purple striae, and easy bruising, due to altered protein metabolism
- Muscle weakness and wasting, due to protein catabolism
- Suppression of growth in children.

Corticosteroid therapy suppresses endogenous secretion of adrenal hormones via negative feedback on the hypothalamic–pituitary–adrenal axis.

Adrenal atrophy can persist for years after withdrawal from prolonged corticosteroid therapy. Replacement corticosteroid therapy is needed to compensate for the lack of sufficient adrenocortical response in times of stress (e.g. illness, surgery). Steroid therapy must be withdrawn slowly after long-term treatment, as sudden withdrawal can lead to an acute adrenal insufficiency crisis.

With glucocorticoid therapy, the modification of inflammatory and immune reactions leads to an increased susceptibility to infections. This can progress unnoticed because of the suppression of normal indicators of infection, such as inflammation. Increased susceptibility occurs to usually pathogenic and opportunistic bacterial, viral and fungal organisms. Re-activation of latent infections (e.g. tuberculosis, herpesviruses) can occur.

The effects are most serious when corticosteroids are being used systemically, although topical use can exacerbate superficial skin infections, and inhaled corticosteroids can encourage oropharyngeal thrush etc.

The other effects of glucocorticoids include mood changes – euphoria and, rarely, psychosis, peptic ulceration due to inhibition of gastrointestinal prostaglandin synthesis, and eye problems such as cataracts and exacerbation of glaucoma.

Fluid retention, hypokalaemia and hypertension can all be side-effects of any corticosteroids that possess significant mineralocorticoid activity.

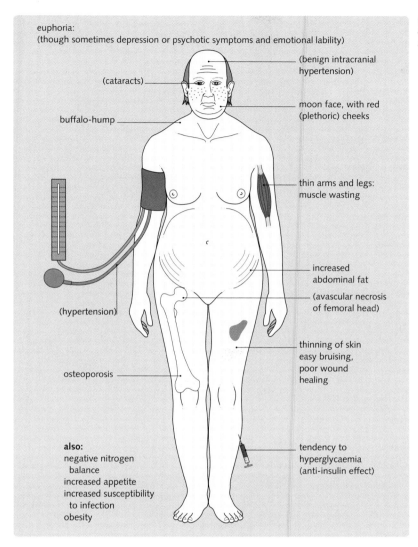

euphoria:
(though sometimes depression or psychotic symptoms and emotional lability)

(cataracts)

buffalo-hump

(benign intracranial hypertension)

moon face, with red (plethoric) cheeks

thin arms and legs: muscle wasting

increased abdominal fat

(avascular necrosis of femoral head)

(hypertension)

thinning of skin easy bruising, poor wound healing

osteoporosis

also:
negative nitrogen balance
increased appetite
increased susceptibility to infection
obesity

tendency to hyperglycaemia (anti-insulin effect)

Fig. 6.15 Effects of prolonged corticosteroid use – the Cushingoid appearance.

You must know the adverse effects of corticosteroid therapy as they are numerous, common and a popular exam question. Some of the adverse effects caused by corticosteroids are logical exaggerations of their normal physiological actions, others are more unexpected and must therefore be learned individually.

Therapeutic notes on specific steroid agents

Glucocorticoids

Hydrocortisone (cortisol):

- Is administered orally for adrenal replacement therapy, and possesses mineralocorticoid activity
- Is administered intravenously in status asthmaticus and anaphylactic shock
- Is applied topically for eczema, inflammatory bowel conditions, etc.

Prednisolone:

- Is predominantly glucocorticoid in activity
- Is the oral drug most widely used in allergic and inflammatory diseases.

Deflazacort:

- Derived from prednisolone, with high glucocorticoid activity
- Administered orally, and indicated in inflammatory and allergic disorders.

Betamethasone and dexamethasone:

- Have very high glucocorticoid activity with insignificant mineralocorticoid activity.
- Are very potent drugs used orally and by injection to suppress inflammatory and allergic disorders, and to reduce cerebral oedema – they do not possess salt- or water-retaining actions.

Beclometasone:

- Is the dipropionate ester of betamethasone
- Is a very potent drug with no mineralocorticoid activity that is useful topically, as it is poorly absorbed through membranes and skin
- Is used as an aerosol in asthma, and as a cream and ointment in eczema to provide high local anti-inflammatory effects with minimal systemic penetration.

Triamcinolone:

- Is a moderately potent drug used in severe asthma
- Is also administered by intra-articular injection for rheumatoid arthritis.

Mineralocorticoids

Fludrocortisone:

- Has such high mineralocorticoid activity that glucocorticoid activity is insignificant
- Is administered orally, in combination with a glucocorticoid, in replacement therapy.

THE REPRODUCTIVE SYSTEM

Hormonal control of the reproductive system

Physiology of the female reproductive tract

The female gonads, or ovaries, are responsible for oogenesis and the secretion of the steroid sex hormones, namely oestrogens (mainly oestradiol) and progesterone. The production of the female

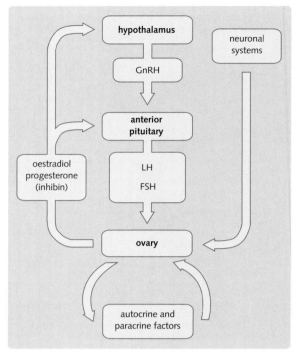

Fig. 6.16 Hypothalamic–pituitary–ovarian axis. (GnRH, gonadotrophin-releasing hormone; LH, luteinizing hormone; FSH, follicle-stimulating hormone.)

sex hormones is controlled by the hypothalamic–pituitary–ovarian axis (Fig. 6.16).

Gonadotrophin-releasing hormone (GnRH) is secreted by the hypothalamus and stimulates the pulsatile secretion of the gonadotrophins, follicle-stimulating hormone (FSH) and luteinizing hormone (LH) by the anterior pituitary. In turn, these act upon the ovaries to stimulate the release of oestradiol, progesterone and other ovarian hormones.

The ovarian hormones are able to exert a negative feedback on the hypothalamus and/or the pituitary. Some of these are selective in their inhibition; for example, inhibin selectively inhibits FSH release from the pituitary, activin selectively stimulates FSH release from the pituitary, and gonadotrophin-surge-attenuating factor selectively inhibits LH secretion from the pituitary.

Menstrual cycle

The menstrual cycle is divided into a follicular phase (days 1–14) and a luteal phase (days 14–28). The cycle proceeds as follows (numbers refer to Fig. 6.17):

Fig. 6.17 The menstrual cycle. (FSH, follicle-stimulating hormone; LH, luteinizing hormone.)

1. Day 1 is the first day of menstruation, which involves the shedding of the uterine endometrium. Plasma oestrogen levels are low and thus little negative feedback occurs. As a result, the secretion of LH and FSH begins to increase.
2. 10–25 pre-antral follicles start to enlarge and secrete oestrogen.
3. FSH stimulates the granulosa cells to secrete oestrogen, the levels of which rise.
4. About 1 week into the cycle, one of the follicles becomes dominant, and the others undergo atresia. The dominant follicle secretes increasingly larger amounts of oestrogen.
5. Plasma oestrogen levels rise significantly as a result of increased sensitivity of the granulosa cells to FSH.
6. Elevated oestrogen levels provide negative feedback, and FSH secretion decreases.
7. Plasma oestrogen levels are now so high (>200 pg/mL) that they exert a positive feedback on gonadotrophin secretion. This

occurs for about 2 days, during which FSH stimulates the appearance of LH receptors on the granulosa cells.

8. An LH surge occurs. This results in a decrease in oestrogen secretion, an increase in progesterone secretion by the granulosa cells, and the resumption of meiosis in the egg.
9. Oestrogen levels decline after ovulation.
10. The first meiotic division is completed.
11. On day 14, ovulation, the release of the ovum, occurs. This is approximately 18 hours after the LH surge.
12. The granulosa cells are transformed into the corpus luteum, which secretes both oestrogen and progesterone in large quantities.
13. There is a rise in the levels of oestrogen and progesterone. As a result, FSH and LH secretion is suppressed, and their levels fall.
14. If fertilization does not take place, the corpus luteum degenerates after about 10 days.
15. Oestrogen and progesterone levels fall; menstruation is imminent.
16. FSH and LH secretion increase once more, and the 28-day cycle begins again.

Physiology of the male reproductive tract

The male gonads, or testes, are responsible for spermatogenesis and the secretion of the steroid sex hormone testosterone. Spermatogenesis takes place in the lumen of the seminiferous tubules of the testis. The production of the male sex hormones is controlled by the hypothalamic–pituitary axis (Fig. 6.18).

The Sertoli cells are connected to one another by tight junctions, and extend from the basement membrane of the seminiferous tubules into the lumen. Under the influence of FSH, these synthesize testosterone receptors and inhibin.

The Leydig cells are found in the connective tissue between the tubules. Under the influence of LH, these synthesize testosterone. Testosterone acts locally to increase sperm production, and also peripherally on the testosterone-sensitive tissues of the body.

Testosterone and inhibin are able to exert negative feedback control over the anterior pituitary, the former decreasing LH secretion and the latter decreasing FSH secretion. In addition, testosterone and inhibin act on the hypothalamus to decrease GnRH secretion.

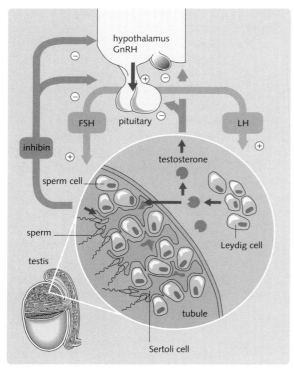

Fig. 6.18 Hormonal control of Sertoli, Leydig and sperm cell function. (FSH, follicle-stimulating hormone; GnRH, gonadotrophin-releasing hormone; LH, luteinizing hormone.) (Redrawn from Page et al. 2002.)

Drugs that affect the reproductive system

Oral contraceptives

Combined oral contraceptive pill

The combined oral contraceptive pill (COCP) contains both an oestrogen (usually ethinylestradiol, 20–50 µg) and a progestogen (an analogue of progesterone).

COCPs provide a highly effective form of contraception. Their efficacy is reduced by some broad-spectrum antibiotics, which reduce enterohepatic recirculation of oestrogen by killing gut flora.

Mechanism of action: The levels of steroids mimic the luteal phase of the menstrual cycle, and suppress, via negative feedback effects, the secretion of gonadotrophins. As a result, follicular selection and maturation, the oestrogen surge, the LH surge, and thus ovulation, do not take place.

Route of administration: Oral.

Indications: Contraception and menstrual symptoms.

Contraindications: Pregnancy, breastfeeding, or to those with a history of heart disease or hypertension, hyperlipidaemia or any prothrombotic coagulation abnormality, diabetes mellitus, migraine, breast or genital tract carcinoma or liver disease.

Adverse effects: Nausea, vomiting and headache, weight gain, breast tenderness, impaired liver function, impaired glucose tolerance in diabetic women, 'spotting' (slight bleeding at the start of the menstrual cycle), thrombosis and hypertension, a slightly increased risk of cervical cancer, and a possibly increased risk of breast cancer.

Therapeutic regimen: COCPs are taken for 21 days (starting on the first day of the menstrual cycle) at about the same time each day, with a 7-day break to induce a withdrawal bleed. If the delay in taking the pill is greater than 12 hours, the contraceptive effect may be lost.

Progesterone-only pill (minipill)

The minipill consists of low-dose progestogen; ovulation still takes place and menstruation is normal. The minipill is not as effective as the COCP.

Mechanism of action: The minipill causes thickening of cervical mucus preventing sperm penetration. It also causes suppression of gonadotrophin secretion, and occasionally ovulation, but the latter effect does not occur in the majority of women.

Route of administration: Oral.

Indications: Contraception. It is more suitable for heavy smokers and patients with hypertension or heart disease, diabetes mellitus and migraine, or in those who have other contraindications for oestrogen therapy.

Contraindications: Pregnancy, arterial disease, liver disease, breast or genital tract carcinoma.

Adverse effects: Menstrual irregularities, nausea, vomiting and headache, weight gain, breast tenderness.

Therapeutic regimen: The minipill is taken as one tablet daily, at the same time, starting on day 1 of the menstrual cycle and then continuously. If the delay in taking the pill is greater than 3 hours, the contraceptive effect may be lost.

Many female patients forget to mention the oral contraceptive pill when they list their medications, so ensure to ask specifically as numerous important drug interactions may need to be considered.

Mrs Hayat, 29 years old, recently had pulmonary embolism on return from her holiday to Egypt. On admission and investigation, colon cancer was detected. A few weeks later, she goes to her GP to enquire about oral contraception. Since she has a predisposition to venous thrombosis, the GP advises her to take oral progestogen-only contraceptives, rather than a COCP.

Other contraceptive regimens

Depot-progesterone

Examples of depot-progesterone drugs include medroxyprogesterone acetate and the etonogestrel-releasing implant. These provide long-term contraception.

Mechanism of action: Depot-progesterone causes thickening of cervical mucus. It also causes suppression of gonadotrophin secretion, and occasionally ovulation, but the latter effect does not occur in the majority of women.

Route of administration: Medroxyprogesterone acetate is administered intramuscularly. The etonogestrel-releasing implant system relies on a hormone rod placed subdermally.

Indications: Contraception.

Contraindications: Pregnancy, arterial disease, liver disease, osteoporosis, breast or genital tract carcinoma.

Adverse effects: Menstrual irregularities, nausea, vomiting and headache, weight gain, breast tenderness.

Therapeutic notes: Medroxyprogesterone acetate provides protection for about 12 weeks. The etonogestrel-implant system provides protection for 3 years.

Post-coital ('morning-after' pill/emergency contraception)

The post-coital or 'morning-after' pill, levonorgestrel, provides a form of emergency contraception.

Mechanism of action: High doses of a progestogen alone, or a progestogen with an oestrogen prevent implantation of the fertilized egg. This is 75% effective. Contractions of the smooth muscle are induced, and these accelerate the movement of the fertilized egg into the unprepared uterine endometrium.

Route of administration: Oral.

Indications: The morning-after pill is used for emergency contraception after unprotected intercourse.

Contraindications: Preparations containing oestrogens should not be used in patients who have contraindications to oestrogens (see above).

Adverse effects: Nausea, vomiting and headache, dizziness, menstrual irregularities.

Therapeutic regimen: The morning-after pill regimen depends upon the type of pill being taken, but commonly consist of one or two tablets within 72 hours of intercourse, and one or two tablets 12 hours later. Consult the *British National Formulary* (*BNF*) for details.

Possible contraceptives for males

Male contraceptives remain purely experimental.

Oestrogens and antioestrogens

Oestrogen agonists

The adverse symptoms of the menopause can be attributed to decreased levels of oestrogen that occur as the ovaries being to fail. Evidence suggests that oestrogen given in low doses to menopausal women will reduce postmenopausal osteoporosis, vaginal atrophy and the incidence of stroke and myocardial infarction.

A progestogen is co-administered with oestrogen to inhibit oestrogen-stimulated endometrial growth and thus reduce the risk of uterine cancer and fibroids.

Examples of oestrogen agonists include estradiol and estriol.

Mechanism of action: Oestrogen agonists mimic premenopausal endogenous oestrogen levels.

Route of administration: Oral, or by transdermal patches, gels or subcutaneous implants.

Indications: Oestrogen agonists are used alone for hormone replacement therapy (HRT) in menopausal women who have undergone a hysterectomy, and in conjunction with a progestogen if the patient has a uterus.

Contraindications: Pregnancy, oestrogen-dependent cancer, active or previous thromboembolic disease.

Adverse effects: Increased risk of endometrial cancer and possibly an increased risk of breast cancer after many years of treatment.

Therapeutic regimen: Oestrogen agonists are given for several years, starting in the perimenopausal period.

Oestrogen antagonists

Examples of oestrogen antagonists include tamoxifen, clomifene and toremifene.

Mechanism of action: Anti-oestrogens act at oestrogen receptors in oestrogen-sensitive tissues, such as the breast, bone endometrium, and also feedback to the pituitary, antagonizing endogenous oestrogen.

Route of administration: Tamoxifen is administered orally or by intravenous or subcutaneous injection whereas clomifene is administered orally.

Indications: Oestrogen antagonists are used for female infertility and breast cancer.

Contraindications: Hepatic disease, ovarian cysts, endometrial carcinoma.

Adverse effects: Multiple pregnancies and hot flushes. Withdrawal causes visual disturbances and ovarian hyperstimulation.

Progestogens and anti-progestogens

Progestogen agonists

Examples of progestogen agonists include progesterone, medroxyprogesterone, dydrogesterone, hydroxyprogesterone and norethisterone.

Mechanism of action: Progestogen agonists mimic endogenous progesterone.

Route of administration: Oral, or by transdermal patches, gels or subcutaneous implants.

Indications: Progestogen agonists are given for premenstrual symptoms, severe dysmenorrhoea, menorrhagia, endometriosis, contraception and as part of HRT.

Contraindications: Pregnancy or to those with arterial disease, liver disease or breast or genital tract carcinoma.

Adverse effects: Menstrual irregularities, nausea, vomiting and headache, weight gain, breast tenderness.

Progestogen antagonists

Mifepristone is an example of a progestogen antagonist.

Mechanism of action: Progestogen antagonists bind to progesterone receptors but exert no effect. They sensitize the uterus to prostaglandins and can therefore be used in combination with prostaglandins in the termination of early pregnancy.

Route of administration: Oral.

Indications: Progestogen antagonists are used in the termination of pregnancy.

Contraindications: Progestogen antagonists should not be given to pregnant women (64 days' gestation or more), to women with adrenal failure or haemorrhagic disorders, or to those on anticoagulant or long-term corticosteroid treatment, or to smokers aged 35 years and over.

Adverse effects: Vaginal bleeding, faintness, nausea and vomiting.

Androgens and antiandrogens

Androgen agonists

Testosterone and mesterolone are examples of androgen agonists.

Mechanism of action: Androgen agonists mimic endogenous androgens.

Route of administration: Oral, intramuscularly or by implant or cutaneous patch.

Indications: Androgen agonists are given as androgen-replacement therapy in castrated men, for pituitary or testicular disease causing hypogonadism, and for breast cancer.

Contraindications: Androgen agonists should not be given to men with breast or prostate cancer, to people with hypercalcaemia, or to women who are pregnant or breast-feeding.

Adverse effects: Sodium retention causing oedema, hypercalcaemia, suppression of spermatogenesis, virilism in women and premature closure of epiphyses in prepubertal boys. The incidence of prostate abnormalities and prostate cancer is also increased.

Androgen antagonists
Cyproterone is an androgen antagonist that is a progesterone derivative. Both oestrogens and progestogens have anti-androgenic properties.

Mechanism of action: Androgen antagonists are partial agonists at androgen receptors, and act on the hypothalamus to reduce the synthesis of gonadotrophins. They inhibit spermatogenesis, causing reversible infertility, but are not contraceptives.

Route of administration: Oral.

Indications: Androgen antagonists are used for male hypersexuality and sexual deviation, prostate cancer, acne, female hirsutism, and precocious puberty.

Contraindications: Androgen antagonists should not be given to people with hepatic disease or severe diabetes, or to those aged 18 and under as their bones are not fully matured.

Adverse effects: Fatigue and lethargy, and hepatotoxicity.

Therapeutic notes: Finasteride is technically an anti-androgen, although inhibits the enzyme 5α-reductase which metabolizes testosterone to the more potent androgen dihydrotestosterone. Finasteride is indicated in benign prostatic hyperplasia and is administered orally.

Like breast cancer in women, prostate cancer in men is most often hormone dependent. Exogenous androgens can promote and anti-androgens can suppress tumour growth.

Anabolic steroids
Nandrolone and stanozolol are examples of anabolic steroids.

Mechanism of action: Anabolic steroids are androgenic; stimulate protein synthesis and promote wound and fracture healing.

Route of administration: Nandrolone is administered by deep intramuscular injection, and stanozolol orally.

Indications: Anabolic steroids can be used for osteoporosis in post-menopausal women, aplastic anaemias and chronic biliary obstruction.

Contraindications: Hepatic impairment, men with prostate or breast cancer, pregnant women.

Adverse effects: Acne, sodium retention causing oedema, virilization in women, amenorrhoea, inhibition of spermatogenesis, liver tumours.

GnRH agonists and antagonists
Agonists
Goserelin, leuprolide and buserelin are examples of GnRH agonists.

Mechanism of action: GnRH agonists are given intermittently, and mimic endogenous GnRH. Continuous use desensitizes the GnRH receptors on the gonadotrophs and inhibits gonadotrophin synthesis.

Route of administration: Buserelin is administered intranasally whereas goserelin and leuprolide are administered by subcutaneous injection.

Indications: GnRH agonists are used for ovulation induction in those with GnRH deficiency, endometriosis, precocious puberty, and sex-hormone-dependent cancers and prostate cancer.

Adverse effects: Menopause-like symptoms, including hot flushes, palpitations, and decreased libido due to hypo-oestrogenism, and breakthrough bleeding.

Therapeutic regimen: Pulsatile administration of GnRH agonists is every 90 minutes for a few minutes. The treatment must not exceed 6 months, and should not be repeated.

Antagonists
Danazol and gestrinone are examples of a GnRH antagonists.

Mechanism of action: GnRH antagonists inhibit the release of GnRH and the gonadotrophins. They bind to the sex steroid receptors, displaying androgenic, anti-oestrogenic, and anti-progestogenic effects.

Route of administration: Oral.

Indications: GnRH antagonists are given for endometriosis, menstrual disorders, including menorrhagia, cystic breast disease, gynaecomastia.

Contraindications: Pregnancy, hepatic, renal or cardiac impairment, vascular disease.

Adverse effects: Nausea and vomiting, weight gain, androgenic effects such as acne and hirsutism.

Therapeutic notes: Cetrorelix and ganirelix are luteinizing hormone releasing hormone antagonists, inhibiting the release of the gonadotrophins. They are administered parenterally and are used for infertility in specialist centres.

Oxytocic drugs

The oxytocic drugs, oxytocin, ergometrine, prostaglandins E and F (e.g. gemeprost [PGE_1 analogue], dinoprostone [PGE_2] and carboprost [15-methyl PGF_{2a}]). All cause uterine contractions.

Oxytocin is a posterior pituitary hormone that acts on uterine muscle to induce powerful contractions. It does this directly and also indirectly by stimulating the muscle to synthesize prostaglandins.

In addition, prostaglandins ripen and soften the cervix, further aiding the expulsion of a uterine mass.

Mechanism of action: Oxytocin acts on oxytocin receptors. The mechanism for ergometrine is not well understood, but may be via partial agonist action at α-adrenoceptors or 5-hydroxytryptamine receptors. The prostaglandins act at prostaglandin receptors.

Route of administration: Gemeprost and dinoprostone are administered by vaginal pessary; dinoprostone can also be administered extra-amniotically; oxytocin is administered by slow intravenous infusion, and oxytocin and ergometrine together are injected intramuscularly. Prostaglandins can be administered by intravenous infusion.

Indications: Prostaglandins are used to induce abortion. Oxytocin and dinoprostone are used for the induction of labour while oxytocin, ergometrine and carboprost (in those unresponsive to oxytocin and ergometrine) are used for the management of the third-stage of labour and prevention and treatment of postpartum haemorrhage.

Contraindications: Oxytocic drugs should not be given to women with vascular diseases; ergometrine should not be used to induce labour.

Adverse effects: Nausea and vomiting, vaginal bleeding, uterine pain. Oxytocin can cause hypotension and tachycardia.

BONE AND CALCIUM

Bone and calcium physiology

Bone is a tissue comprised mainly of calcium, phosphates and a protein meshwork, in addition to the components of the bone marrow.

Bone functions to provide support and enables us to carry out various physiological processes such as respiration and movement. Bone is also an active tissue and crucial in the homeostasis of calcium and phosphate.

Serum calcium is ultimately controlled by the peptide, parathyroid hormone (PTH), derived from the parathyroid glands. PTH maintains serum calcium by acting on the kidney to reabsorb calcium from the tubular filtrate, and to stimulate the activation of vitamin D. PTH also acts directly on bone, mobilizing calcium. Activated vitamin D (1,25-dihydroxycholecalciferol) promotes absorption of calcium from the gut. PTH is secreted in response to low serum calcium.

Calcitonin, from the thyroid gland, inhibits calcium mobilization from bone, and decreases reabsorption from the renal tubules.

Disorders of bone and calcium

Osteoporosis is an overall loss of bone mass, and commonly occurs in women after the menopause, when oestrogens fall, and bone mobilisation slowly increases. Other common causes of osteoporosis include thyrotoxicosis, and excessive glucocorticoids (exogenous or endogenous).

Osteodystrophy occurs in renal failure and is driven by secondary hyperparathyroidism. Rickets (vitamin D deficiency) is now rare in the West, although the adult variant, osteomalacia, is not uncommon. Hypercalcaemia is a medical emergency, and is most often due to malignancy.

Rehydration therapy is as important in hypercalcaemia as it is in ketoacidosis (hyperglycaemia), as fluid will be lost in the urine due to osmotic diuresis.

Drugs used in bone and calcium disorders

Mrs Price, 73 years old, weighing 44 kg, presents with a painful, swollen and 'dinner fork-like' deformity of her wrist. Radiography shows she has fractured both radial and ulnar styloid processes (Colles' fracture). The doctor was concerned that she had poor bone density and sent her for a DEXA (dual energy X-ray absorptiometry) scan. The scan indicated Mrs Price had developed early osteoporosis. Her bones are manually aligned and put in a cast to be reviewed in 6 weeks. She is put on alendronate, a bisphosphonate, to increase her bone density and thus help prevent further fractures. Also, she is put on calcium and vitamin D supplements.

Bisphosphonates
Disodium etidronate, alendronate and disodium pamidronate are examples of bisphosphonates.

Mechanism of action: Bisphosphonates inhibit and potentially destroy osteoclasts, which are responsible for mobilizing calcium from bone.

Route of administration: Oral, parenteral.

Indications: Prevention of postmenopausal osteoporosis and corticosteroid-induced osteoporosis, and for the management of hypercalcaemia of malignancy.

Contraindications: Renal impairment, hypocalcaemia.

Adverse effects: Nausea, oesophageal reactions (with oral preparations), hypocalcaemia.

Calcium salts
Calcium gluconate and calcium lactate are calcium salts.

Mechanism of action: Calcium supplementation replace calcium deficiencies.

Route of administration: Oral, intravenous.

Indications: Hypocalcaemia, calcium deficiency, osteoporosis.

Contraindications: Hypercalcaemia.

Adverse effects: Mild gastrointestinal disturbance, bradycardia, arrhythmias.

Therapeutic notes: If calcium is given parenterally, serum calcium should be repeatedly monitored.

Vitamin D
Vitamin D can be administered in its inactive form as ergocalciferol, or in its active form as calcitriol.

Mechanism of action: Vitamin D acts on the gut to absorb calcium from the diet.

Route of administration: Oral, parenteral.

Indications: Vitamin D deficiency, hypocalcaemia secondary to hypoparathyroidism, renal failure and postmenopausal osteoporosis.

Contraindications: Hypercalcaemia.

Adverse effects: Symptoms of overdosage include anorexia, lassitude, nausea and vomiting, weight loss, hypercalcaemia.

Therapeutic notes: Serum calcium should be monitored closely once vitamin D therapy has started, and if symptoms of hypercalcaemia appear.

Calcitonin
Mechanism of action: Calcitonin binds specific receptors on osteoclasts inhibiting their mobilisation of bone, and acts on the kidney to limit calcium reabsorption from the proximal tubules.

Route of administration: Subcutaneous or intramuscular.

Indications: Hypercalcaemia, Paget's disease of bone, bone pain in neoplastic disease.

Contraindications: Caution if history of allergy, or renal impairment.

Adverse effects: Nausea, vomiting, flushing, diarrhoea, tingling of hands.

Selective oestrogen receptor modulator
The drug is called raloxifene.

Mechanism of action: Raloxifene has both oestrogen antagonistic (uterine endometrium and breast tissue) and agonistic properties (bone and lipid metabolism).

Route of administration: Oral.

Indications: Treatment and prevention of postmenopausal osteoporosis.

Contraindications: History of venous thromboembolism, undiagnosed uterine bleeding, hepatic or severe renal impairment, pregnancy, breastfeeding.

Adverse effects: Venous thromboembolism, thrombophlebitis, hot flushes, leg cramps, peripheral oedema, flu-like symptoms.

Therapeutic notes: It may reduce the incidence of oestrogen-receptor positive breast cancer and cardiovascular events but there is no clear evidence of this as yet.

Kidney and urinary system

7

Objectives

After reading this chapter, you will:

- Understand the function of the kidney and urinary system
- Know which drugs affect kidney and urinary function and how they do so
- Be aware of drug indications, contraindications and adverse reactions.

BASIC CONCEPTS

Despite making up only 1% of total body weight, the kidneys receive approximately 25% of the cardiac output.

The volume of plasma filtered by the kidneys is termed the glomerular filtration rate (GFR) and is equal to approximately 180 L/day for a person weighing 70 kg. This means that the entire plasma volume is filtered about 60 times a day. The kidneys have a large functional reserve and the loss of one kidney normally produces no ill-effects. The ureters transport the urine from the kidney to the bladder, where urine is stored. Urine leaves the bladder through the urethra. In women, this is a short tube that opens just in front of the vagina. In men, the tube is longer, passing through the prostate and the penis. The kidneys have the most complex functions (see below), the bladder functions as a storage sac, and the ureter and urethra mainly act as conduits for the transportation of urine (Fig. 7.1).

THE KIDNEY

Functions of the kidney

The kidney has several functions. These include:

- Regulation of body water content
- Regulation of body mineral content and composition
- Regulation of body pH
- Excretion of metabolic waste products, e.g. urea, uric acid and creatinine
- Excretion of foreign material, e.g. drugs
- Secretion of renin, erythropoietin and 1,25-dihydroxyvitamin D_3
- Gluconeogenesis.

The nephron

Each kidney is made up of approximately one million functional units, known as 'nephrons' (Fig. 7.2). Each nephron consists of:

- A renal corpuscle which comprises a glomerulus and a Bowman's capsule.
- A tubule which comprises a proximal tubule, loop of Henle, distal convoluted tubule and collecting duct system.

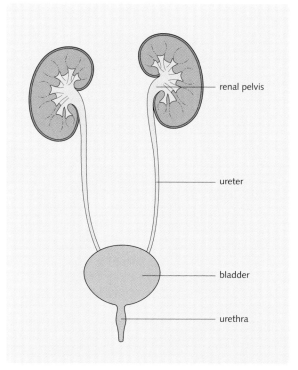

Fig. 7.1 Structure of the kidney and urinary system.

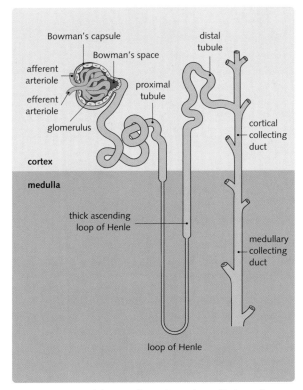

Fig. 7.2 Structure of the juxtaglomerular nephron. (Redrawn from Page et al. 2002.)

Blood supply

Blood reaches each kidney via the renal artery, which divides into numerous branches before forming the afferent arterioles. These afferent arterioles enter the glomerular capillaries (the glomeruli) and leave as the efferent arterioles.

The efferent arteriole leaving most nephrons immediately branches into a set of capillaries known as the 'peritubular capillaries'. These branch extensively and form a network of capillaries surrounding the tubules in the cortex into which reabsorption from the tubule occurs, and from which various substances are secreted into the tubule.

Glomerular filtration

During glomerular filtration, the fluid fraction of blood in the glomerulus is forced through the capillary endothelium, a basement membrane, and the epithelium of the Bowman's capsule, to enter a fluid-filled space known as the 'Bowman's space'.

Approximately 20% of the plasma entering the glomerulus is filtered. The filtered fluid is known as the glomerular filtrate and consists of protein-free plasma.

Tubular function

The tubules are involved in reabsorption and secretion. Important components of plasma tend to be reabsorbed more or less completely, e.g. sodium and glucose are 99–100% reabsorbed. Waste products are only partially reabsorbed, e.g. approximately 45% of urea is reabsorbed.

The tubules secrete hydrogen and potassium ions, as well as organic species such as creatinine, and drugs such as penicillin.

Sodium and water reabsorption

Approximately 99% of filtered water and sodium is reabsorbed, but none is secreted.

Sodium is pumped out of tubular cells into the interstitium by the Na^+/K^+ ATPase pump in their basolateral membrane. This forms a concentration gradient of sodium; high concentration within the filtrate of the tubule lumen, and a low concentration of sodium within the cytoplasm of the tubular cells. This gradient forms the basis of most reabsorption and secretion processes that subsequently occur. Sodium reabsorption from the lumen varies according to the section of the tubule (see Figs 7.3–7.6 below).

Water is reabsorbed by passive diffusion, following the movement of sodium ions, and through specific water channels (aquaporins) in the collecting tubules, which greatly increases the reabsorption of water.

Proximal tubule

The Bowman's capsule extends into the proximal tubule, which is made up of an initial convoluted section and a straight section. The proximal tubule is:

- The site into which many drugs are secreted
- Permeable to water and ions.

Approximately two-thirds of the filtrate volume is reabsorbed back into the blood in the proximal tubule.

Sodium movement into the cell is coupled with that of glucose and amino acids, whereas chloride movement is by passive diffusion (Fig. 7.3). Reabsorption of bicarbonate also takes place in the proximal tubule.

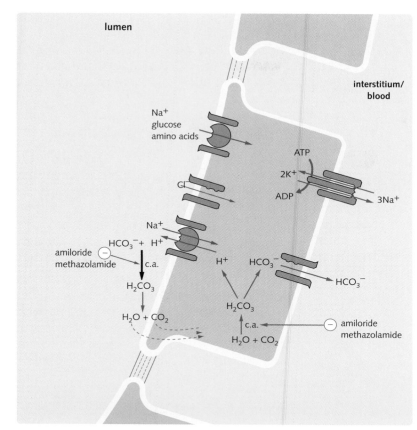

lumen

interstitium/
blood

Na+
glucose
amino acids

ATP

2K+

ADP

Cl⁻

3Na+

Na+

HCO₃⁻ + H+

amiloride
methazolamide

c.a.

H+

HCO₃⁻

HCO₃⁻

H₂CO₃

H₂CO₃

H₂O + CO₂

c.a.

amiloride
methazolamide

H₂O + CO₂

Fig. 7.3 The proximal tubule is one of the sites of bicarbonate (HCO_3^-) reabsorption. Carbonic acid (H_2CO_3) is formed in the cytoplasm from the action of carbonic anhydrase (c.a.) on carbon dioxide (CO_2) and water. H_2CO_3 immediately dissociates into HCO_3^-, which moves down its concentration gradient across the basolateral membrane, and H^+, which is secreted into the lumen in exchange for Na^+. In the lumen, H^+ combines with filtered HCO_3^- to form H_2CO_3 and subsequently CO_2 and water, which are able to diffuse back into the cell. (Redrawn from Page et al. 2002.)

Loop of Henle

The loop of Henle is shaped like a hairpin and consists of a descending limb, a thin ascending limb and a thick ascending limb.

Twenty-five per cent of filtered sodium is reabsorbed in the thick ascending limb (see Fig. 7.4 below), but this portion of the tubule is impermeable to water. Increase in the solute load (sodium) in the interstitium between the ascending loop and the collecting tubules sets up an osmotic gradient which subsequently permits water reabsorption from the collecting tubules – the countercurrent multiplier system.

Juxtaglomerular apparatus

Where the afferent and efferent arterioles enter the glomerulus, a group of specialized cells, the macula densa, are situated, in what is named the juxtaglomerular apparatus. These cells secrete renin, which is a fundamental part of renin–angiotensin system. The renin–angiotensin system is involved directly in vascular tone and in the release of aldosterone (Ch. 2).

Distal convoluted tubule and collecting tubule

The distal tubule is continuous with the collecting duct. The collecting duct is the site at which the tubules of many nephrons merge before draining into the renal pelvis. The renal pelvis is continuous with the ureter.

The late distal tubule and collecting duct contain two cell types (see Fig. 7.6 later):

- Principal cells, which incorporate sodium and potassium channels
- Intercalated cells, which incorporate H^+ATPases that secrete hydrogen ions.

Sodium movement into the principal cells exceeds potassium movement out of the cells, so that a negative potential difference is established. Sodium is transported across the basolateral membrane by Na^+/K^+ ATPase and potassium is moved into the cell before being forced out by the negative potential.

This part of the tubule is the major site for potassium secretion.

The late distal tubule and collecting duct also contain mineralocorticoid receptors. When aldosterone binds to these, it produces an increase in the synthesis of Na^+ and K^+ channels, Na^+/K^+ ATPase, and ATP, so that Na^+ reabsorption is increased, and K^+ and H^+ secretion are also increased.

The collecting tubule is also the site for water reabsorbing via specific water channels named aquaporins. Fine-tuning of the amount of water to be reabsorbed is controlled by the hypothalamus, which governs how much anti-diuretic hormone (ADH or vasopressin) is released from the pituitary gland. Release of ADH results in more aquaporins being inserted into the luminal membrane, and more water being reabsorbed (Ch. 2).

Atrial natriuretic peptide, derived from the atria of the heart in response to fluid overload, is believed to act on the distal nephron causing a water and solute diuresis. This is a potential target for future therapeutic manipulation.

> Several different sodium channels exist in the renal tubule, which is why the various diuretic drugs act at different sites along its course, and have different molecular actions and clinical side-effects.

DIURETICS

> Mrs Hurst, 77 years old, has developed increasing dyspnoea and fatigue. She has also noticed ankle swelling preventing her from wearing her favourite wellington boots. She has a past medical history of angina, takes aspirin regularly and glyceryl trinitrate when required. Following ECG and B type natriuretic peptide testing, she was diagnosed as having heart failure.
>
> Her symptoms, being caused by pulmonary and peripheral oedema, were treated with the loop diuretic furosemide with the aim of decreasing her fluid overload. Enalapril (an angiotensin-converting enzyme [ACE] inhibitor) and carvedilol (a β-blocker) were started concurrently, because they have been shown to improve symptoms and decrease mortality.

Diuretics are drugs that work on the kidneys to increase urine volume by reducing salt and water reabsorption from the tubules. They are prescribed in the treatment of oedema, where there is an increase in interstitial fluid volume leading to tissue swelling.

Underlying causes of oedema

Oedema occurs when the rate of fluid formation exceeds that of fluid reabsorption from the interstitial fluid into the capillaries. Oedema has many causes. The commoner causes for systemic oedema are:

- Congestive cardiac failure
- Hypoalbuminaemia (including liver failure and the nephrotic syndrome).

Loss of fluid from the intravascular space into the interstitial compartment results in an apparent hypovolaemic state. Poor perfusion of the kidneys activates the renin–angiotensin system, which causes sodium and water retention. This exacerbates the problem of oedema.

Types of diuretics

Loop diuretics
Furosemide, bumetanide, torsemide are examples of loop diuretics.

Loop diuretics cause the excretion of 15–25% of filtered sodium as opposed to the normal 1% or less. This can result in a profound diuresis.

Site of action: Loop diuretics act at the thick ascending segment of loop of Henle.

Mechanism of action: Loop diuretics inhibit the $Na^+/K^+/2Cl^-$ co-transporter in the luminal membrane (Fig. 7.4). This increases the amount of sodium reaching the collecting duct and thereby increases K^+ and H^+ secretion. Calcium and magnesium reabsorption is also inhibited, owing to the decrease in potential difference across the cell normally generated from the recycling of potassium.

Loop diuretics additionally have a venodilator action, which often brings about relief of clinical symptoms prior to the onset of diuresis.

Route of administration: Oral, intravenous or intramuscular. Intravenous route is used in emergencies as therapeutic effect is much quicker

lumen

loop
diuretics

interstitium/
blood

Fig. 7.4 Transport mechanism in the thick ascending loop of Henle. Loop diuretics block the Na⁺/K⁺/2Cl⁻ co-transporter (1) thereby increasing the excretion of Na⁺ and Cl⁻. These drugs also decrease the potential difference across the tubule cell, which arises from the recycling of K⁺ (2), and this leads to increased excretion of Ca²⁺ and Mg²⁺ by inhibiting paracellular diffusion (3). (Redrawn from Page et al. 2002.)

(about 30 minutes compared with 4–6 hours for an oral dose).

Indications: Acute pulmonary oedema, oliguria due to acute renal failure, and resistant congestive heart failure (CHF) and hypertension.

Contraindications: Loop diuretics should not be given to those with severe renal impairment. They should be given only with extreme caution to patients receiving:

- cardiac glycosides (as the hypokalaemia caused by loop diuretics potentiates the action of

cardiac glycosides and consequently increases the risk of cardiac glycoside-induced arrhythmias)
- aminoglycoside antibiotics, as these interact with loop diuretics and increase the risk of ototoxicity and potential hearing loss.

Adverse effects: Hypokalaemia, hyponatraemia, hyperuricaemia, hypotension, hypovolaemia. Metabolic alkalosis may occur due to increased hydrogen secretion and thus excretion. Hypocalcaemia and hypomagnesaemia are also possible.

> Most diuretics drugs block sodium reabsorption from the renal tubule. High solute load in the tubule results in an osmotic diuresis.

Thiazide and related diuretics

Bendroflumethiazide, chlortalidone, metolazone and indapamide are examples of thiazide or related diuretics.

Thiazides produce a moderately potent diuresis, causing the excretion of 5–10% of filtered sodium

Site of action: Thiazide diuretics act on the early distal tubule.

Mechanism of action: Thiazide diuretics inhibit the Na⁺/Cl⁻ co-transporter in the luminal membrane (Fig. 7.5). Like loop diuretics, they increase the secretion of K⁺ and H⁺ into the collecting ducts but, in contrast, they decrease Ca²⁺ excretion by a mechanism possibly involving the stimulation of a Na⁺/Ca²⁺ exchange across the basolateral membrane; this is due to reduced tubular cell sodium concentration.

Route of administration: Oral, peak effect at 4–6 hours.

Indications: Hypertension, and oedema secondary to CHF, liver disease or nephrotic syndrome. Occasionally used for prophylaxis of calcium-containing renal stones.

Contraindications: Hypokalaemia, hyponatraemia, hypercalcaemia. Caution when prescribing to those taking cardiac glycosides, or to those with diabetics mellitus (thiazides may cause hyperglycaemia).

Adverse effects: Hypokalaemia, hyperuricaemia, hyponatraemia, and hypermagnesaemia, hypercalcaemia, metabolic alkalosis.

Fig. 7.5 Transport mechanisms in the early distal tubule. Thiazide diuretics increase the excretion of Na^+ and Cl^- by inhibiting the Na^+/Cl^- co-transporter (1). The reabsorption of Ca^{2+} (2) is increased by these drugs by a mechanism that may involve stimulation of Na^+/Ca^{2+} countertransport (3) due to an increase in the concentration gradient for Na^+ across the basolateral membrane. (Redrawn from Page et al. 2002.)

Fig. 7.6 Transport mechanisms in the late distal tubule and collecting duct. Amiloride and triamterene block the luminal Na^+ channels, which reduces the lumen-negative potential difference across the principal cell and decreases the driving force for K^+ secretion from the principal cell and H^+ secretion from the intercalated cell. The net effect is increased Na^+ excretion and decreased K^+ and H^+ excretion. Aldosterone binds to a cytoplasmic mineralocorticoid receptor (MR) stimulating the production of aldosterone-induced proteins (AIP), which (1) activate and increase the synthesis of Na^+ and K^+ channels; (2) increase the synthesis of Na^+/K^+ ATPase, and (3) increase mitochondrial production of adenosine triphosphate (ATP). The effect of aldosterone is to decrease Na^+ excretion and increase K^+ and H^+ excretion in urine, whereas spironolactone, an aldosterone antagonist, has the opposite effects. (Redrawn from Page et al. 2002.)

Potassium-sparing diuretics

Spironolactone, amiloride and triamterene are all potassium-sparing diuretics.

Potassium-sparing diuretics produce mild diuresis and cause the excretion of 2–3% of filtered sodium.

Site of action: Potassium-sparing diuretics work at the late distal tubule and collecting duct (Fig. 7.6).

Mechanism of action: There are two classes of potassium-sparing diuretics:

148

- Sodium-channel blockers, e.g. amiloride and triamterene. These drugs block sodium reabsorption by the principal cells, thus reducing the potential difference across the cell and reducing K^+ secretion. Secretion of H^+ from the intercalated cells is also decreased.
- Aldosterone antagonists, e.g. spironolactone. Spironolactone is a competitive antagonist at aldosterone receptors, and thus reduces Na^+ reabsorption and therefore K^+ and H^+ secretion. The degree of diuresis depends on aldosterone levels.

Route of administration: Oral.

Indications: In conjunction with other diuretics (thiazides, loop diuretics) in managing heart failure or hypertension, to maintain normal serum potassium levels.

Aldosterone antagonists are used in the treatment of hyperaldosteronism, which can be primary (Conn's syndrome) or secondary (as a result of CHF, liver disease or nephrotic syndrome).

Contraindications: Potassium-sparing diuretics interact with angiotensin-converting enzyme inhibitors, increasing the risk of hyperkalaemia. They should not be given to patients with renal failure.

Adverse effects: Gastrointestinal disturbances, hyperkalaemia, hyponatraemia. Aldosterone antagonists have a wide range of adverse effects, including gynaecomastia, menstrual disorders and male sexual dysfunction.

Therapeutic notes: Low-dose spironolactone has beneficial effects in CHF. Several preparations exist which combine a potassium-sparing diuretic with either a thiazide or a loop diuretic, for example co-amilofruse which contains amiloride and furosemide; such drugs are listed in the *British National Formulary* (*BNF*).

Osmotic diuretics
Mannitol is an osmotic diuretic.

Site of action: Osmotic diuretics exert their effects in tubular segments that are water permeable; proximal tubule, descending loop of Henle, and the collecting ducts.

Mechanism of action: Osmotic diuretics are freely filtered at the glomerulus, but only partially, if at all, reabsorbed. Passive water reabsorption is reduced by the presence of this non-reabsorbable solute within the tubule lumen. The net effect is increased water loss, with a relatively smaller loss of sodium.

Route of administration: Mannitol is administered intravenously.

Indications: Osmotic diuretics are used mainly for raised intracranial, and rarely raised intraocular, pressure (glaucoma).

Contraindications: Congestive cardiac failure, pulmonary oedema.

Adverse effects: Chills and fever.

Therapeutic notes: Osmotic diuretics are seldom used in heart failure as expansion of blood volume can be greater than the degree of diuresis produced.

THE URINARY SYSTEM

Urinary retention
Acute urinary retention is treated with urethral catheterization. Chronic urinary retention is usually painless, and management depends upon the underlying cause. In men, the commonest cause for chronic urinary retention is benign prostatic hyperplasia (BPH). Surgery is the definitive treatment, though many patients can be treated medically. Three classes of drugs can be used to treat bladder outflow obstruction secondary to BPH. These are:

- α-Blockers
- Parasympathomimetics
- Anti-androgens

α-Blockers
Doxazosin and prazosin are examples of α-blockers, and act by relaxing the smooth muscle at the urethra opening of the bladder, increasing the flow of urine. Since the α-blockers are also used as vasodilators in cardiovascular disease (Ch. 2), hypotension can be a side-effect, though are otherwise well tolerated.

Parasympathomimetics
Parasympathomimetics, such as bethanechol, act by increasing detrusor muscle contraction. Their effect is most marked when there is bladder outlet obstruction, and they have no role in the relief of acute urinary retention. Side-effects include sweating, bradycardia and intestinal colic. They are now used infrequently, being superseded by catheterization.

Anti-androgens

Finasteride is a specific inhibitor of the enzyme 5α-reductase, which converts testosterone to the more potent androgen dihydrotestosterone. This inhibition loads to a reduction in prostate size, and improvement of urinary flow. The anti-androgens are described in Chapter 6.

Urinary incontinence

Mr Raheem, 80 years old, presents with a history of increasing nocturia, urgency and reduced urinary flow for the past 2 years. Urinalysis was negative. Renal function and ultrasound were normal. His urine flow rate showed moderate impairment. Digital rectal examination revealed a smooth, enlarged prostate, suggestive of benign prostatic hyperplasia. Prostate serum antigen was normal, supporting a diagnosis of benign prostatic hyperplasia (rather than prostatic cancer). Since the patient was reluctant to undergo an operation and declined transurethral resection of the prostate (TURP), he was managed medically by tamsulosin, an α-adrenergic blocker.

Urinary incontinence by definition is the inability to prevent the discharge of urine. There are three main types of urinary incontinence:

- True incontinence
- Stress incontinence
- Urge incontinence.

Urge incontinence is the only type that is practically amenable to pharmacological intervention, mostly with antimuscarinic drugs.

Antimuscarinics

Oxybutynin is the most widely used antimuscarinic for urge incontinence.

Mechanism of action: Oxybutynin relaxes the detrusor muscle of the bladder.

Route of administration: Oral, transdermal (patches).

Indications: Urinary frequency, urgency, urge incontinence.

Contraindications: Intestinal obstruction, significant bladder outflow obstruction, glaucoma.

Adverse effects: Dry mouth, constipation, blurred vision, nausea and vomiting.

Therapeutic notes: The main side-effects are typically the anticholinergic ones, and are commonly dose related.

Erectile dysfunction

Erectile dysfunction (impotence) is a common problem worldwide and has numerous causes.

The penis is innervated by autonomic (involuntary) and somatic (voluntary) nerves. Parasympathetic innervation brings about erection, and sympathetic innervation is responsible for ejaculation. Nonadrenergic, noncholinergic neurotransmission (NANC) also appears to promote erection.

Nitric oxide is believed to be the principal mediator of inducing and sustaining an erection. This highly reactive species activates the guanylyl cyclase enzyme, which subsequently generates cyclic guanosine monophosphate (cGMP).

The synthesis of cGMP in turn activates a protein kinase, which phosphorylates ion channels in the plasma membrane, and causes hyperpolarisation of the smooth muscle cell. Intracellular calcium ions are consequently sequestered into the endoplasmic reticulum, and further calcium influx into the cell inhibited by the closure of calcium channels. The overall effect of a fall in intracellular calcium is a relaxation of the smooth muscle, and increased blood flow to the penis.

While nitric oxide has a very short half-life and is molecularly unstable, cGMP is broken down by a specific group of enzymes, the phosphodiesterases, which subsequently results in the penis returning to its flaccid state. Phosphodiesterase type 5 is thought to be the principal species within the penis, and clearly a target for therapeutic manipulation.

Phosphodiesterase inhibitors

Sildenafil is a selective inhibitor of phosphodiesterase type 5.

Mechanism of action: Inhibition of phosphodiesterase-mediated degradation of cGMP. Higher intracellular levels of cGMP result in continual relaxation of penile smooth muscle and maintenance of an erection.

Route of administration: Oral.

Indications: Erectile dysfunction. There are strict guidelines in the UK as to which groups of patients can be prescribed sildenafil on the National Health

Service. These include patients with: diabetes, multiple sclerosis, Parkinson's disease, poliomyelitis, prostate cancer, severe pelvic injury, single gene neurological disease, spina bifida or spinal cord injury. For a comprehensive list of criteria, consult the *BNF*.

Contraindications: Concurrent treatment with nitrates. Conditions in which vasodilation or sexual activity inadvisable.

Adverse effects: Dyspepsia, headache, flushing, visual disturbances.

Therapeutic notes: Non-specific inhibition of phosphodiesterase type 6 in the retina is responsible for occasional colour disturbances in some patient's vision. Erection will not occur unless there is sexual stimulation.

Prostaglandin E$_1$

Alprostadil is a synthetic prostaglandin E$_1$ analogue.

Mechanism of action: It has a similar effect to on penile smooth muscle as nitric oxide.

Route of administration: Direct injection into the corpus cavernosum of the penis, or applied into the urethra.

Indications: Erectile dysfunction.

Contraindications: Predisposition to prolonged erection, urethral stricture and use of other agents for erectile dysfunction.

Adverse effects: Penile pain, priapism.

Therapeutic notes: Any erection lasting longer than four hours should be reported.

Phosphodiesterase enzymes degrade the cyclic nucleotides cAMP and cGMP. Inhibitors of the phosphodiesterases, such as sildenafil, and the less specific xanthines such as theophylline, result in accumulation of these mediators, which brings about the physiological effects of these drugs.

Gastrointestinal system 8

Objectives

After reading this chapter, you will:

- Understand the function of the gastrointestinal system
- Know which drugs affect gastrointestinal function
- Be aware of drug indications, contraindications and adverse reactions.

THE STOMACH

Basic concepts

The stomach not only acts as a sac to store food, but also helps in its breakdown both mechanically and chemically (through hydrochloric acid and digestive enzymes). Peptic ulceration and gastro-oesophageal reflux disease (GORD) are two of the common problems that can occur in the stomach.

Peptic ulceration

The gastric epithelium secretes several substances – hydrochloric acid (HCl) (parietal cells), digestive enzymes (peptic cells), and mucus (mucus-secreting cells). The acid and enzymes convert food into a thick semi-liquid paste called chyme, whereas the mucus protects the stomach from its own corrosive secretions.

Peptic ulceration results from a breach in the mucosa lining the alimentary tract caused by acid and enzyme attack (Fig. 8.1). Unprotected mucosa

Weakened mucosal defence	Normal	Increased attack
weakened defences vulnerable to being breached by normal acid/enzyme levels	acid/enzyme attack is adequately balanced by mucosal and other defences	increased attack breaks down the defences that would normally be adequate
e.g. • *Helicobacter pylori* infection. • loss of normal mucosal defences, e.g. NSAIDs (see Chapter 10)	e.g. • healthy state	e.g. • hyperacidity (Zollinger–Ellison syndrome)

Fig. 8.1 Peptic ulceration. (NSAID, non-steroidal anti-inflammatory drug.) (Adapted from Underwood J. *General and Systematic Pathology*, 2nd edition, Churchill Livingstone, Edinburgh, 1996.)

rapidly undergoes autodigestion leading to a range of damage – inflammation or gastritis, necrosis, haemorrhage, and even perforation as the erosion deepens.

Gastric and duodenal ulcers differ in their location, epidemiology, incidence and aetiology but present with similar symptoms and treatment is based on similar principles. Peptic ulcer disease is chronic, recurrent and common, affecting at least 10% of the population in developed countries. *Helicobacter pylori* plays a role in the pathogenesis of a significant proportion of peptic ulcer disease.

Sir Francis Avery-Jones said: 'An ulcer represents the adverse outcome of a conflict between the aggressive forces in the stomach or duodenum (acid/enzymes) and the defence mechanisms (mucus-bicarbonate barrier/ surface epithelium)'. This concept can be used as a way to rationalize your thinking of the causes and thus appropriate treatment of peptic ulcers.

Mr Springfields is a 40-year-old city worker, who presents to accident and emergency with epigastric pain relieved by eating, smelling heavily of alcohol and smoke. He has vomited dark-coloured blood and this is evident on his shirt. He admits to melaena and recent weight loss. Mr Springfields has a 20-pack year smoking history and a 1-year past medical history of back pain, for which he takes ibuprofen. He is pale and tachycardic, with a blood pressure of 110/65 mmHg. Upper gastrointestinal flexible endoscopy reveals a shallow ulcer overlying a blood clot. Biopsy is taken to test for *H. pylori* and returns positive. His management includes being given oxygen and blood transfusions. He is also given *H. pylori* eradication therapy (a proton pump inhibitor and antibiotics) consisting of omeprazole, amoxicillin and metronidazole.

Protective factors

The mucosal defences against acid/enzyme attack consist of:

- The mucous barrier (approximately 500 mm thick), a mucous matrix into which bicarbonate ions are secreted, producing a buffering gradient.

- The surface epithelium, which requires prostaglandins E_2 and I_2, synthesized by the gastric mucosa. These are thought to exert a cytoprotective action by increasing mucosal blood flow.

Acid secretion

The regulation of acid secretion by parietal cells is especially important in peptic ulceration and constitutes a major target for drug action (Fig. 8.2). Acid is secreted from gastric parietal cells by a unique proton pump that catalyses the exchange of intracellular H^+ for extracellular K^+. The secretion of HCl is controlled by the activation of three main receptors on the basolateral membrane of the parietal cell. These are:

- Gastrin receptors, which respond to gastrin secreted by the G cells of the stomach antrum
- Histamine (H_2) receptors, which respond to histamine secreted from the enterochromaffin-like paracrine cells that are adjacent to the parietal cell
- Muscarinic (M_1, M_3) receptors on the parietal cell, which respond to acetylcholine (ACh) released from neurons innervating the parietal cell.

Although the parietal cells possess muscarinic and gastrin receptors, both ACh and gastrin mainly exert their acid secretory effect indirectly, by stimulating nearby enterochromaffin-like cells to release histamine. Histamine then acts locally on the parietal cells where activation of the H_2 receptor results in the stimulation of adenylyl cyclase and the subsequent secretion of acid. Excessive production of gastrin from a rare tumour, a gastrinoma, can result in excess acid production, and in peptic ulceration, a condition known as Zollinger–Ellison syndrome.

Gastro-oesophageal reflux

Stomach contents are normally prevented from re-entering the oesophagus by the lower oesophageal sphincter (LOS). Loss of tone of the LOS, or a rise in intra-abdominal pressure are the commonest causes of GORD, of which heartburn is the major symptom. Conservative treatment options include weight loss, and raising the head of the patient's bed. Precipitating factors should be avoided, as should excess smoking and alcohol. The drugs used in GORD are the same as for other acid-related disorders (Fig. 8.3).

Fig. 8.2 Acid secretion from parietal cells is reduced by muscarinic antagonists, histamine (H_2) antagonists and the proton pump inhibitors. Gastrin (G) and acetylcholine (Ach) stimulate the parietal cell directly to increase acid secretion and also stimulate enterochromaffin-like cells to secrete histamine, which then acts upon the H_2 receptors of the parietal cell. Antacids raise the luminal pH by neutralizing hydrogen ions. Mucosal strengtheners adhere to and protect ulcer craters and may kill *Helicobacter pylori*. (Redrawn from Page et al. 2002.)

Prevention and treatment of acid-related disease

Drugs that are effective in the treatment of peptic ulcers either reduce/neutralize gastric acid secretion or increase mucosal resistance to acid-pepsin attack. Peptic ulcers thus treated will heal rapidly, but recurrence is common unless *H. pylori* is eliminated.

Reduction of acid secretion

Proton pump inhibitors (PPI)

Omeprazole and lansoprazole are examples of PPIs.

Mechanism of action: PPIs cause irreversible inhibition of H^+/K^+ ATPase that is responsible for H^+ secretion from parietal cells (see Fig. 8.2). They are inactive prodrugs and are converted at acidic pH to sulphonamide, which combines covalently and thus irreversibly with -SH groups on H^+/K^+ ATPase. This inhibition is highly specific and localized.

Route of administration: Oral. Some PPIs can be given intravenously.

Indications: Short-term treatment of peptic ulcers, eradication of *H. pylori*, severe GORD, confirmed oesophagitis, Zollinger–Ellison syndrome.

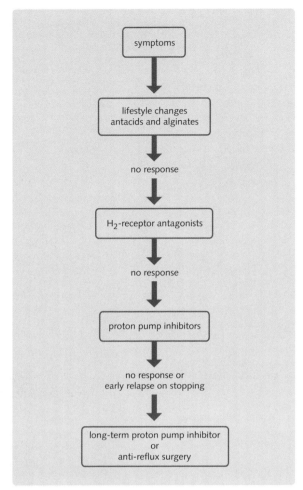

symptoms

↓

lifestyle changes
antacids and alginates

↓

no response

↓

H₂-receptor antagonists

↓

no response

↓

proton pump inhibitors

↓

no response or
early relapse on stopping

↓

long-term proton pump inhibitor
or
anti-reflux surgery

Fig. 8.3 Treatment of gastro-oesophageal reflux disease: a stepwise approach. (Adapted from Haslett et al. *Davidson's Principles and Practice of Medicine*, 18th edition, Churchill Livingstone, Edinburgh, 1999.)

Contraindications: No important contraindications are reported.

Adverse effects: Gastrointestinal upset, nausea, headaches. There might be a risk of gastric atrophy with long-term treatment.

Histamine H₂-receptor antagonists

Examples of H₂-receptor antagonists include cimetidine and ranitidine.

Mechanism of action: H₂-receptor antagonists competitively block the action of histamine on the parietal cell by their antagonism of H₂ receptors (Fig. 8.2).

Route of administration: Oral. Some antihistamines can be given intravenously.

Indications: H₂-receptor antagonists are the first-line treatment of peptic ulcer disease and GORD.

Contraindications: Cimetidine should be avoided by patients stabilized on warfarin, phenytoin and theophylline.

Adverse effects: Dizziness, fatigue, gynaecomastia, rash.

Therapeutic notes: H₂-receptor antagonists do not reduce acid production to the same extent as proton pump inhibitors, but do relieve the pain of ulcer and promote healing. The drugs are administered at night-time when acid buffering by food is at its lowest. The usual regimen is twice daily for 4–8 weeks. Cimetidine inhibits the P_{450} enzyme system, reducing the metabolism of drugs such as warfarin, phenytoin, theophylline and MDMA ('ecstasy'), potentiating their pharmacological effect.

Mucosal strengtheners

Misoprostol

Mechanism of action: Misoprostol is a synthetic analogue of prostaglandin E. It imitates the action of endogenous prostaglandins (PGE_2 and PGI_2) in maintaining the integrity of the gastroduodenal mucosal barrier, and promotes healing (Fig. 8.2).

Route of administration: Oral.

Indications: Ulcer healing and ulcer prophylaxis with non-steroidal anti-inflammatory drug (NSAID) use.

Contraindications: Misoprostol should not be given to people with hypotension, or to women who are pregnant or breastfeeding.

Adverse effects: Diarrhoea, abdominal pain.

Therapeutic notes: Misoprostol is most effective at correcting the deficit caused by NSAIDs that inhibit cyclooxygenase-1 and reduce prostaglandin synthesis (Ch. 10). Misoprostol can prevent NSAID-associated ulcers, and therefore is particularly useful in elderly people in whom NSAIDs cannot be withdrawn.

Chelates

Bismuth chelate and sucralfate appear to help protect the gastric mucosa by several means, including inhibiting the action of pepsin, promoting synthesis of protective prostaglandins and stimulating the secretion of bicarbonate. They are administered orally and are generally well tolerated.

Antacids

Examples of antacids include aluminium hydroxide and magnesium carbonate.

Mechanism of action: Antacids consist of alkaline Al^{3+} and Mg^{2+} salts that are used to raise the luminal pH of the stomach. They neutralize acid and, as a result, may reduce the damaging effects of pepsin, which is pH dependent (Fig. 8.2). Additionally, Al^{3+} and Mg^{2+} salts bind and inactivate pepsin.

Route of administration: Oral.

Indications: Symptomatic relief of ulcers, non-ulcer dyspepsia, and GORD.

Contraindications: Aluminium hydroxide and magnesium hydroxide should not be given to people with hypophosphataemia.

Adverse effects: Constipation, diarrhoea.

Therapeutic notes: Antacids are still useful for the relief of symptoms of ulceration; frequent high dosing can promote ulcer healing but this is rarely practical.

Alginates

Alginate-containing antacids are administered orally, and form an impenetrable raft which floats on the surface of the gastric contents. This layer prevents gastric acid from refluxing into the oesophagus, and is therefore most useful in GORD. This class of drug is very well tolerated, but does not have any effect on acid secretion, or on preventing or healing of peptic ulcers.

Helicobacter pylori **eradication regimens**

H. pylori plays a significant role in the pathogenesis of peptic ulcer disease. It does not cause ulcers in everyone it infects (50–80% of the population) but, of those who develop ulcers, 90% can be found to have an *H. pylori* infection in their antrum.

Treatment of peptic ulcer disease should include eradication of *H. pylori*. The rate of recurrence of duodenal ulcer after healing can be as high as 80% within 1 year when *H. pylori* eradication is not part of the treatment, but less than 5% when *H. pylori* is eradicated.

The ideal treatment for *H. pylori* eradication is not yet clear. Current regimens under evaluation include:

- The 'classic' triple therapy – 1 or 2 weeks' treatment with omeprazole, metronidazole and amoxicillin or clarithromycin. This eliminates *H. pylori* in 90% of patients but adverse effects, compliance and resistance can be problematic.
- Dual therapy – omeprazole is given in combination with a single antibiotic, usually either amoxicillin or clarithromycin, although it is less effective at *H. pylori* eradication and is not recommended.

> Peptic ulcer disease is very common, and potentially life-threatening. Always check with patients if they have an ulcer or ulcer-like symptoms before prescribing NSAIDs.

NAUSEA AND VOMITING

Basic concepts

Nausea is an unpleasant feeling in the upper abdomen and throat, which usually precedes vomiting, though for many patients nausea is experienced without vomiting. Nausea alone can be as distressing as the act of vomiting itself. The commoner causes for nausea and vomiting are shown in Figure 8.4. The act of vomiting is coordinated in the vomiting centre within the brainstem. This centre receives neuronal input from several sources, though fibres from the chemoreceptor trigger zone (CTZ) of the fourth ventricle appear fundamental in

Fig. 8.4 Commoner causes of nausea and vomiting

- Gastrointestinal irritation
- Motion sickness
- Vestibular disease
- Hormone disturbance
- Drugs and radiation
- Exogenous toxins
- Pain
- Psychogenic factors
- Intracranial pathology

bringing about emesis. The CTZ lies outside the blood–brain barrier, and is sensitive to many stimuli, such as drugs and endogenous and potentially exogenous chemical mediators. The CTZ contains numerous dopamine receptors, which partially explains why anti-Parkinsonian drugs (dopaminergic drugs) often induce nausea and vomiting, whereas some antidopaminergic drugs are used as antiemetics.

Emetic drugs

It is advantageous, occasionally, to induce emesis (vomiting) to empty the stomach of an ingested toxic substance. Ipecacuanha is given as a liquid, and causes gastric irritation resulting in emesis. There is no evidence to support its use, however, and gastric lavage is the preferred method.

Antiemetic drugs

H_1-receptor antagonists

Cyclizine and cinnarizine are antiemetic antihistamines.

Mechanism of action: These antihistamines have little effect on nausea and vomiting induced by substances acting directly upon the CTZ, though appear effective antiemetics in motion sickness and vestibulocochlear disease.

Route of administration: Cyclizine – oral, intramuscular, intravenous.

- Cinnarizine – oral.

Indications: Motion sickness, vestibular disorders, vertigo.

Adverse effects: Drowsiness, dry mouth, blurred vision.

Therapeutic notes: Antihistamines have significant antimuscarinic activity, and should be used with caution in prostatic hypertrophy, urinary retention and glaucoma.

Phenothiazines

Prochlorperazine is the most widely used antiemetic drug in this class, though the phenothiazines are also used for their antipsychotic properties (Ch. 5).

Mechanism of action: Numerous effects. Block dopamine, histamine and muscarinic receptors.

Route of administration: Oral, rectal, intramuscular.

Indications: Nausea and vomiting, vertigo, psychosis (Ch. 5).

Contraindications: May exacerbate existing parkinsonian symptoms.

Adverse effects: Sedation, postural hypotension, increased prolactin levels, extrapyramidal effects.

Dopamine antagonists

Domperidone and metoclopramide are examples of the antiemetic dopamine antagonists.

Mechanism of action: Domperidone and metoclopramide block dopamine receptors, and act on the CTZ. Their central antiemetic effect is enhanced as they also promote gastric emptying and small intestine peristalsis.

Route of administration: Metoclopramide – oral, intramuscular, intravenous.

- Domperidone – oral, rectal.

Indications: Nausea and vomiting, functional dyspepsia.

Contraindications: Metoclopramide is not routinely given to patients under the age of 20 as there is an increased risk of extrapyramidal side-effects in the young.

Adverse effects: Extrapyramidal effects, hyperprolactinaemia.

5-HT_3 receptor antagonists

Ondansetron is an example of 5-HT_3 receptor antagonists.

Mechanism of action: Antagonism of the 5-HT_3 (serotonin) receptor in the CTZ is believed to be responsible for the antiemetic effects of this class of drugs.

Route of administration: Oral, rectal, intramuscular, intravenous.

Indications: Nausea and vomiting, especially associated with administration of cytotoxic drugs.

Adverse effects: Constipation, headache.

Others antiemetics

The synthetic cannabinoid nabilone has antiemetic properties where there is direct stimulation of the CTZ. Hyoscine is a muscarinic-receptor antagonist, and like the antihistamines is most effective in the treatment of motion sickness. Betahistine dihydrochloride is used in Ménière's disease, though its prime effects are assumed to be on the vestibulocochlear nerve.

Nausea is one of the most distressing symptoms for the patient, and whereas antiemetic drugs only control symptoms, prescribing them really does bring about immediate relief.

THE INTESTINES

Basic concepts

Intestinal motility

Normal motility, or peristalsis, of the intestinal tract acts to mix bowel contents thoroughly and to propel them in a caudal direction. Regulation of normal intestinal motility is under neuronal and hormonal control.

Neuronal control

Two principal intramural plexuses form the enteric nervous system. These are:

- The myenteric plexus (Auerbach's plexus) – located between the outer longitudinal and middle circular muscle layers.
- The submucous (Meissner's) plexus – on the luminal side of the circular muscle layer.

Together, these autonomic ganglionated plexuses control the functioning of the gastrointestinal tract through complex local reflex connections between sensory neurons, smooth muscle, mucosa and blood vessels.

Extrinsic parasympathetic fibres from the vagus are excitatory and extrinsic sympathetic fibres are inhibitory. The enteric autonomic nervous system is a major target in the pharmacological therapy of gastrointestinal disorders.

Hormonal control

The activity of the gastrointestinal tract is influenced both by endocrine (e.g. gastrin) and paracrine (e.g. histamine, secretin, cholecystokinin, vasoactive intestinal peptide) secretions. Other than in the context of local control of acid secretion in the stomach (p. 154), an understanding of these other hormones is not of immediate relevance to an understanding of the pharmacological therapy of gastrointestinal disorders.

Drugs that affect intestinal motility

Four classes of drug are used clinically for their effects on gastrointestinal motility (Fig. 8.5). These are:

- Motility stimulants
- Antispasmodics
- Laxatives (purgatives)
- Antidiarrhoeals.

Motility stimulants

Agents that increase the motility of the gastro-intestinal tract without a laxative effect are used for motility disorders such as GORD and gastric stasis (slow stomach emptying), or for diagnostic techniques such as duodenal intubation. Domperidone and metoclopramide in addition to their antiemetic effects, both act to increase gastric and intestinal motility, though their mechanism of action for the latter remains unclear.

Antispasmodics

The smooth muscle relaxant properties of antispasmodic drugs may be useful as adjunctive treatment in non-ulcer dyspepsia, irritable bowel syndrome and diverticular disease.

There are two classes of antispasmodic drug. These are:

- Antimuscarinics
- Drugs acting directly on smooth muscle.

Antimuscarinics

Examples of antimuscarinics include atropine, propantheline and dicyclomine.

Mechanism of action: Antimuscarinics act by inhibiting parasympathetic activity, causing relaxation of gastrointestinal smooth muscle.

Route of administration: Oral.

Indications: Non-ulcer dyspepsia, irritable bowel syndrome, diverticular disease.

Contraindications: Antimuscarinics tend to relax the lower oesophageal sphincter and should be avoided in GORD. Other contraindications include angle-closure glaucoma, myasthenia gravis, paralytic ileus and prostatic enlargement.

Adverse effects: Anticholinergic effects – dry mouth, blurred vision, dry skin, tachycardia, urinary retention.

Fig. 8.5 Intestinal motility: control and site of drug action.

Drugs acting directly on smooth muscle

Mebeverine, alverine and peppermint oil are examples of drugs that act directly on smooth muscle.

Mechanism of action: Mebeverine, alverine and peppermint oil are believed to be direct relaxants of smooth muscle.

Route of administration: Oral.

Indications: Irritable bowel syndrome and diverticular disease.

Contraindications: Paralytic ileus.

Adverse effects: Nausea, headache, heartburn are occasional problems.

> Irritable bowel syndrome is extremely common in all age groups and in both sexes, and is often self-limiting over time. Sinister pathology should be excluded, and the patient reassured. Dietary modification and antispasmodics form the mainstay of treatment.

Laxatives

Laxatives are drugs used to hasten transit time in the gut and encourage defecation. Laxatives are used to relieve constipation (an infrequent or difficult passage of stool) and to clear the bowel prior to medical and surgical procedures.

It should be remembered that individual bowel habit can vary considerably – the passage of stools twice a day to once every 3 days is normal. The frequency and volume of stool are best regulated by diet, but drugs may be necessary. The passage of food through the intestine can be hastened by:

- Bulk-forming laxatives
- Osmotic laxatives
- Stimulant laxatives
- Faecal softeners.

Bulk-forming laxatives

Bran, methylcellulose and ispaghula husk are examples of bulk-forming laxatives.

Mechanism of action: Bulk-forming laxatives increase the volume of the non-absorbable solid residue in the gut, distending the colon and stimulating peristaltic activity.

Route of administration: Oral.

Indications: Constipation, particularly when small hard stools are present.

Contraindications: Dysphagia, intestinal obstruction, colonic atony, faecal impaction.

Adverse effects: Flatulence, abdominal distension and gastro-intestinal obstruction.

Therapeutic notes: Adequate fluid intake should be encouraged, and clinical effects may take several days to develop.

Osmotic laxatives

Examples of osmotic laxatives include lactulose and saline purgatives.

Mechanism of action: Osmotic laxatives are poorly absorbed compounds that increase the water content of the bowel by osmosis. Lactulose is a semi-synthetic disaccharide that is not absorbed from the gastro-intestinal tract. Similarly, magnesium and sodium salts are poorly absorbed and are osmotically active.

Route of administration: Oral.

Indications: Constipation, hepatic encephalopathy.

Contraindications: Intestinal obstruction.

Adverse effects: Flatulence, cramps, abdominal discomfort.

Stimulant laxatives

Senna, danthron, bisacodyl and sodium picosulphate are examples of stimulant laxatives.

Mechanism of action: Stimulant laxatives increase gastrointestinal peristalsis and water and electrolyte secretion by the mucosa possibly by stimulating enteric nerves.

Route of administration: Oral.

Indications: Constipation and bowel evacuation prior to medical/surgical procedures.

Contraindications: Intestinal obstruction.

Adverse effects: In the short term, side-effects of stimulant laxatives include intestinal cramp. Prolonged use can lead to damage to the nerve plexuses resulting in the deterioration of intestinal function and atonic colon. Danthron is potentially carcinogenic, hence its limited use.

Therapeutic notes: Stimulant laxatives should be given for short periods only, and danthron is indicated for use only in the terminally ill.

Faecal softeners

Liquid paraffin and docusate sodium are examples of faecal softeners.

Mechanism of action: Faecal softeners promote defaecation by softening (e.g. docusate sodium) and/or lubricating (e.g. liquid paraffin) faeces to aid their passage through the gastrointestinal tract.

Route of administration: Oral. Docusate sodium can be administered rectally.

Indications: Constipation, faecal impaction, haemorrhoids, anal fissures.

Contraindications: Should not be given to children younger than 3 years.

Adverse effects: The prolonged use of liquid paraffin may impair the absorption of fat-soluble vitamins A and D and cause 'paraffinomas'.

Therapeutic notes: Prolonged use of faecal softeners is not recommended.

Antidiarrhoeal drugs

Diarrhoea is the passage of frequent, liquid stools. Causes of diarrhoea include infections, toxins, drugs, chronic disease and anxiety.

Acute secretory diarrhoea usually results from an infection, is extremely common, and causes much preventable mortality, especially in children younger than 2 years in developing countries. The vigour with which diarrhoea should be treated depends very much on the cause and the clinical evaluation of patient risk.

There are four approaches to the treatment of severe acute diarrhoea. These are:

- Maintenance of fluid and electrolyte balance through oral rehydration therapy (ORT)
- Use of antimicrobial drugs
- Use of opiate-like antimotility drugs
- Use of stool modifiers/adsorbents.

Maintenance of fluid and electrolyte balance through ORT

ORT should be the first priority in the treatment of acute diarrhoea of all causes, and can be life-saving.

ORT solutions are isotonic or slightly hypotonic; they vary in their composition but a standard formula would contain NaCl, KCl, sodium citrate and glucose in appropriate concentrations.

Intravenous rehydration therapy is needed if dehydration is severe.

Use of antimicrobial drugs

Antibiotic treatment of diarrhoea is useful only when a pathogen has been identified or is highly suspected. Acute infectious diarrhoea is usually self-limiting. Antibiotic therapy itself carries certain risks:

- Spreading antibiotic resistance among enteropathogenic bacteria
- Destroying normal commensal gut flora, allowing overgrowth of the bacterium *Clostridium difficile*, which can result in pseudomembranous colitis, a potentially fatal condition.

Antibiotic treatment is indicated in:

- Severe cholera or *Salmonella typhimurium* infection – tetracycline
- *Shigella* species infections – ampicillin
- *Campylobacter jejuni* – erythromycin or ciprofloxacin.

Antibiotics are discussed in detail in Chapter 11.

Use of opiate-like antimotility drugs

Examples of opiate-like antimotility drugs include loperamide and codeine.

Mechanism of action: Opiate-like antimotility drugs act on μ-opiate receptors in the myenteric plexus, which increases the tone and rhythmic contraction of the intestine, but lessens propulsive activity. Loperamide and codeine also have an antisecretory action.

Route of administration: Oral.

Indications: Opiate-like antimotility drugs have a limited role as an adjunct to fluid and electrolyte replacement in acute diarrhoea. They are also used as adjunctive therapy in some chronic diarrhoeal conditions.

Contraindications: Opiate-like antimotility drugs should not be given to people with diarrhoeal conditions such as acute ulcerative colitis or antibiotic-associated colitis. They are not recommended for children.

Adverse effects: Nausea, vomiting, abdominal cramps, constipation, drowsiness.

Therapeutic notes: Loperamide is the most appropriate opioid for local effects on the gut.

Mr Sandhu, a 27-year-old medical student, went to India for 2 weeks and developed cramps in his lower abdomen, loose, watery and explosive stools, a feeling of general malaise, nausea and occasional vomiting. He self-diagnosed himself with traveller's diarrhoea. Mr Sandhu started taking loperamide, which he had brought with him and noticed some improvement almost immediately. However, he stayed unwell and went to seek medical advice. He was given oral rehydration therapy because he had lost a lot of fluid through diarrhoea and vomiting. This helped and he was well again after 4 days.

Use of stool modifiers/adsorbents

Examples of stool modifiers/adsorbents include kaolin, chalk, charcoal and methylcellulose.

Mechanism of action: It has been suggested that stool modifiers/adsorbents act by absorbing toxins or by coating and protecting the intestinal mucosa, though there is no evidence to support this.

Route of administration: Oral.

Indications: There is little evidence to recommend adsorbents at all.

Contraindications: Adsorbents are not recommended for acute diarrhoeas.

Adverse effects: Stool modifiers/adsorbents may reduce the absorption of other drugs.

Therapeutic notes: Adsorbents are popular 'remedies' for the treatment of diarrhoea, although there is little evidence of their benefits.

> Diarrhoea can be life-threatening, especially in children. Management in most cases relies on fluid replacement, prior to treating the underlying cause.

Inflammatory bowel disease

The inflammatory bowel diseases fall into two categories that share a number of common features. Symptoms often relapse and remit, and their aetiology remains unclear. Crohn's disease can affect the entire gut, and inflammation occurs throughout the full thickness of the bowel wall, while ulcerative colitis affects only the large bowel, and inflammation is limited to bowel mucosa.

Treatment of these conditions is not only pharmacological but also depends on psychological support, correction of nutritional deficiencies, and often surgical resection.

Drug treatment is aimed at controlling inflammation and bringing about remission, and the mainstay of drug treatment for these diseases are:

* Glucocorticoids
* Aminosalicylates
* Immunosuppressives, cytotoxics and antibiotics.

Glucocorticoids
Examples of glucocorticoids include prednisolone, budesonide and hydrocortisone.

Mechanism of action: Glucocorticoids have an anti-inflammatory effect (Ch. 10).

Route of administration: In localized disease glucocorticoids may be administered rectally as enemas, suppositories or foams. In extensive or severe disease, oral or intravenous therapy may be required.

Indications: Glucocorticoids are given for acute relapses of inflammatory bowel disease.

Contraindications: Bowel obstruction or perforation, or for prolonged periods.

Adverse effects: Cushingoid side-effects may occur with long-term glucocorticoid use (Ch. 10).

Therapeutic notes: Budesonide is locally acting and poorly absorbed, so has fewer systemic side-effects.

Aminosalicylates
Sulfasalazine, mesalazine and olsalazine are examples of aminosalicylates.

Mechanism of action: Sulfasalazine is broken down in the gut to the active component 5-aminosalicylate (5-ASA) and sulfapyridine which acts as a vehicle to transport the drug to the colon. Mesalazine is 5-ASA, and olsalazine is two molecules of 5-ASA. The mechanism of action of the active molecule 5-ASA is unknown, though is postulated to act by scavenging free radicals, or interfering with cytokine networks.

Route of administration: Oral, rectal.

Indications: Maintenance therapy of inflammatory bowel conditions.

Contraindications: Aminosalicylates should not be given to people with salicylate hypersensitivity and renal impairment.

Adverse effects: Sulfapyridine is responsible for the majority of this drugs side-effects. Nausea, vomiting, headache and rashes. Blood disorders and oligospermia have been reported.

Immunosuppressives, cytotoxics and antibiotics
When steroids are needed to control symptoms, and side-effects are troublesome or potentially so, the immunosuppressant azathioprine (Ch. 10) is used as an adjunct to other therapies. In addition, cytotoxic drugs such as methotrexate (Ch. 12), anticytokine antibodies such as infliximab (Chapter 10) and the antibiotic metronidazole (Ch. 11) have all been used to modulate the disease process with varying degrees of success.

Obesity

Obesity is becoming increasingly common in the West, and is associated with many disease, such as:

* Cardiovascular disease
* Diabetes mellitus

- Gallstones
- Osteoarthritis.

Dietary restriction and an exercise programme should be explored prior to surgical or pharmacological intervention. The most widely used anti-obesity drugs act directly upon the gastrointestinal tract. There are also centrally acting appetite suppressants.

Drugs acting on the gastrointestinal tract

Orlistat and methylcellulose are examples of such anti-obesity drugs.

Mechanism of action: Orlistat is a pancreatitic lipase inhibitor, and reduces the breakdown and subsequent absorption of fat from the gut. Methylcellulose is believed to act as a bulk-forming agent, and reduces food intake by promoting early satiety (fullness).

Route of administration: Oral.

Adverse effects: Orlistat often results in oily, frequent stools, flatulence, abdominal and rectal pain.

- Methylcellulose may produce flatulence and abdominal distension.

Other anti-obesity drugs

The centrally acting appetite suppressant sibutramine is licensed for adjunctive management of obesity but for no more than 1 year's usage; weight loss may return after cessation. Numerous other drugs are being evaluated for their anti-obesity properties, including the endogenous mammalian peptide leptin, which appears to induce satiety and counteract the properties of another transmitter, neuropeptide Y, which is believed to promote feeding.

Anal disorders

Haemorrhoids, anal fissures and pruritus are commonly encountered problems. Bland ointments are the best treatment option, with careful attention to cleanliness. When necessary, topical preparations containing a local anaesthetic (Ch. 9) or corticosteroid (Ch. 10) may provide symptomatic relief. Perianal thrush can be treated with nystatin (Ch. 11). Haemorrhoids are often treated by injection with a sclerosant, commonly oily phenol.

Stoma care is simple, though requires a thoughtful, practical approach, and empathy with the patient. Details of specific stoma care options can be obtained from the *British National Formulary*.

THE PANCREAS AND GALL BLADDER

Pancreatic supplements

Pancreatic exocrine secretions contain important enzymes that break down proteins (trypsin, chymotrypsin), starch (amylase), and fats (lipase). These are essential for efficient digestion.

Pancreatin is an extract of pancreas containing protease, lipase and amylase, that is given by mouth to compensate for reduced or absent exocrine secretions in cystic fibrosis, and following pancreatectomy, total gastrectomy or chronic pancreatitis. Pancreatin is inactivated by gastric acid and so precautions must be taken to optimize delivery of the pancreatin to the duodenum.

Pancreatin preparations are best taken with food; histamine H_2 antagonists (e.g. cimetidine) may be taken an hour before ingestion of the pancreatin to reduce gastric acid secretion, although acid-resistant (enterically coated formulations) are now available.

Even though pancreatin contains peptides, which would normally be degraded in the stomach, these tablets are coated in an acid resistant layer, and the enzymes and proenzymes within them have endogenous resistance to both acid and proteases, and become active in the small intestine.

Gall bladder

Bile is secreted by the liver and is stored in the gall bladder. Bile contains cholesterol, phospholipids, and bile salts. Bile salts are important for keeping cholesterol in solution. The formation of 'stones' in the bile is relatively common (cholelithiasis), and can result in blockage of the draining duct, with subsequent infection and inflammation (cholecystitis). Surgical removal of the gall bladder (cholecystectomy) has largely replaced the use of drugs in the management of symptomatic gallstones, although this is suitable for patients not treatable by other means.

The dissolution of small cholesterol stones is carried out by prolonged oral administration of the bile acid ursodeoxycholic acid.

Ursodeoxycholic acid

The bile salt ursodeoxycholic acid is administered orally, and handled by the body in the same fashion as endogenous bile salt. It works by:

- Decreasing secretion of cholesterol into the bile
- Decreasing cholesterol absorption from the intestine.

The net effect is a reduced cholesterol concentration in the bile and a tendency for the dissolution of existing stones.

Colestyramine

This orally administered anion-exchange resin binds bile acids in the gut and prevents their reabsorption and enterohepatic recirculation. It is used in the treatment of pruritus associated with partial biliary obstruction and primary biliary cirrhosis, and in hypercholesterolaemia.

Pain and anaesthesia

9

Objectives

After reading this chapter, you will:

- Have a basic understanding of the pain system and the principles of pain relief
- Have a basic understanding of the usage of local and general anaesthesia
- Have good knowledge of the different drug classes, their mechanism of action and adverse effects.

BASIC CONCEPTS

Pain is a common everyday experience that performs an essential defensive function. However, uncontrolled pain can severely diminish quality of life, and it may then be amenable to pharmacotherapy.

Pain, which may be acute or chronic, is defined as an unpleasant sensory and emotional experience associated with actual or potential tissue damage. Pain is a subjective experience, as there are currently no means of accurately and objectively assessing the degree of pain a patient is experiencing.

An analgesic drug is one that effectively removes (or at least lessens) the sensation of pain. The principles of pain relief are:

1. Careful assessment
2. Diagnosis of the cause of the pain
3. Use of analgesics in accordance with the analgesic ladder
4. Regular review of the effectiveness of the prescribed drug.

According to the analgesic ladder (Fig. 9.1), if optimal use of a drug from the non-opioid class (e.g. 1000 mg of paracetamol 6-hourly) (see Ch. 10) does not result in satisfactory pain relief, the prescription should be increased one step to a weak opioid (eg. 60 mg of co-proxamol 4-hourly). If this is not enough the patient will require a strong opioid (e.g. morphine).

Pain perception

Pain perception is best viewed as a three-stage process – activation of nociceptors, followed by the transmission and onward passage of pain information.

Activation of nociceptors in the peripheral tissues

Noxious thermal, chemical or mechanical stimuli can trigger the firing of primary afferent fibres (type

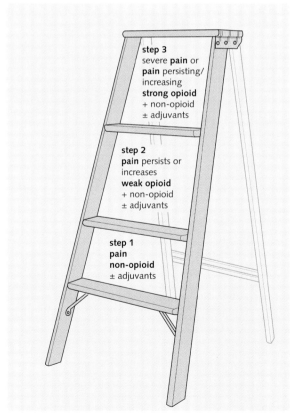

step 3
severe **pain** or **pain** persisting/ increasing
strong opioid
+ non-opioid
± adjuvants

step 2
pain persists or increases
weak opioid
+ non-opioid
± adjuvants

step 1
pain
non-opioid
± adjuvants

Fig. 9.1 The World Health Organization (WHO) analgesic ladder for chronic pain.

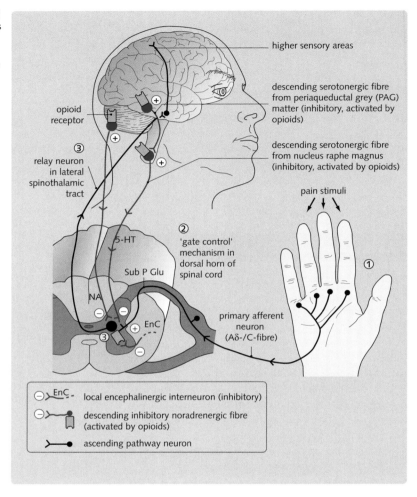

Fig. 9.2 Nociceptive pathways and sites of opioid action. (1). Activation of nociceptors in the peripheral tissues; (2). transmission of pain information; (3). onward passage of pain information to higher centres. (Glu, glutamate; 5-HT, 5-hydroxytryptamine (serotonin); NA, noradrenaline; Sub P, substance P.)

C/Aδ), through the activation of nociceptors (pain-specific receptors) in the peripheral tissues (Fig. 9.2).

Transmission of pain information

Transmission of pain information from the periphery to the dorsal horn of the spinal cord is inhibited or amplified by a combination of local (spinal) neuronal circuits and descending tracts from higher brain centres. This constitutes the 'gate-control mechanism'. In the gate-control mechanism:

- The primary afferent fibres synapse in lamina I and II of the dorsal horn of the spinal cord.
- Transmitter peptides (substance P, calcitonin gene-related peptide, bradykinin, glutamate) and nitric oxide are involved in the ascending pain pathways, though the interactions are complex and have not yet been fully defined.

- The activity of the dorsal horn relay neurons is modulated by several inhibitory inputs. These include: local inhibitory interneurons, which release opioid peptides; descending inhibitory noradrenergic fibres from the locus ceruleus area of the brainstem, which are activated by opioid peptides; and descending inhibitory serotonergic fibres from the nucleus raphe magnus and periaqueductal grey areas of the brainstem, which are also activated by opioid peptides (Fig. 9.2).

Onward passage of pain information

The onward passage of pain information is via the spinothalamic tract, to the higher centres of the brain. The higher centres of the brain coordinate the cognitive and emotional aspects of pain and control appropriate reactions. Opioid peptide release in both the spinal cord and the brainstem can reduce the activity of the dorsal horn relay neurons and cause analgesia, known as 'shutting the gate' (Fig. 9.2).

Opioid receptors

All opioids, whether endogenous peptides, naturally occurring drugs, or chemically synthesized drugs, interact with specific opioid receptors to produce their pharmacological effects.

Drugs interact with opioid receptors as either full agonists, partial agonists, mixed agonists (full agonists on one opioid receptor but partial agonists on another) or as antagonists. Opioid analgesics are agonists.

There are three major opioid receptor subtypes: μ, δ and κ. The existence of a fourth receptor(s) remains controversial.

Generally speaking:

- μ receptors are thought to be responsible for most of the analgesic effects of opioids and for some major adverse effects, e.g. respiratory depression. Most of the analgesic opioids in use are μ receptor agonists.
- δ receptors are probably more important in the periphery, but they may also contribute to analgesia.
- κ receptors contribute to analgesia at the spinal level, and may elicit sedation and dysphoria, but they produce relatively few adverse effects, and do not contribute to physical dependence.
- σ receptors are not selective opioid receptors, but they are the site of action of psychomimetic

drugs, such as phencyclidine (PCP). They may account for the dysphoria produced by some opioids.

Opioid receptor activation has an inhibitory effect on synapses in the central nervous system (CNS) and in the gut (Fig. 9.3).

Secondary-messenger systems associated with opioid receptor activity include:

- μ/δ receptors, the activation of which causes hyperpolarization of a neuron by opening potassium channels and inhibiting calcium channels
- κ receptors, the activation of which inhibits calcium channels.

Activation of all opioid receptors by endogenous or exogenous opioids results in:

- Inhibition of the enzymes adenylase cyclase and thus a reduction in cAMP production
- Inhibition of voltage-gated calcium-channel opening
- Potassium-channel activation which causes hyperpolarization of the cell membrane.

Endogenous opioids

Physiologically, the CNS has its own 'endogenous opioids' that are the natural ligands for opioid receptors. There are three main families of endogenous opioid peptides occurring naturally in the CNS:

- Endorphins
- Dynorphins
- Enkephalins.

Fig. 9.3 Actions mediated by opioid receptor subtypes			
Action	**μ/δ**	**κ**	**σ**
Analgesia	Supraspinal and spinal	Spinal	—
Respiratory depression	Marked	Slight	—
Pupil	Constricts	—	Dilates
GIT mobility	Reduced (constipating)	—	—
Mood/effect	Euphoria inducing but also sedating	Dysphoria inducing mildly sedating	Marked dysphoric and psychomimetic actions
Physical dependence	+++	+	—

GIT, gastrointestinal tract

Fig. 9.4 Endogenous opioid peptides

Precursor molecules	Products	Relative opioid receptor affinity
Pro-opiomelanocortin (POMC)	Endorphins e.g. β-endorphin and other non-opioid peptides e.g. ACTH	μ
Proenkephalin	Enkephalins e.g. Leu^5 enkephalin, Met^5 enkephalin, extended Met^5 enkephalins	δ μ μ
Prodynorphin	Dynorphins e.g. dynorphin A	κ

ACTH, adrenocorticotrophic hormone

They are derived from three separate gene products (precursor molecules), but all possess homology at their amino end.

The expression and anatomical distribution of the products of these three precursor molecules within the CNS is varied, and each has a distinct range of affinities for the different types of opioid receptor (Fig. 9.4).

Though it is known that the endogenous opioids possess analgesic activity, their precise function in the CNS and elsewhere is poorly defined. They are not used therapeutically.

> Mrs Moore is a 60-year-old patient with advanced breast cancer who is receiving chemotherapy. She suffers with bone pain due to metastases. She has been on several analgesics for the pain since its onset, including non-steroidal anti-inflammatory drugs (NSAIDs). NSAIDs were effective to start off with, however the pain sharply increased in severity over the following months and so a decision was made to give her co-proxamol. Co-proxamol is an example of a compound analgesic, containing dextropropoxyphene and paracetamol. Compound analgesics contain both an opioid and a non-opioid. Co-proxamol was more effective in controlling the pain and she was able to continue doing more of the daily activities she used to do, until now. She has increasingly been feeling the pain and is suffering terribly. Review of her pain management and symptoms is taken and she is put on regular morphine as part of her palliative care management.

Fig. 9.5 Opioid analgesics

Weak opioid analgesics	Strong opioid analgesics
Pentazocine	Morphine
Codeine	Diamorphine
Dihydrocodeine	Phenazocine
Dextropropoxyphene	Pethidine
	Buprenorphine
	Nalbuphine

OPIOID ANALGESIC DRUGS

Opioid analgesics are drugs, either naturally occurring (e.g. morphine) or chemically synthesized, that interact with specific opioid receptors to produce the pharmacological effect of analgesia.

The first opioid drug was opium, the crude exudate of the seed head of the opium poppy *Papaver somniferum*; simple extraction yields morphine. Subsequently, many synthetic and semisynthetic opioids have been created by pharmacologists. Examples of opioid analgesics are given in Figure 9.5.

Mechanism of action: Opioid analgesic drugs work by agonist action at opioid receptors (see above).

Note that the sense of euphoria produced by strong opioids undoubtedly contributes to their analgesic activity by helping to reduce the anxiety and stress associated with pain. This effect also accounts for the illicit use of these drugs.

Route of administration: Oral, rectal, intravenous, intramuscular, transdermal and transmucosal (as lozenges).

Oral absorption is irregular and incomplete, necessitating larger doses; 70% is removed by first-pass hepatic metabolism. Fentanyl is available in a transdermal drug delivery system as a self-adhesive patch, which is changed every 72 hours. Transdermal fentanyl is particularly useful in patients prone to nausea, sedation or severe constipation with morphine. Morphine is the drug of choice for severe nociceptive pain.

Indications: Strong opioids are used in moderate to severe pain, particularly visceral, postoperative or cancer-related; in myocardial infarction and acute pulmonary oedema; and in perioperative analgesia (p. 177).

Weak opioids are used in the relief of 'mild to moderate' pain, as antitussives (Ch. 3), and as antidiarrhoeal agents (Ch. 8), taking advantage of these 'side-effects' of opioid analgesics.

Contraindications: Opioid analgesics should not be given to people in acute respiratory depression, with acute alcoholism, at risk of paralytic ileus, and with head injuries prior to neurological assessment (interferes with assessment of the level of consciousness).

Adverse effects: Opioid analgesics share many side-effects, though qualitative and quantitative differences exist. These can be subdivided into central adverse actions and peripheral adverse actions.

Central adverse actions include the following:

- Drowsiness and sedation, in which initial excitement is followed by sedation and finally coma (on overdose)
- Reduction in sensitivity of the respiratory centre to carbon dioxide, leading to shallow and slow respiration
- Tolerance and dependence (Ch. 5)
- Suppression of cough, an effect exploited clinically in antitussives (Ch. 3)
- Vomiting due to stimulation of the chemoreceptor trigger zone (CTZ)
- Pupillary constriction due to stimulation of the parasympathetic third cranial nerve nucleus
- Hypotension and reduced cardiac output, which are partly due to reduced hypothalamic sympathetic outflow.

Peripheral adverse actions include the following:

- Constipation, which is partly due to stimulation of cholinergic activity in gut wall ganglia that results in smooth wall spasm
- Contraction of smooth muscle in the sphincter of Oddi and in the ureters, which results in an increase in blood amylase and lipase due to pancreatic stasis
- Histamine release, which produces bronchospasm, flushing and arteriolar dilatation
- Lowered sympathetic discharge and direct arteriolar dilatation, which results in lowered cardiac output and hypotension.

Adverse effects of opioids tend to limit the dose that can be given, and the level of analgesia that can be maintained. The most serious of all these effects is respiratory depression, which is the most common cause of death from opioid overdose.

Constipation and nausea are also common problems and clinically it is common to co-administer laxatives and an antiemetic (Ch. 8).

Tolerance and dependence: Tolerance to opioid analgesics can be detected within 24–48 hours from the onset of administration, and it results in larger and larger doses of the drug being needed to achieve the same clinical effect.

Dependence involves μ receptors and is both physical and psychological in nature and is discussed in Chapter 5. If physical dependence develops, it is characterized by a definite withdrawal syndrome following cessation of drug treatment. This syndrome comprises a complex mixture of irritable, and sometimes aggressive, behaviour combined with extremely unpleasant autonomic symptoms such as fever, sweating, yawning and pupillary dilatation. The withdrawal syndrome is relieved by the administration of μ receptor agonists, and worsened by the administration of μ receptor antagonists.

Psychological dependence of opioid analgesics is based on the positive reinforcement provided by euphoria.

In the clinical context, especially in terminal care, where tolerance and dependence can be monitored, they are not inevitably problematic. However, the fear of tolerance and dependence often leads to over-caution in the use of opioid analgesics, and inadequate pain control in some patients. It is not uncommon for palliative care patients to take over 1000 mg of morphine sulphate twice daily and remain alert and active.

Therapeutic notes: Strong opioid analgesics include morphine, diamorphine (heroin), phenazocine, pethidine, buprenorphine and nalbuphine:

- Morphine remains the most valuable drug for severe pain relief, though it frequently causes nausea and vomiting. It is the drug of choice for severe pain in terminal care. Morphine is the standard against which other opioid analgesics are compared.
- Diamorphine (heroin) is twice as potent as morphine, owing to its greater penetration of the blood–brain barrier. It is metabolized to 6-acetylmorphine and thence morphine in the body. Diamorphine causes less nausea and hypotension than morphine, but more euphoria.

- Phenazocine has a more prolonged action than morphine, and it can be administered sublingually. It can be useful in biliary colic as it has less of a tendency to increase biliary spasm than other opioids.
- Pethidine is more lipid soluble than morphine, and it has a rapid onset and short duration of action, making it useful in labour. Pethidine is equianalgesic compared with morphine, but it produces less constipation. Interaction with monoamine inhibitors is serious, causing fever, delirium and convulsions or respiratory depression.
- Buprenorphine has both agonist and antagonist actions at opioid receptors, and it may precipitate withdrawal symptoms in patients dependent on other opioids. It has a longer duration of action than morphine and its lipid solubility allows sublingual administration. Vomiting may be a problem. Unlike most opioid analgesics, the effects of buprenorphine are only partially antagonized by naloxone owing to its high-affinity attraction to opioid receptors.
- Nalbuphine is an agonist at κ receptors and an antagonist at μ receptors. It is equianalgesic compared with morphine, but it produces less nausea and vomiting. High doses cause dysphoria.

Weak opioid analgesics include pentazocine, codeine, dihydrocodeine and dextropropoxyphene:

- Pentazocine has both κ/σ receptor agonist and μ antagonist actions, and it may precipitate withdrawal symptoms in patients dependent on other opioids. Pentazocine is weak orally, but, by injection, it has a potency between that of morphine and codeine. It is not recommended because of the side-effects of thought disturbances and hallucinations, which probably are due to its action on σ receptors.
- Codeine has about one-twelfth of the analgesic potency of morphine. The incidence of nausea and constipation limit the dose and duration that can be used. Codeine is also used for its antitussive and antidiarrhoeal effects.
- Dihydrocodeine has an analgesic efficacy similar to that of codeine. It may cause dizziness and constipation.
- Dextropropoxyphene has an analgesic efficacy about half that of codeine (i.e. very mild), and so it is often combined with aspirin or

paracetamol. Such mixtures can be dangerous in overdose, with dextropropoxyphene causing respiratory depression and acute heart failure and the paracetamol being hepatotoxic.

Opioid antagonists

Examples of opioid antagonists include naloxone and naltrexone.

Mechanism of action: These drugs act by specific antagonism at opioid receptors: μ, δ and κ receptors are blocked more or less equally. They block the actions of endogenous opioids as well as of morphine-like drugs.

Naloxone is short acting (half-life: 2–4 hours) while naltrexone is long acting (half-life: 10 hours).

Route of administration: Intravenous.

Indications: Opioid antagonists are given to reverse opioid-induced analgesia and respiratory depression rapidly, mainly after overdose, or to improve breathing in newborn babies who have been affected by opioids given to the mother.

Adverse effects: Precipitation of withdrawal in those with physical dependence on opioids. Reversal of analgesic effects of opiate agonist.

HEADACHE AND NEURALGIC PAIN

Headache

Headache is a very common presenting symptom, yet one which can be difficult to manage. The most common causes of headache include:

- Tension-type headache
- Migraine
- Headache associated with eye or sinus disease.

More sinister causes of headache (including meningitis and neoplasia) are less common, and these can often be confidently excluded by the history and by examination.

The pathophysiology underlying headache is unclear, though symptomatic relief is often obtained from NSAIDs and paracetamol (see p. 184). Some headaches are related to stress and anxiety, and these patents may benefit from antidepressant drugs (Ch. 5).

The management of migraine addresses the acute attacks or attempts to prevent migrainous episodes (prophylaxis) in those who experience frequent attacks. Drugs used for acute migrainous attacks:

- NSAIDs and paracetamol (see p. 184)
- Antiemetics (Ch. 8)
- Serotonin (5-HT$_1$) agonists.

Drugs used in migraine prophylaxis are:

- Antihistamine/serotonin (5-HT) antagonists
- β-antagonists (Ch. 3)
- Tricyclic antidepressants (Ch. 5).

Serotonin (5-HT$_1$) agonists
- Sumatriptan and rizatriptan are serotonin agonists.

Mechanism of action: Serotonin agonists are believed to reverse the dilatation of cerebral blood vessels in the acute attack, which may be responsible for some of the symptoms of migraine.

Route of administration: Oral, intranasal, subcutaneous.

Indications: Acute migrainous attacks.

Contraindications: Caution in coronary artery disease (may cause vasoconstriction or coronary vessels), hepatic impairment, pregnancy and breastfeeding.

Adverse effects: Sensations of tingling, heat, chest tightness.

Antihistamine/serotonin antagonists
Pizotifen is the main drug in this class.

Mechanism of action: Unlike the serotonin agonists, pizotifen appears to limit the initial pro-inflammatory and vascular changes which precede migrainous episodes.

Route of administration: Oral.

Indications: Prevention of vascular headache.

Contraindications: Cautions in urinary retention, angle-closure glaucoma, renal impairment, pregnancy, breastfeeding.

Adverse effects: Antimuscarinic effects, drowsiness, increased appetite.

Headache is a common complaint, and more often than not it does not represent a sinister pathology. Analgesia will simply help control the symptoms so, if a patient frequently returns with pain, be sure to look for a treatable underlying cause.

Neuralgic pain

Neuralgic pain is classically nerve pain, in the distribution of a particular nerve or nerve root. The more common pathologies, which come into this category, include sciatica and trigeminal neuralgia.

Neuralgia commonly occurs because of compression or entrapment of the nerve or nerve root, and definitive management relies on surgical release of the nerve.

Pharmacological options can be employed when surgery is ill advised, or ineffective, or as an adjunct. NSAIDs are not particularly effective for neuralgic pain, and they have usually been self-prescribed prior to the patient consulting a professional opinion.

Antidepressants, in particular amitriptyline, often have an 'analgesic' effect in neuralgic pain, and often at a dose lower than their antidepressant effect (Ch. 4).

The other main class of drug used orally in neuralgic pain are the antiepileptics, notably carbamazepine, phenytoin and more recently lamotrigine (Ch. 4). These potentially stabilize the neurons involved, and limit their activation.

Local anaesthesia of the nerve in question can provide relief for some patients, though nerve ablation with drugs or by surgical means can be performed to alleviate symptoms.

LOCAL ANAESTHESIA

Basic concepts

History

Local anaesthetics are drugs used to inhibit pain sensation. These drugs work by reversibly blocking nerve conduction.

South American Indians have been chewing the leaves of the coca plant, *Erythroxylum coca*, for thousands of years. When they chewed the plant, they found that their mouths and tongues went numb, and that euphoria and excitement were induced. Cocaine was found to be the active ingredient, and it was first isolated from the coca plant in 1860.

Freud was the first to use cocaine clinically to treat patients, but this was unsuccessful. In 1884, however, Koller obtained some cocaine from Freud and was able to demonstrate its local anaesthetic effects on the cornea.

Procaine was first synthesized in 1905 as a synthetic substitute for cocaine.

Chemistry

All local anaesthetics have the same basic structure:

- An aromatic group (lipophilic end) linked to a basic side chain (hydrophilic end) by an ester or amide bond (Fig. 9.6)
- The basic side chain (usually a secondary or tertiary amine) is important because only the uncharged molecule can enter the nerve axoplasm.

Potency and duration of action are correlated with high lipid solubility.

Pharmacokinetics

Elimination of local anaesthetics depends on the nature of the chemical bond:

- Local anaesthetics with ester bonds are inactivated by plasma cholinesterases
- Local anaesthetics with amide bonds are degraded by N-dealkylation in the liver.

Metabolites can often be pharmacologically active.

Mechanism of block

Importance of pH and ionization

Local anaesthetics are weak bases ($pK_a = 8-9$). Only the uncharged form can penetrate lipid membranes; thus, quaternary ammonium compounds, which are fully protonated, must be injected directly into the nerve axon if they are to work.

The proportion of uncharged local anaesthetic is governed by the pH, the pK_a and the Henderson–Hasselbalch equation (Ch. 1):

$$B + H^+ = BH^+$$
$$pK_a = pH + \log [BH^+]/[B]$$

A local anaesthetic with a pK_a of 8.0 will be 10% uncharged at pH 7.0, 50% uncharged at pH 8.0, and 5% uncharged at pH 6.0.

Routes of block

The majority of local anaesthetics block by two routes (Fig. 9.7):

- By the hydrophobic route, the uncharged form enters the membrane and blocks the channel from a site in the protein membrane interface.
- By the hydrophilic route, the uncharged form crosses the membrane to the inside where the charged form blocks the channel. This pathway depends on the channel being open and, therefore, this type of block is use dependent. Use dependency is especially important in the antiarrhythmic action of local anaesthetics.
- Nerve block occurs when the number of non-inactivated channels (those unaffected by the drug) is insufficient to bring about depolarization to threshold.

Fig. 9.6 General structure of ester- and amide-linked local anaesthetics.

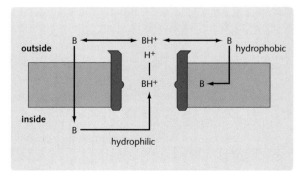

Fig. 9.7 Hydrophobic and hydrophilic routes of block for local anaesthesia.

Mr Hadeed is a 34-year-old metal grinder who presents to Moorfields Eye Hospital accident and emergency with an acute onset of left eye pain, which occurred while at work. He has never had any pain like this before. Slit-lamp examination revealed a fairly superficial foreign body in his left eye. In order to remove the foreign body, the eye is prepared with the application of lidocaine (local anaesthetic) eye drops and then the foreign body is removed with a needle.

Routes of administration

Surface anaesthesia

In surface anaesthesia, the local anaesthetic is applied directly to the mucous membranes, e.g. cornea, bronchial tree, oesophagus and genitourinary tract. The local anaesthetic, e.g. lidocaine, must be able to penetrate the tissues easily. For skin tetracaine (amethocaine) is used to anaesthetize the skin prior to venepuncture, especially in children and anxious adults.

Problems occur when large areas, e.g. the bronchial tree, are anaesthetized.

Infiltration anaesthesia

Infiltration anaesthesia involves direct injection of a local anaesthetic into tissue. Often, a vasoconstrictor such as adrenaline is used with the local anaesthetic to prevent the spread of the local anaesthetic into the systemic circulation. Vasoconstrictors must never be used at extremities as ischaemia could result.

Intravenous regional anaesthesia (IVRA) involves the injection of the local anaesthetic distal to a cuff inflated above arterial pressure. It is important that the cuff is not released prematurely as this could cause the release of a potentially toxic bolus into the circulation. This type of local anaesthetic block is now seldom used.

Nerve block anaesthesia

In nerve block anaesthesia, local anaesthetic is injected close to the appropriate nerve trunk, e.g. the brachial plexus. The injection must be accurate in location.

Spinal and epidural anaesthesia

Spinal anaesthesia involves the injection of a local anaesthetic into the cerebrospinal fluid (CSF) in the subarachnoid space. A certain amount of spread can be controlled by increasing the specific gravity of the solution and tilting the patient.

In epidural anaesthesia, the local anaesthetic is injected into the space between the dura mater and the spinal cord.

In both spinal and epidural anaesthesia, the local anaesthetic acts by blocking mainly spinal roots, as opposed to the spinal cord itself. Problems arise from the block of preganglionic sympathetic fibres supplying the vasculature (causing vasodilatation) and the heart (causing bradycardia), both leading to hypotension. Rostral spread can lead to the blocking of intercostal and phrenic nerves and result in respiratory depression.

In inflamed tissues, the pH is acidic, resulting in a greater proportion of the charged form of the anaesthetic, thus delaying or preventing onset of action of the anaesthetic.

Unwanted effects

Unwanted effects of local anaesthetics are mainly associated with the spread of the drug into the systemic circulation. These include:

- Effects on the CNS, such as restlessness, tremor, confusion, agitation. At high doses, CNS depression can occur. Procaine is worse than lidocaine or prilocaine for causing CNS depression, and is seldom used. The exception is cocaine, which, owing to its monoamine-uptake blocking activity, produces euphoria
- Respiratory depression
- Possible effects on the cardiovascular system, including myocardial depression and vasodilatation
- Visual disturbances and twitching
- Severe toxicity causes convulsions and coma.

Fentanyl is related to pethidine and should not be used in patients who have been on monoamine inhibitors in the previous 14 days. Interaction between these drugs is thought to produce an accumulation of serotonin and the patient may become delirious and violent, or may develop fatal respiratory depression, severe hypertension and dysrhythmias.

Fig. 9.8 Properties and uses of the main local anaesthetics

	Rate of onset	Duration	Tissue penetration	Chemistry	Common use
Cocaine	Rapid	Moderate	Rapid	Ester bond	ENT
Procaine	Moderate	Short	Slow	Ester bond	Little used, CNS effects
Tetracaine (amethocaine)	Slow	Long	Moderate	Ester bond	Topical, pre-venepuncture
Oxybuprocaine (benoxinate)	Rapid	Short	Rapid	Ester bond	Surface, ophthalmology
Benzocaine	Very slow	Very long	Rapid	Ester bond, no basic side chin	Surface ENT
Lidocaine (lignocaine)	Rapid	Moderate	Rapid	Amide bond	Widely used in all applications, EMLA
Prilocaine	Moderate	Moderate	Moderate	Amide bond	Many uses, IVRA, EMLA. Low toxicity
Bupivacaine	Slow	Long	Moderate	Amide bond	Epidural and spinal anaesthesia

ENT, ear, nose and throat; IVRA, intravenous regional anaesthetic

Fig. 9.9 Naturally occurring and synthetic sodium-channel blockers

Compound	Source	Type of block
Tetrodotoxin	Puffer fish	Outside only
Saxitoxin	Plankton	Outside only
μ-conotoxins	Piscivorous marine snail	Affects inactivation
μ-agatoxins	Funnel web spider	Affects inactivation
α-, β-, and γ-toxins	Scorpions	Complex
QX314 and QX222	Synthetic, permanently charged local anaesthetics	Inside only (hydrophobic pathway)
Benzocaine	Synthetic, uncharged local anaesthetic	From within the membrane (hydrophilic pathway)
Local anaesthetics	Plant (cocaine), others synthetic	Inside and from within the membrane

Properties and uses

Figure 9.8 shows the properties and uses of the main local anaesthetics, and Figure 9.9 lists other compounds that block sodium channels.

GENERAL ANAESTHESIA

Basic concepts

General anaesthesia is the absence of sensation associated with a reversible loss of consciousness.

Fig. 9.10 General anaesthetic agents

Premedication	Induction/ intravenous agents	Maintenance/ inhalation agents
• Relief from anxiety e.g. diazepam, lorazepam • Reduction of parasympathetic bradycardia and secretions e.g. atropine, hyoscine • Analgesia e.g. NSAIDs, fentanyl • Postoperative antiemesis e.g. metoclopramide, prochlorperazine	• Barbiturates e.g. thiopental • Non-barbiturates e.g. propofol, ketamine	Nitrous oxide Halothane Enflurane Isoflurane

NSAID, non-steroidal anti-inflammatory drug

General anaesthetics are used as an adjunct to surgical procedures in order to render the patient unaware of, and unresponsive to, painful stimuli. Modern anaesthesia is characterized by the so-called balanced technique, in which drugs and anaesthetic agents are used specifically to produce:

- Analgesia
- Sleep/sedation
- Muscle relaxation and abolition of reflexes.

No one drug or anaesthetic agent can produce all these effects, and so a combination of agents is used in the three clinical stages of surgical general anaesthesia. The three stages are:

- Premedication
- Induction
- Maintenance.

Some may argue that a fourth stage exists, in which drugs are used to reverse the action of agents given in the previous three stages.

Premedication

Premedication is often given on the ward before the patient is taken to the operating theatre (Fig. 9.10), and it has four component aims:

- Relief from anxiety
- Reduction of parasympathetic bradycardia and secretions
- Analgesia
- Prevention of postoperative emesis.

Relief from anxiety

Oral benzodiazepines, e.g. diazepam and midazolam (p. 87), are most effective and they perform three useful functions:

- Relieve apprehension and anxiety before anaesthesia
- Lessen the amount of general anaesthetic required to achieve and to maintain unconsciousness
- Possibly, sedate postoperatively.

Reduction of parasympathetic bradycardia and secretions

Muscarinic antagonists, e.g. atropine and hyoscine (Ch. 4), are used to prevent salivation and bronchial secretions, and more importantly to protect the heart from arrhythmias, particularly bradycardia caused by some inhalation agents and neuromuscular blockers.

Analgesia

Opioid analgesics, e.g. fentanyl, are often given prior to an operation: although the patient is unconscious during surgery, adequate analgesia is important to stop physiological stress reactions to pain. NSAIDs are useful alternatives and adjuncts to opiates, though are likely to be inadequate for severe postoperative pain used alone.

Postoperative antiemesis

Drugs that provide postoperative antiemesis include metoclopramide and prochlorperazine. Nausea and vomiting are common after general anaesthesia, often because of the administration of opioid drugs peri- and postoperatively. Antiemetic drugs can be given with the premedication to inhibit this.

Induction

Intravenous agents (see Fig. 9.10) are used to produce a rapid induction of unconsciousness.

Intravenous agents are preferred by patients, since injection lacks the menacing quality of having a mask placed over the face.

Prevention of acid aspiration in emergency and obstetric operations is crucial, and it relies on the administration of either an H_2-receptor antagonist or a proton pump inhibitor prior to induction (Ch. 8).

Maintenance

Inhalation anaesthetic agents (Fig. 9.10) are used to maintain a state of general anaesthesia after induction in most patients, though intravenous agents can be used via a continuous pump.

Anaesthetic agents

Anaesthetic agents depress all excitable tissues including central neurons, cardiac muscle and smooth and striated muscle. Different parts of the CNS have different sensitivities to anaesthetics, and the reticular activating system, which is responsible for consciousness, is among the most sensitive. Hence, it is possible to use anaesthetics at a concentration that produces unconsciousness without unduly depressing the cardiovascular or respiratory centres of the brain, or the myocardium. However, for the majority of anaesthetics the margin of safety is small.

Intravenous anaesthetics

Intravenous anaesthetics, e.g. thiopental, propofol and ketamine, are all CNS depressants. They produce anaesthesia by relatively selective depression of the reticular activating system of the brain. They may be used alone for short surgical procedures, but they are used mainly for the induction of anaesthesia, and, therefore, it is rapidity of onset that is the desirable feature.

Intravenous anaesthetics are all highly lipid-soluble agents and cross the blood–brain barrier rapidly; their rapid onset (<30 seconds) results from this rapid transfer into the brain, and high cerebral blood flow. Duration of action is short (minutes) and terminated by redistribution of the drug from the CNS into less-well-perfused tissues (Fig. 9.11); drug metabolism is irrelevant to recovery.

Thiopental

Mechanism of action: Thiopental is a highly lipophilic member of the barbiturate group of CNS

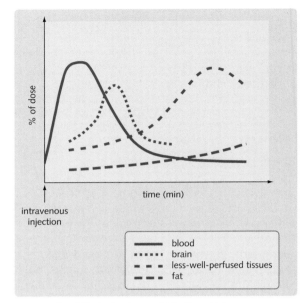

Fig. 9.11 Graph illustrating how redistribution of intravenous anaesthetic agents causes a short central duration of action. (Adapted from Rang H, Dale M, Ritter J. *Pharmacology*, 4th edn. Churchill Livingstone, 1995.)

depressants that act to potentiate the inhibitory effect of GABA on the $GABA_A/Cl^-$ receptor channel complex.

Route of administration: Intravenous.

Indications: Rapid induction of general anaesthesia.

Contraindications: Thiopental should not be given to a patient with a previous allergy to it; porphyria.

Adverse effects: Respiratory depression, myocardial depression (bradycardia), vasodilatation, anaphylaxis. There is a risk of severe vasospasm if it is accidentally injected into an artery.

Therapeutic notes: Thiopental is a widely used induction agent, but it has no analgesic properties. It provides smooth and rapid (<30 seconds) induction but, owing to its narrow therapeutic margin, overdosage with consequent cardiorespiratory depression can occur. Thiopental is given as the sodium salt, which is unstable in solution and so it must be made up immediately before use.

Propofol

Mechanism of action: Propofol is similar to thiopental in its mechanism of action.

Route of administration: Intravenous.

Indications: Induction or maintenance of general anaesthesia or sedation in intensive care units.

Contraindications: Propofol should not be given to patients with a previous allergy to it or sedation of ventilated children.

Adverse effects: Convulsions, anaphylaxis, and delayed recovery from anaesthesia have occasionally been reported as side-effects.

Therapeutic notes: Propofol is associated with rapid recovery without nausea or hangover, and it is very widely used. Propofol is the drug of choice if an intravenous agent is to be used to maintain anaesthesia by a continuous infusion.

> Dina is a 17-year-old student who presents to accident and emergency, looking very unwell and with severe pain in her right iliac fossa (lower right corner of her abdomen). Her mother told doctors that the pain had originally started around her belly button about a couple of hours ago and that she has vomited twice since. Examination reveals a tender abdomen with guarding. A computed tomography scan shows an inflamed appendix. She is rushed to theatre. Midazolam is given as sedation because she is rather anxious about the sudden forthcoming operation. Hyoscine is given prior to the operation, since it dries bronchial and salivary secretions. Domperidone is also given beforehand for antiemesis. General anaesthesia is induced by propofol and maintained with isoflurane. The muscle relaxant rocuronium and the analgesic fentanyl (intravenous) are also given for the operation. Rocuronium is stopped before completion of the operation, but a small dose of neostigmine is required to fully reverse the effect of rocuronium.

Etomidate
Mechanism of action: The mechanism of action of etomidate is similar to that of thiopental.

Route of administration: Intravenous.

Indications: Rapid induction of general anaesthesia.

Contraindications: Etomidate should not be given to patients with a previous allergy to it.

Adverse effects: Extraneous muscle movement and pain on injection, possible adrenocortical suppression.

Therapeutic notes: Etomidate is an induction agent that gained favour over thiopental because of its larger therapeutic margin and faster metabolism leading to fewer hangover effects. Etomidate is more prone to causing extraneous muscle movement and pain on injection compared with other agents.

Ketamine
Mechanism of action: Ketamine produces full surgical anaesthesia but the form of the anaesthesia is known as dissociative anaesthesia, as the patient may remain conscious though amnesic and insensitive to pain. This effect is probably related to an action on *N*-methyl-D-aspartate (NMDA)-type glutamate receptors.

Ketamine is a derivative of the street drug PCP (angel dust).

Route of administration: Intravenous, intramuscular.

Indications: Ketamine is used in the induction and maintenance of anaesthesia, especially in children.

Contraindications: Ketamine should not be given to people with hypertension or psychosis.

Adverse effects: These include cardiovascular stimulation, tachycardia and raised arterial blood pressure, as well as transient psychotic sequelae such as vivid dreams and hallucinations.

Therapeutic notes: Ketamine is not often used as an induction agent, owing to the high incidence of dysphoria and hallucinations during recovery in adults. These effects are much less marked in children, and ketamine, in conjunction with a benzodiazepine, is often used for minor procedures in paediatrics.

Inhalation anaesthetics

Examples of inhalation anaesthetics include halothane, enflurane, isoflurane, sevoflurane and desflurane. Nitrous oxide also has anaesthetic properties.

Inhalation anaesthetics may be gases or volatile liquids. They are commonly used for the maintenance of anaesthesia after induction with an intravenous agent.

Mechanism of action: It is not known exactly how inhalation anaesthetic agents produce their effects. Unlike most drugs, inhalation anaesthetics do not all belong to one recognizable chemical class. The shape and electronic configuration of the molecule are evidently unimportant. A distinct anaesthetic 'receptor' is, therefore, unlikely; it would seem that the pharmacological action of inhalation anaesthetics is dependent on the physicochemical properties of the molecule.

Three theories of anaesthesia have received the most attention–the lipid, hydrate and protein theories.

The lipid theory arose because a close correlation was noticed between anaesthetic potency and lipid solubility. It has been suggested that anaesthetics dissolve in membrane lipid and affect its physical state by two possible mechanisms. These are:

- Volume expansion – which is supported by pressure reversal of anaesthesia, but qualitative inconsistencies exist
- Membrane fluidization – although the high concentrations required and weak effect of temperature make this difficult to accept.

The hydrate theory arose because anaesthetic molecules stabilize water molecules in their vicinity. It has been suggested that this alteration of the membrane accounts for the effects of anaesthetics.

Although there is some correlation between potency and the ability to form hydrates, anomalous compounds such as sulphur hexafluoride do not form hydrates, but they do have anaesthetic properties.

The protein theory arose because there is increasing evidence that anaesthetics may act by binding to discrete hydrophobic domains of membrane proteins. This would explain the 'cut-off' phenomenon and the stereoselectivity of anaesthetics, whereby the size of the domain excludes molecules above a certain size or that are the wrong shape. The protein theory is currently popular, but the nature of the target protein(s) in the CNS has not been identified. Possible targets include voltage-operated channels, receptor-operated channels, or secondary-messenger systems.

Like the benzodiazepines and barbiturates, thiopental and propofol act via the $GABA_A/Cl^-$ receptor in causing CNS depression.

Pharmacokinetic aspects

The depth of anaesthesia produced by inhalation anaesthetics is directly related to the partial pressure (tension) of the agent in the arterial blood, as this determines the concentration of agent in the CNS. The concentration of anaesthetic in the blood is in turn determined by:

- The concentration of anaesthetic in the inspired gas (alveolar concentration)
- The solubility of the anaesthetic in blood (blood/gas partition coefficient)
- Cardiac output
- Alveolar ventilation.

Rapid induction and recovery are important properties of an anaesthetic agent, allowing flexible control over the arterial tension (and hence brain tension) and, therefore, the depth of anaesthesia. The speed at which induction of anaesthesia occurs is determined by two properties of the anaesthetic: its solubility in blood (blood/gas partition coefficient) and its solubility in fat (lipid solubility). Therefore:

- Agents of low blood solubility (e.g. nitrous oxide, enflurane) produce rapid induction and recovery because relatively small amounts are required to saturate the blood, and so the arterial tension (and hence brain tension) rises and falls quickly (Fig. 9.12).
- Agents of high blood solubility (e.g. halothane) have much slower induction and recovery times because much more anaesthetic solution is

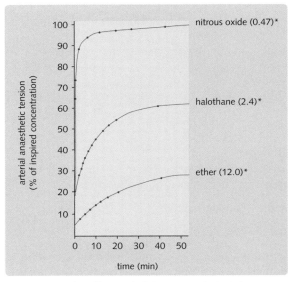

Fig. 9.12 Rate of equilibrium of inhalation anaesthetics in humans. (Adapted from Papper EM, Kitz R. *Uptake and Distribution of Anaesthetic Agents.* McGraw-Hill, 1963.)

required before the arterial anaesthetic tension approaches that of the inspired gas (see Fig. 9.12).

- Agents with high lipid solubility (e.g. ether) accumulate gradually in the body fat during prolonged anaesthesia, and so may produce a prolonged hangover if used for a long operation (see Fig. 9.12).

Nitrous oxide

Mechanism of action: See above.

Route of administration: Inhalation.

Indications: Nitrous oxide is used in the maintenance of anaesthesia (in combination with other agents), and for analgesia (50% mixture in oxygen: Entonox®).

Contraindications: Pneumothorax. Nitrous oxide diffuses into air containing closed spaces resulting in an increased pressure, in the case of pneumothorax, this may compromise breathing.

Adverse effects: Nitrous oxide was thought to be relatively free of side-effects – it has little effect on cardiovascular and respiratory systems – but the risk of bone marrow suppression is now a known factor.

Therapeutic notes: Nitrous oxide cannot produce surgical anaesthesia when administered alone, because of a lack of potency. It is commonly used as a non-flammable carrier gas for volatile agents, allowing their concentration to be reduced. As a 50% mixture in oxygen, nitrous oxide is a good analgesic, and it is used in childbirth and by paramedics.

Halothane

Mechanism of action: See above.

Route of administration: Inhalation.

Indications: Halothane is used in the maintenance of anaesthesia.

Contraindications: Halothane should not be given to people with a previous reaction to halothane or exposure to halothane in the previous 3 months.

Adverse effects: Like most volatile anaesthetics, halothane causes cardiorespiratory depression.

Respiratory depression results in elevated pCO_2 and perhaps ventricular arrhythmias. Halothane also depresses cardiac muscle fibres and may cause bradycardia. The result of this is a concentration-dependent hypotension.

The most significant toxic effect of halothane is severe hepatic necrosis, which occurs in 1 in 35 000 cases. Lesser degrees of liver damage may occur more frequently. The damage is caused by metabolites of the 20% of administered halothane that is biotransformed in the liver (80% of an administered dose is excreted by the lungs).

Therapeutic notes: Halothane is a halogenated hydrocarbon, and it is probably the most widely used inhalation agent.

Enflurane

Mechanism of action: See above.

Route of administration: Inhalation.

Indications: Enflurane is used in the maintenance of anaesthesia.

Contraindications: Enflurane should not be given to people with epilepsy.

Adverse effects: Enflurane causes cardiorespiratory depression similar to that with halothane, although the incidence of arrhythmias is much lower than with halothane.

Enflurane undergoes only 2% metabolism in the liver, so it is much less likely than halothane to cause hepatotoxicity. The disadvantage of enflurane is that it may cause electroencephalogram (EEG) changes and muscle twitching, and special caution is needed in epileptic subjects.

Therapeutic notes: Enflurane is a volatile anaesthetic similar to, but less potent than, halothane, about twice the concentration being necessary for maintenance. Induction and recovery times are faster than for halothane.

Isoflurane

Mechanism of action: See above.

Route of administration: Inhalation.

Indications: It is used in the maintenance of anaesthesia.

Contraindications: Susceptibility to malignant hyperthermia.

Adverse effects: Isoflurane has actions similar to those of halothane, but it has fewer effects upon the cardiorespiratory system. Hypotension is caused by a dose-related decrease in systemic vascular resistance rather than a marked fall in cardiac output. Less hepatic metabolism (0.2%) occurs than with enflurane, so hepatotoxicity is even rarer.

Therapeutic notes: Isoflurane is an isomer of enflurane. It has a potency intermediate between that of halothane and enflurane.

Nitrous oxide is used as an adjunct to other inhaled agents, as it reduces the dose required to maintain anaesthesia, thus limiting side-effects, and allowing more rapid recovery.

Use of neuromuscular blockers in anaesthesia

For some operations, e.g. intra-abdominal, complete relaxation of skeletal muscle is essential. Some general anaesthetic agents have significant neuromuscular blocking actions, but drugs that specifically block the neuromuscular junction are frequently employed, e.g. suxamethonium, rocuronium, vecuronium and atracurium (Ch. 4).

Inflammation, allergic diseases and immunosuppression

10

Objectives

After reading this chapter, you will:

- Understand the basic principles behind inflammation, allergies and immunosuppression
- Know the different drug classes used to treat these conditions and their mechanism of action
- Be aware of the indications, contraindications and adverse drug reactions.

INFLAMMATION

Inflammation describes the changes seen in response to tissue injury or insult, as originally defined by the five Latin words *dolor*, *rubor*, *calor*, *tumor* and *functio laesa*, meaning pain, redness, heat, swelling and loss of function, respectively. These changes occur because of alterations in local blood vessels, that is dilatation of the blood vessels, which lead to increased permeability, and increased receptiveness for leucocytes, resulting in the accumulation of inflammatory cells at the site of injury. The main cells seen in an acute inflammatory response are neutrophils and macrophages. Lymphocytes, as well as basophils and eosinophils, also accumulate, especially in certain types of inflammation.

Inflammatory responses are produced and controlled by the interaction of a wide range of inflammatory mediators, some derived from leucocytes, some from the damaged tissues. Examples include histamine, kinins (bradykinin), neuropeptides (substance-P, calcitonin gene-related peptide), cytokines (e.g. interleukins [ILs]) and the arachidonic acid metabolites (eicosanoids).

Arachidonic acid metabolites: the eicosanoids

Of the inflammatory mediators mentioned above, the eicosanoids are of special importance because:

- They are involved in the majority of inflammatory reactions
- Most anti-inflammatory therapy (i.e. non-steroidal anti-inflammatory drugs (NSAIDs) and steroidal anti-inflammatory drugs

([glucocorticoids]) is based on the manipulation of their biosynthesis.

The eicosanoids are a family of polyunsaturated fatty acids formed from arachidonic acid. The biosynthetic pathway is shown in Figure 10.1. Arachidonic acid is derived mainly from phospholipids of cell membranes, from which it is mobilized by the action of the enzyme phospholipase A_2. Arachidonic acid is then further metabolized:

- By cyclooxygenase to produce the 'classic prostaglandins', thromboxane and prostacyclin, collectively known as the prostanoids
- By lipoxygenase to produce the leukotrienes
- The actions of eicosanoids in inflammatory reactions are listed in Figure 10.2.

Anti-inflammatory drugs

The main drugs used for their broad-spectrum anti-inflammatory effects are:

- Non-steroidal anti-inflammatory drugs (p. 184).
- Steroidal anti-inflammatory drugs (glucocorticoids) (Ch. 6 and p. 187).

Both these classes of anti-inflammatory drug exert their effect by inhibiting the formation of eicosanoids (see Fig. 10.1).

In addition, a number of other drug classes, used clinically under certain circumstances, have more restricted anti-inflammatory actions. These are:

- Disease-modifying antirheumatic drugs (DMARDs) (p. 187)
- Drugs used to treat gout (p. 189)
- Antihistamines (p. 195)
- Drugs used to treat skin disorders.

Fig. 10.1 Biosynthetic pathway of the eicosanoids. (LT, leukotrienes; HETE, hydroxyeicosatetraenoic acid; PG, prostaglandin; HPETE, hydroperoxyeicosatetraenoic acid; NSAID, non-steroidal anti-inflammatory drug.)

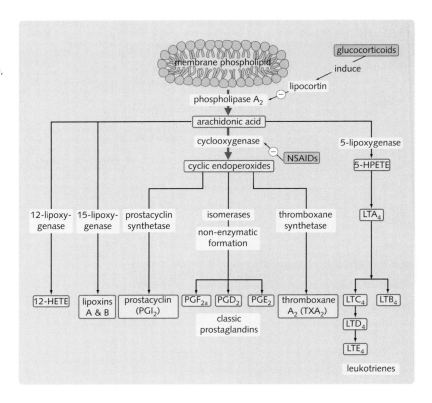

Fig. 10.2 Actions of the eicosanoids in the inflammatory reaction	
Eicosanoid	**Actions in inflammation**
• Prostanoids	
'Classic prostaglandins' e.g. PGD_2, PGE_2, PGF_2	Produce increased vasodilatation, vascular permeability and oedema in an inflammatory reaction; prostaglandins also sensitize nociceptive fibres to stimulation by other inflammatory mediators
Thromboxane A_2 (TXA_2)	Platelet aggregation and vasoconstriction
Prostacyclin (PGI_2)	Inhibition of platelet aggregation and vasodilatation
• Leukotrienes	
e.g. LTB_4, LTC_4	Increase vascular permeability, promote leucocyte chemotaxis (and cause contraction of bronchial smooth muscle)

NSAIDs

NSAIDs are a chemically diverse group of drugs that all possess the ability to inhibit both forms of the enzyme cyclooxygenase (see Fig. 10.1), an action that is responsible for their pharmacological effects (see Fig. 10.4 below).

The first drugs of this type were the salicylates (e.g. aspirin), extracted from the bark of the willow tree. Subsequently, many synthetic and semi-synthetic NSAIDs have been created by pharmacologists. Chemically and structurally heterogeneous, they are related through their common mechanism of action (Fig. 10.3).

Mechanism of action: The main action of all the NSAIDs is inhibition of the enzyme cyclooxygenase. This enzyme is involved in the metabolism of arachidonic acid to form the prostanoids, i.e. the 'classic prostaglandins', prostacyclin and thromboxane A_2. Inhibition of cyclooxygenase can occur by several mechanisms:

- Irreversible inhibition – e.g. aspirin causes acetylation of the active site.
- Competitive inhibition – e.g. ibuprofen acts as a competitive substrate.
- Reversible, non-competitive inhibition – e.g. paracetamol has a free radical trapping action that interferes with the production of

Fig. 10.3 Classes of non-steroidal anti-inflammatory drugs and comparison of their main actions

Chemical class	Examples	Analgesic	Antipyretic	Anti-inflammatory
Salicylic acids	Aspirin	+	+	+
Propionic acids	Ibuprofen Fenuprofen	+	+	+
Acetic acids	Indometacin	+	+	++
Oxicams	Piroxicam	+	+	++
Pyrazolones	Phenylbutazone	+/-	+	++
Fenemates	Mefenamic acid	+	+	+/-
para-Aminophenols	Paracetamol	+	+	-

hydroperoxidases, which are believed to have an essential role in cyclooxygenase activity.

Cyclooxygenase exists in two enzyme isoforms:

- COX-1 – expressed in most tissues, especially platelets, gastric mucosa and renal vasculature, and involved in physiological cell signalling. Most adverse effects of NSAIDs are caused by inhibition of COX-1.
- COX-2 – induced at sites of inflammation and produces the prostanoids involved in inflammatory responses. Analgesic and anti-inflammatory effects of NSAIDs are largely due to inhibition of COX-2.

COX-2-specific inhibitors licensed for use in several countries for symptomatic relief in osteoarthritis and rheumatoid arthritis, have a reduced incidence of gastric side-effects. However, they are associated with an increased incidence of adverse cardiovascular events (such as myocardial infarction). If a patient cannot tolerate another drug, a COX-2 specific inhibitor can be considered after calculating the individual patient's risk to benefit ratio (including their risk factors for cardiovascular disease).

Always remember the reasons behind the conflict over NSAIDs. The cardiologist will want every patient on aspirin – for its anti-platelet action. The gastroenterologist and the nephrologist will want to stop aspirin – as it causes gastrointestinal upset and ulceration, and potentially worsens renal blood flow.

Clinical effects: NSAIDs work by the inhibition of cyclooxygenase and resulting inhibition of prostaglandin synthesis, producing three major clinical actions of potential therapeutic benefit: analgesia, an anti-inflammatory action and an antipyretic (fever reducing) action (Fig. 10.4).

Not all NSAIDs possess these three actions to exactly the same extent, an example being the lack of anti-inflammatory activity possessed by paracetamol (see Fig. 10.3).

In addition to these three main categories of effect, aspirin has a pronounced effect on inhibiting platelet aggregation, due to reduced thromboxane synthesis. This has led to its successful use in primary and secondary prevention of cardiovascular and cerebrovascular events (Ch. 2).

Indications: NSAIDs are widely used for a variety of complaints. They are available on prescription and 'over the counter'. Their use includes musculoskeletal and joint diseases (strains, sprains, rheumatic problems, arthritis, gout etc.), analgesia for mild to moderate pain relief including headaches and dysmenorrhoea, and symptomatic relief in fever.

Contraindications: NSAIDs should not be given to people with gastrointestinal ulceration or bleeding, or a previous hypersensitivity to any NSAID. Caution should be used in asthma and when renal function is impaired.

Adverse effects: Generalized adverse effects of NSAIDs are common, especially in the elderly and in chronic users, and mostly arise from the non-selective inhibition of COX-1 and COX-2 (Fig. 10.5).

Fig. 10.4 Three major clinical actions of non-steroidal anti-inflammatory drugs (NSAIDs)

Clinical action	Mechanism of action
Analgesic action	• The analgesic effect is largely a peripheral effect that is due to the inhibition of prostaglandin synthesis at the site of pain and inflammation • Prostaglandins do not produce pain directly, but sensitize nociceptive fibre nerve endings to other inflammatory mediators (bradykinin, histamine, 5-HT), amplifying the basic pain message; prostaglandins of the E and F series are implicated in this sensitizing action • Thus NSAIDs are most effective against pain where there is an inflammatory component • A small component of the analgesic action of NSAIDs is a consequence of a central effect in reducing prostaglandin synthesis in the CNS; paracetamol especially works in this manner
Anti-inflammatory action	• Prostaglandins produce increased vasodilatation, vascular permeability and oedema in an inflammatory reaction • Inhibition of prostaglandin synthesis therefore reduces this part of the inflammatory reaction • NSAIDs do not inhibit the numerous other mediators involved in an inflammatory reaction; thus inflammatory cell accumulation, for example, is not inhibited
Antipyretic action	• During a fever leucocytes release inflammatory pyrogens (e.g. interleukin-1) as part of the immune response; these act on the thermoregulatory centre in the hypothalamus to cause an increase in body temperature • This effect is believed to be mediated by an increase in hypothalamic prostaglandins (PGEs), the generation of which is inhibited by NSAIDs • NSAIDs do not affect temperature under normal circumstances or in heat stroke

Fig. 10.5 General adverse effects of non-steroidal anti-inflammatory drugs (NSAIDs)

System	Adverse effect	Cause
GI	Dyspepsia, nausea, vomiting	Inhibition of the normal protective actions of prostaglandins on the gastric mucosa
	Ulcer formation and potential haemorrhage risk in chronic users	PGE_2 and PGI_2 normally inhibit gastric acid secretion, increase mucosal blood flow, and have a cytoprotective action
Renal	Renal damage/nephrotoxicity	Inhibition of PGE_2- and PGI_2-mediated vasodilatation in the renal medulla and glomeruli
	Renal failure can occur after years of chronic misuse	
Other	Bronchospasm, skin rashes, other allergic-type reactions	Hypersensitivity reaction/allergy to drug

GI, gastrointestinal; PG, prostaglandin

Less commonly, liver disorders and bone marrow depression are seen. Other unwanted effects that are relatively specific to individual compounds are also seen (see below).

Therapeutic notes on individual NSAIDs
Salicylic acids, e.g. aspirin, which:

• Is cheap, and is still the drug of choice for many sorts of mild pain despite a relatively high incidence of gastrointestinal side-effects. It is also used for its antiplatelet action
• Produces tinnitus in toxic doses.

Propionic acids, e.g. ibuprofen, which:

- Is effective and well tolerated
- Is the drug of choice for inflammatory joint disease, owing to its low incidence of side-effects.

Acetic acids, e.g. indometacin, which:

- Is a highly potent inhibitor of COX that is effective but associated with a high incidence of side-effects
- Commonly causes neurological effects such as dizziness and confusion, as well as gastrointestinal upsets.

Oxicams, e.g. piroxicam, which:

- Is a potent drug widely used for chronic inflammatory conditions
- Is given only once daily, but causes a relatively high incidence of gastrointestinal problems.

Pyrazolones, e.g. phenylbutazone, which:

- Is an extremely potent agent but can produce a fatal bone marrow aplasia. For this reason it is reserved for the treatment of intractable pain in ankylosing spondylitis.

Fenemates, e.g. mefenamic acid, which:

- Is a moderately potent drug
- Commonly causes gastrointestinal upsets and occasionally skin rashes.

para-Aminophenols, e.g. paracetamol, which:

- Is used as an analgesic and antipyretic but is not considered an anti-inflammatory drug
- Is effective for pain, especially headaches, and fever. This is probably due to its mechanism of action in trapping free radicals and interfering with the production of hydroperoxidases, which are believed to have an essential role in cyclooxygenase activity. In areas of inflammation, phagocytic cells produce high levels of peroxide that swamp this effect. For more information see Chapter 9.

COX-2 specific inhibitors, e.g. lumiracoxib and celecoxib, which:

- Preferentially inhibit the inducible COX-2 enzyme, limiting COX-1-mediated side-effects observed with other, non-specific NSAIDs.

The COX-2 inhibitors are licensed in the UK for symptomatic relief in osteoarthritis and rheumatoid arthritis. They are contraindicated in inflammatory bowel disease, ischaemic heart disease or cerebrovascular disease.

Steroidal anti-inflammatory drugs (glucocorticoids)

There are two main groups of corticosteroids, the glucocorticoids and the mineralocorticoids. It is the glucocorticoids (such as cortisone and cortisol), which posses powerful anti-inflammatory actions that make them useful in several diseases, e.g. rheumatoid arthritis, inflammatory bowel conditions, bronchial asthma (see Ch. 3) and inflammatory conditions of the skin.

Their profound generalized inhibitory effects on inflammatory responses result from the effects of corticosteroids in altering the activity of certain corticosteroid-responsive genes. The anti-inflammatory action results from:

- Reduced production of acute inflammatory mediators, especially the eicosanoids (see Fig. 10.1). Corticosteroids prevent the formation of arachidonic acid from membrane phospholipids by inducing the synthesis of a polypeptide called lipocortin. Lipocortin inhibits phospholipase A_2, the enzyme normally responsible for mobilizing arachidonic acid from cell membrane phospholipids, and thus inhibits the subsequent formation of both prostaglandins and leukotrienes.
- Reduced numbers and activity of circulating immunocompetent cells, neutrophils and macrophages.
- Decreased activity of macrophages and fibroblasts involved in the chronic stages of inflammation, leading to decreased inflammation and decreased healing. Glucocorticoids are discussed in detail in Ch. 6.

Rheumatoid arthritis

DMARDs are a diverse group of agents that are mainly used in the treatment of rheumatoid arthritis, which is a chronic, progressive and destructive inflammatory disease of the joints (Fig. 10.6).

The mechanism of action of the DMARDs is often unclear – they appear to have a long-term depressive effect on the inflammatory response as well as possibly modulating other aspects of the immune system.

Fig. 10.6 Disease-modifying antirheumatic drugs (DMARDs)

Class	Example
Gold salts	Sodium aurothiomalate, auranofin
Penicillamine	Penicillamine
Antimalarials	Chloroquine, hydroxyquinine
Sulfasalazine	Sulfasalazine
Immunosuppressants	Cytotoxic drugs: methotrexate, azathioprine, ciclosporin

All DMARDs have a slow onset of action, with clinical improvement not becoming apparent until 4–6 months after the initiation of treatment. DMARDs have been shown to improve symptoms and reduce disease activity. They are believed to retard erosive damage at joints, as judged radiologically.

DMARDs are generally indicated for use in severe, active, progressive rheumatoid arthritis when NSAIDs alone have proved inadequate. DMARDs are frequently used in combination with an NSAID and/or low-dose glucocorticoids.

Gold salts
Examples of gold salts include sodium aurothiomalate and auranofin.

Mechanism of action: The mechanism of action of gold salts is unknown – they may be taken up by, and inhibit, mononuclear macrophages, or may affect the production of free radicals.

Route of administration: Sodium aurothiomalate is given by intramuscular injection, and auranofin orally.

Adverse effects: Rashes, proteinuria, ulceration, diarrhoea, bone marrow suppression.

Therapeutic notes: When administering gold salts, careful patient monitoring, including blood counts and urine analysis, is necessary. If any serious adverse effects develop, treatment must be stopped.

Penicillamine
Mechanism of action: The mechanism of action of penicillamine is unknown. It chelates metals and has immunomodulatory effects, including suppression of immunoglobulin production and effects on immune complexes. Penicillamine may also decrease synthesis of interleukin (IL)-1.

Route of administration: Oral.

Adverse effects: Rashes, proteinuria, ulceration, gastrointestinal upsets, fever, transient loss of taste, bone marrow suppression.

Therapeutic notes: When administering penicillamine, careful patient monitoring, including blood counts and urine analysis, is necessary. If any serious adverse effects develop, treatment must be stopped.

Antimalarials
Examples of antimalarials include chloroquine and hydroxychloroquine (Ch. 11).

Mechanism of action: The mechanism of antimalarials is unclear. They interfere with a wide variety of leucocyte functions, including IL-1 production by macrophages, lymphoproliferative responses and T-cell cytotoxic responses.

Route of administration: Oral.

Adverse effects: At the low doses currently recommended for antimalarials, toxicity is rare. The major adverse effect is retinal toxicity.

Therapeutic notes: People on antimalarials should have their vision monitored.

Sulfasalazine
Mechanism of action: Sulfasalazine is broken down in the gut into its two component molecules, 5-aminosalicylate (5-ASA) and sulfapyridine. The 5-ASA moiety is believed to be a free radical scavenger and responsible for most of this drug's antirheumatic effects.

Route of administration: Oral.

Adverse effects: Side-effects of sulfasalazine are mainly due to sulfapyridine; they are common, but rarely serious. These include nausea, vomiting, headache and rashes. Rarely, blood disorders and oligospermia are reported.

Therapeutic notes: People on sulfasalazine should have their blood counts monitored.

Immunosuppressants
Certain drugs with immunosuppressive actions have been shown to be effective in rheumatoid arthritis. These include azathioprine, ciclosporin and corticosteroids which may work by suppressing the autoimmune component of rheumatoid arthritis (p. 196).

DMARDs are prescribed by a specialist. Their mechanism of action is largely unknown, but remember most patients taking these agents need regular blood tests to assess their renal and liver function, and to monitor their red and white blood cell counts.

Cytokine inhibitors

Cytokine inhibitors are also thought to retard destruction of joints caused by rheumatoid arthritis. They are usually used for highly active rheumatoid arthritis in those who have failed to respond to at least two standard DMARDs. The primary pro-inflammatory cytokines are tumour necrosis factor (TNF)-α and IL-1. Thus, their inflammatory role in diseases, such as rheumatoid arthritis can be reduced via cytokine inhibitors.

Monoclonal antibodies

Examples of monoclonal antibodies include adalimumab and infliximab.

Mechanism of action: The monoclonal antibodies bind TNF-α, preventing its interaction with cell surface receptors and the subsequent proinflammatory events.

Indications: Moderate to severe rheumatoid arthritis, after DMARDs have not provided an adequate response.

Contraindications: Pregnancy, breastfeeding, severe infections, heart failure.

Route of administration: Subcutaneous injection.

Adverse effects: Tuberculosis, septicaemia, gastro-intestinal disturbance, worsening heart failure, hypersensitivity reactions, blood disorders.

Interactions: Avoid concomitant use of live vaccines.

Therapeutic notes: Monitor for infections, discontinue if active tuberculosis is suspected.

Soluble TNF-α blocker

An example is etanercept.

Mechanism of action: Contains the ligand-binding component of the human TNF receptor. It, therefore, competes with the patient's own receptors, thereby acting like a sponge to remove most of the TNF-α molecules from the joints and blood.

Indications: Moderate to severe rheumatoid arthritis, after DMARDs have not provided an adequate response.

Contraindications: Pregnancy, breastfeeding, severe infections, heart failure.

Route of administration: Subcutaneous injection.

Adverse effects: Predisposition to infections, exacerbation of heart failure or demyelinating central nervous system (CNS) disorders, blood disorders.

Interactions: Avoid concomitant use of live vaccines.

Therapeutic notes: Monitor for infections.

The -mab of adalimumab and infliximab stands for their being Monoclonal AntiBodies! The -rcept of etanercept is a useful clue to remember it is the soluble ReCEPTor for TNF-α!

Mrs Arlington, a 50-year-old secretary, presented at her GP because of worsening pain in her left and right wrists and fingers, causing her increasing difficulty to type. Tender swelling is noted at those joints. A diagnosis of rheumatoid arthritis is made following X-ray showing erosions and blood tests showing that she is positive for IgM rheumatoid factor. Initially, she is given daily aspirin but is unable to tolerate it and returns 3 weeks later complaining of gastrointestinal pain. When planning alternative treatment, her hypertension and mild angina (cardiovascular risk factors) are taken into account. The aspirin is replaced by ibuprofen and she is given omeprazole (a proton pump inhibitor) to protect her stomach. This helps to begin with, however, 3 months later she presents with worsening symptoms. A diagnosis of progressive rheumatoid arthritis is made. The ibuprofen is replaced by prednisolone (a glucocorticoid) and she is put on the DMARD, sulfasalazine.

Gout

Gout is a condition in which uric acid (monosodium urate) crystals are deposited in tissues, especially in the joints, provoking an inflammatory response that

Fig. 10.7 Drugs used in the treatment of gout

• Treatment of an acute attack	Example
NSAIDs	Indometacin
Immunosuppressive	Colchicine
• Prophylaxis against recurrent attacks (reduction of plasma uric acid concentration)	
Agents that reduce uric acid synthesis	Allopurinol
Agents that increase uric acid excretion (Uricosurics)	Sulfinpyrazone, probenecid

NSAID, non-steroidal anti-inflammatory drug

manifests as an extremely painful acute arthritis. Uric acid crystallizes in the tissues when plasma urate levels are high, due to either excessive production or reduced renal excretion.

There are two treatment strategies for gout – treatment of an acute attack and prophylaxis against further attacks (Fig. 10.7).

Treatment of an acute attack

Non-steroidal anti-inflammatory drugs
At the onset of an acute attack of gout, NSAIDs are used for their general anti-inflammatory and analgesic effects (p. 184).

Aspirin and other salicylates are not used in gout as they inhibit uric acid excretion in the urine, exacerbating serum concentrations.

Colchicine
Mechanism of action: Colchicine helps in gouty arthritis by inhibiting the migration of leucocytes such as neutrophils into the inflamed joint. This effect is achieved as a result of the action of colchicine binding to tubulin, the protein monomer of microtubules, resulting in their depolymerization. The end result is that cytoskeletal movements and cell motility are severely inhibited.

The inhibition of microtubular function inhibits mitotic spindle formation, giving colchicine a cytotoxic effect on dividing cells. This cytotoxic effect is responsible for side-effects of colchicine.

Route of administration: Oral, rarely intravenously.

Adverse effects: Side-effects of colchicine include gastrointestinal toxicity, with nausea, vomiting and

diarrhoea, occurring in 80% of people. Rarely, bone marrow suppression and renal failure occur.

Therapeutic notes: Colchicine is rapidly effective. It is given for the first 24 hours of an attack and then for no more than 7 days. Nausea and vomiting are common side-effects.

Prophylaxis against recurrent attacks

Preventative management of gout includes diet and lifestyle changes, as well as the use of drugs that reduce plasma uric acid concentration. These drugs should not be used during an acute attack, as they will initially worsen symptoms. NSAIDs or colchicine should be co-administered for the first 3 months of treatment, as initiation of prophylactic treatment may precipitate an acute attack.

Agents that reduce uric acid synthesis
Allopurinol is an example of a drug that reduces uric acid synthesis.

Mechanism of action: Allopurinol inhibits the enzyme xanthine oxidase, which converts purines (from DNA breakdown) into uric acid, thus reducing uric acid production.

Route of administration: Oral.

Adverse effects: Headaches, dyspepsia, diarrhoea, rash, drug interactions and acute exacerbation of gout initially. Rarely, life-threatening hypersensitivity occurs.

Agents that increase uric acid excretion
Uricosurics are drugs that increase uric acid excretion. Examples of uricosurics include sulfinpyrazone and probenecid.

Mechanism of action: Uricosurics compete with uric acid for reabsorption in the proximal tubules, preventing uric acid reabsorption and resulting in uricosuria.

Route of administration: Oral.

Adverse effects: Gastrointestinal upset, deposition of uric acid crystals in the kidney, interference with excretion of certain drugs, and acute exacerbation of gout initially.

Therapeutic notes: Uricosurics should not be used during an acute attack of gout. NSAIDs or colchicine should be co-administered for the first 3 months of treatment, as initiation of treatment may precipitate an acute attack.

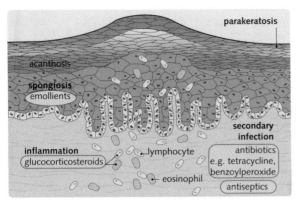

Fig. 10.8 Characteristics of eczema and its drug treatment. (Redrawn from Page et al. 2002.)

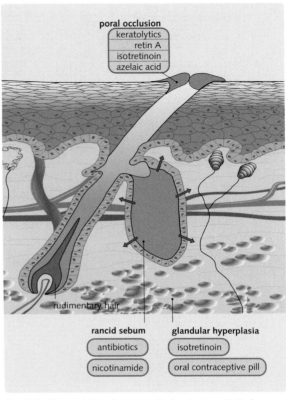

Fig. 10.9 Characteristics of acne and its drug treatment. (Redrawn from Page et al. 2002.)

Skin disorders

The most common skin diseases are eczema, acne, psoriasis, skin cancer (usually managed surgically), viral warts and urticaria.

Eczema (dermatitis)

Eczema is an inflammatory disease of the skin, defined by the presence of epidermal intercellular oedema or spongiosis. It can occur because of a number of factors, such as:

- Exogenous irritants and contact allergens
- Infections
- Atopy
- Drugs
- Certain environmental conditions such as low humidity and ultraviolet light.

Drugs used to treat eczema and their targets are shown in Figure 10.8.

Acne

Acne affects the pilosebaceous unit and occurs where these are numerous, such as on the face, back and chest. It is characterized by the presence of keratin plugs in the sebaceous duct openings, known as comedones. Other signs of acne of worsening degrees of severity include inflammatory papules, pustules, nodules, cysts and scars.

Acne is stimulated by androgens, which is why it is related to puberty, and why the anti-androgen cyproterone is often used in females with acne (Ch. 6).

The drugs used to treat acne and their targets are shown in Figure 10.9.

Psoriasis

Psoriasis is a genetic skin disorder that manifests under certain conditions including stress, infection, damage from ultraviolet light, or trauma. In psoriasis, the turnover rate of skin is eight times that of normal skin (7 days instead of 56 days). Psoriasis is characterized by:

- Thickened skin plaques
- Superficial scales
- Dilated capillaries in the dermis (these might act to initiate psoriasis or as nourishment for hyperproliferating skin)
- An infiltrate of inflammatory cells, especially lymphocytes and neutrophils, in the epidermis and dermis, respectively.

Fig. 10.10 Characteristics of psoriasis and its drug treatment. (Redrawn from Page et al. 2002.)

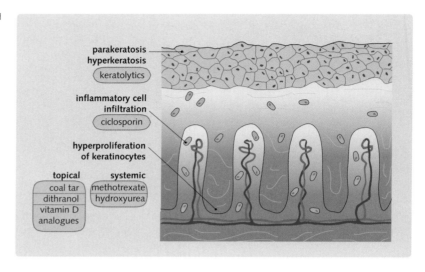

Fig. 10.11 Potency of some topical steroids (UK classification and nomenclature)

Group	Approved name	Proprietary name
I (very potent)	Clobetasol propionate	Dermovate®
II (potent)	Betametasone valerate 0.1%	Betnovate®
	Beclometasone dipropionate	Propaderm®
	Hydrocortisone 17-butyrate	Locoid®
III (moderately potent)	Clobetasone butyrate	Eumovate®
IV (mild)	Hydrocortisone 1%	Various
	Hydrocortisone 2%	Various

Adapted from Graham-Brown et al. Mosby's Color Atlas and Text of Dermatology, 1st edn. 1998

Drugs used to treat psoriasis and their targets are shown in Figure 10.10.

Treatment of skin disorders

Corticosteroids

Examples of corticosteroids include clobetasol propionate, betamethasone, clobetasol butyrate and hydrocortisone (Fig. 10.11).

Mechanism of action: Corticosteroids suppress components of the inflammatory reaction (see Ch. 6 and Fig. 10.8).

Route of administration: Topically; orally, intradermally or intravenously in severe disease.

Indications: Corticosteroids are used for the relief of symptoms due to inflammatory conditions of the skin other than those due to infection, e.g. in eczema.

Contraindications: Rosacea, untreated skin infections.

Adverse effects: Most likely to occur with prolonged, or high dose therapy. Local – spread or worsening of infection, thinning of the skin, impaired wound healing, irreversible striae atrophicae. Systemic – immunosuppression, peptic ulceration, osteoporosis, hypertension, cataracts.

Therapeutic notes: Withdrawal of corticosteroids after high doses or prolonged use should be gradual (Ch. 6). Consult the *British National Formulary* (*BNF*) for up-to-date guidelines.

Dithranol

Dithranol is the most potent topical drug for the treatment of psoriasis.

Mechanism of action: Dithranol modifies keratinization, but the mechanism is unclear (see Fig. 10.10).

Route of administration: Topical.

Contraindications: Dithranol should not be given to people with hypersensitivity or acute and pustular psoriasis.

Adverse effects: Local skin irritation, staining of skin and hair.

Vitamin D analogues
Calcipotriol and tacalcitol are vitamin D analogue derivatives.

Vitamin D analogues are keratolytics, though also used in vitamin D deficiency related to gastrointestinal/biliary disease and renal failure (Ch. 8).

Mechanism of action: The exact mechanism of action is still unclear, but several effects of vitamin D analogues have been observed. These include inhibition of epidermal proliferation and induction of terminal keratinocyte differentiation (see Fig. 10.10).

The anti-inflammatory properties of vitamin D analogues include inhibition of T-cell proliferation and of cytokine release, decreased capacity of monocytes to stimulate T-cell proliferation and to stimulate lymphokine release from T cells, and inhibition of neutrophil accumulation in psoriatic skin.

Route of administration: Topical.

Indications: Psoriasis.

Contraindications: Vitamin D analogues should not be given to people with disorders of calcium metabolism. They should not be used on the face, as irritation may occur.

Adverse effects: Side-effects of vitamin D analogues include local irritation and dermatitis. High doses may affect calcium homoeostasis.

Tar preparations
Coal tar, made up of about 10 000 components, is a keratolytic that is more potent than salicylic acid. It also has anti-inflammatory and antipruritic properties.

Mechanism of action: Coal tar modifies keratinization, but the mechanism is unclear (see Fig. 10.10).

Route of administration: Topical.

Indications: Psoriasis and occasionally eczema.

Contraindications: Coal tar should not be given to people with acute or pustular psoriasis or in the presence of an infection. It should not be used on the face or on broken or inflamed skin.

Adverse effects: Skin irritation and acne-like eruptions, photosensitivity, staining of the skin and hair.

Salicylates
Salicylic acid is keratolytic at a concentration of 3–6%.

Mechanism of action: Salicylic acid causes desquamation via the solubilization of cell-surface proteins that maintain the integrity of the stratum corneum.

Route of administration: Topical.

Indications: Hyperkeratosis, eczema, psoriasis (combined with coal tar or dithranol preparations) and acne, wart and callus eradication.

Contraindications: Sensitivity to the drug, or broken or inflamed skin. High concentrations, such as those needed to treat warts, should not be given to people with diabetes mellitus or peripheral vascular disease, as ulceration may be induced.

Adverse effects: Side-effects of salicylic acid include anaphylactic shock in those sensitive to the drug, skin irritation and excessive drying, and systemic effects if used long term.

Emollients
Emollients are used to soothe and hydrate the skin. A simple preparation is aqueous cream, which is often as effective as more complex drugs.

Most creams are thin emollients, whereas a mixture of equal parts soft white paraffin and liquid paraffin is a thick emollient. Camphor, menthol and phenol preparations have antipruritic effects, whereas zinc- and titanium-based emollients have mild astringent (contracting) effects.

Mechanism of action: Emollients hydrate the skin and reduce transepidermal water loss.

Route of administration: Topical. Many emollients can be added to bath water.

Indications: Emollients are used for the long-term treatment of dry scaling disorders.

Contraindications: None.

Fig. 10.12 Other drugs used in skin disease, their indications and mechanisms of action

Drug	Indication	Mechanism of action
Benzoyl peroxide	Acne vulgaris	Antibacterial/keratolytic
Retinoids (vitamin A derivatives)	Psoriasis/acne	Keratolytic/cyto-inhibitory
Psoralen	Psoriasis	Mutates DNA/cytotoxic
Methotrexate	Psoriasis	Cytotoxic
Ciclosporin (cyclosporin)	Psoriasis	Immunosuppressant
Antibacterial, antiviral, antifungal	Skin infections/warts	Antimicrobial
Antiparasite preparations	Skin/hair infestations	Parasite toxins

From Graham-Brown et al. Mosby's Color Atlas and Text of Dermatology, *1st edn. 1998. By permission of Mosby*

Adverse effects: Some ingredients, such as lanolin or antibacterials, may induce an allergic reaction.

Therapeutic notes: The use of emollients lessens the need for topical steroids, therefore limiting potential side-effects.

Other drugs used in skin disease

Many other drugs are employed in the management of skin disease. Some of the more common drugs are summarized in Figure 10.12.

Preparations of drugs for use on skin

Drugs applied to the skin are delivered by a variety of vehicles such as ointments, creams, pastes, powders, aerosols, gels, lotions and tinctures. Factors affecting the choice of vehicle include:

- The solubility of the active drug
- The ability of the drug to penetration the skin
- The stability of the drug–vehicle complex
- The ability of the vehicle to delay evaporation, this being greatest for ointments and least for tinctures.

Factors that affect the absorption of the drug include:

- Body site – in that absorption is greatest from the scrotum and vulva, high from the scalp and face, and lowest from the palms and soles.
- Skin hydration – as occlusive dressings can increase the absorption of a drug tenfold, for example.
- Skin condition – because damage caused by burns and inflammation increases absorption.
- The concentration gradient across the skin – the greater this is, the greater the rate of absorption.

ALLERGIC DISORDERS AND DRUG THERAPY

Allergic reactions occur when the immune system mounts an inappropriate response to an innocuous foreign substance.

Most common allergic disorders are caused by IgE-mediated type I immediate hypersensitivity reactions that occur in a previously sensitized person re-exposed to the sensitizing antigen. Type I immediate hypersensitivity reactions are also known as atopic disorders.

Patients with atopic diseases have an inherited predisposition to develop IgE antibodies to allergens that are innocuous and non-antigenic in normal people. These specific IgE antibodies become bound to high-affinity IgE receptors (FcεRI) on the surface of tissue mast cells and blood basophils. The cross-linking of this cell-surface-bound IgE by antigens (allergens), on subsequent exposure, induces degranulation and release of mediators such as histamine, leukotrienes and prostaglandins (Fig. 10.13).

The released vasoactive and inflammatory mediators produce many local and systemic effects, including vasodilatation, increased vascular permeability, smooth muscle contraction, oedema, glandular hypersecretion and inflammatory cell infiltration.

Depending on the site of this reaction and release of mediators, a variety of disorders can result (Fig. 10.14).

Drug therapy of allergic disorders

The most effective therapy in hypersensitivity reactions is avoidance of the offending antigen or environment. When this is not possible, drug therapy can be of use (Fig. 10.15).

Adam, a 6-year-old boy, is rushed into accident and emergency with a blood pressure of 65/30 mmHg. He is clearly in distress, breathless and vomiting. Swollen lips and blisters around his mouth are also noted. His father tells the doctor that he had been fine previously and had just started having his lunch, peanut butter sandwiches. Suddenly he became severely unwell. The doctors acted quickly to diagnose anaphylactic shock. Adam is given oxygen and 250 µg adrenaline intramuscularly. Afterwards, he is also given chlorphenamine (H_1- receptor antagonist) and hydrocortisone to prevent relapse. He and his father are advised about the allergic reaction and taught to carry prefilled adrenaline syringes. Adam is also given a MedicAlert bracelet.

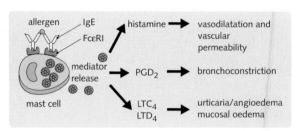

Fig. 10.13 Mechanism of type 1 hypersensitivity (allergic) reaction. (FcεRI, cell surface IgE receptor; LT, leukotriene; PG, prostaglandin.) (Redrawn from Page et al. 2002.)

Histamine and antihistamines

Histamine is a basic amine that is stored in mast cells (fixed in the tissues) and in circulating basophils; it is also found in the stomach and CNS. The effects of histamine are mediated by three different receptor types found on target cells (Fig. 10.16).

As the major chemical mediator released during an allergic reaction, histamine produces a number of effects, mainly via action on H_1-receptors. Therefore H_1 antagonists (antihistamines) are of potential benefit in the treatment of allergic disorders.

H_1-Receptor antagonists: antihistamines

There are two types of H_1-receptor antagonists:

- 'Old' sedative types – e.g. chlorphenamine and promethazine.
- 'New' non-sedative types – e.g. cetirizine and loratadine.

Mechanism of action: Antagonism of histamine H_1-receptors (see Fig. 10.16). In the periphery, their action can inhibit allergic reactions where histamine is the main mediator involved.

The old-style antihistamines are able to cross the blood–brain barrier where both specific and non-specific actions in the CNS produce sedation and antiemetic effects.

Indications: The main use of H_1-receptor antagonists is in the treatment of seasonal allergic rhinitis (hay fever). They are also used for the treatment and prevention of allergic skin reactions such as urticarial rashes, pruritus and insect bites, and in the emergency treatment of anaphylactic shock.

Fig. 10.14 Type I hypersensitivity/allergic disorders			
Disorder	**Site of reaction**	**Response**	**Common allergens**
Anaphylaxis	Circulation	Oedema, circulatory collapse, death	Venoms Drugs
Allergic rhinitis/ hay fever	Nasal passages Conjunctiva	Irritation, oedema, mucosal hypersecretion	Pollen Dust
Asthma	Bronchioles	Bronchoconstriction, mucosal secretion, airway inflammation	Pollen Dust
Food allergy	GIT	Vomiting, diarrhoea, urticaria (hives)	Seafood Milk etc.
Wheal and flare	Skin	Vasodilatation and oedema	Insect venom

GIT, gastrointestinal tract

Fig. 10.15 Drug therapy in allergic disorders

Disorder	Drugs used	Chapter	Mechanism of action
Anaphylaxis	Adrenaline	2 & 4	Vasoconstriction (α_2) Bronchodilation (β_2)
	Antihistamines	3 & 5	Pro-inflammatory mediator antagonism
	Glucocorticoids	2 & 6	Anti-inflammatory
Allergic rhinitis/ hay fever	Antihistamines	3 & 5	Pro-inflammatory mediator antagonism
	Mast-cell stabilizers	5	Inhibition of mast-cell degranulation
	Glucocorticoids	2 & 6	Anti-inflammatory
	Sympathomimetic vasoconstrictors	2, 3 & 4	Decongestion of nasal mucosa
Asthma	See p. 58	4	See p. 57
Food allergies	Antihistamines	4	Pro-inflammatory mediator antagonism
Wheal and flare	Antihistamines	4	Pro-inflammatory mediator antagonism

Fig. 10.16 Effects at histamine receptors

Histamine receptor	Effect
H_1	Responsible for most of the actions of histamine in a type I hypersensitivity reaction: • capillary and venous dilatation (producing 'flare' or systemic hypotension) • increased vascular permeability (producing 'wheal' or oedema) • contraction of smooth muscle (producing bronchial and gastrointestinal contraction)
H_2	Regulation of gastric acid secretion: • H_2-receptors respond to histamine secreted from the enterochromaffin-like cells that are adjacent to the parietal cell (see Chapter 10)
H_3	Involved in neurotransmission: • exact physiological role not clear (presynaptic inhibition of neurotransmitter release in the CNS and autonomic nervous system? role in itch and pain perception?)

The old-style H_1-receptor antagonists can also be used as mild hypnotics (Ch. 5), and to suppress nausea in motion sickness, owing to their actions on the CNS.

Route of administration: Oral, topical, transnasal. Intravenous chlorphenamine can be used in anaphylaxis.

Adverse effects: Old-style antihistamines produce quite pronounced sedation or fatigue, as well as anticholinergic effects such as dry mouth. The newer agents do not do this.

Rare hazardous arrhythmias are associated with a few H_1-receptor antagonists (e.g. terfenadine), especially at high plasma levels or when in combination with imidazole antifungal agents or macrolide antibiotics (Ch. 11). Hypersensitivity reactions, especially to topically applied H_1-receptor antagonists, may occur.

Mast-cell stabilizers, the anti-inflammatory glucocorticoids, and sympathomimetic decongestants are all used in allergy (see Ch. 3).

IMMUNOSUPPRESSANTS

Immunosuppressant drugs are toxic agents, with adverse effects common, serious and frequently dose limiting. Knowledge of these adverse effects and why they occur is therefore important.

Deliberate pharmacological suppression of the immune system is used in the following three main clinical areas:

- To suppress inappropriate autoimmune responses (e.g. systemic lupus erythematosus or rheumatoid arthritis), where the host immune system is 'attacking' host tissue
- To suppress host immune rejection responses to donor organ grafts or transplants
- To suppress donor immune responses against host antigens (prevention of graft versus host disease after bone marrow transplant [GVHD]).

The main pharmacological agents used for immunosuppression are:

- Calcineurin inhibitors
- Anti-proliferatives
- Glucocorticoids (Ch. 6).

Solid organ transplant patients require immunosuppression to prevent organ rejection. They are usually maintained on a corticosteroid combined with a calcineurin inhibitor (ciclosporin) or with an antiproliferative drug (azathioprine or mycophenolate mofetil), or with both.

Mr Isaac, 40 years, has diabetes. He develops end-stage renal failure due to diabetic nephropathy. He is able to receive a renal transplant. The operation is successful and he is started on ciclosporin, mycophenolate mofetil and prednisolone immunosuppression to prevent rejection. When he is discharged, he is also given co-trimoxazole (a mixture of the anti-bacterials, sulfamethoxazole and trimethoprim) and nystatin (anti-fungal) prophylactically. However, 2 months later, he develops an infection. Cytomegalovirus (CMV) is identified as the cause from his symptoms, chest X-ray and detection of CMV DNA by polymerase chain reaction test.

Mr Isaac is treated by two methods:

- A reduction in his immunosuppression (mycophenolate mofetil treatment is suspended). This is vital to allow a better immune response to clear the CMV. Close surveillance of graft function is important during this period.
- Specific anti-viral therapy (ganciclovir).

Mr Isaac responds to this therapy and his symptoms resolve after 6 days.

Calcineurin inhibitors

The main drug in this class is ciclosporin.

Mechanism of action: Ciclosporin is a cyclic peptide, derived from fungi, that has powerful immunosuppressive activity. It has a selective inhibitory effect on T cells by inhibiting the T-cell receptor (TCR)-mediated signal-transduction pathway. It is believed to exert its actions after entering the T cell and preventing the transcription of specific genes (Fig. 10.17).

After entry into the T cell, ciclosporin specifically binds to its cytoplasmic binding protein, cyclophilin. This cyclosporin–cyclophilin complex then binds to a serine/threonine phosphatase called calcineurin, inhibiting its phosphatase activity. Calcineurin is normally activated when intracellular calcium ion levels rise following T-cell-receptor binding to the appropriate major histocompatibility complex: antigen complex. When calcineurin is active it dephosphorylates the cytoplasmic component of the nuclear factor of activated T cells (NF-ATc) into a form that migrates to the nucleus and induces transcription of genes such as IL-2 that are involved in T-cell activation.

Inhibition of calcineurin by the ciclosporin–cyclophilin complex therefore prevents the nuclear translocation of NF-ATc and the transcription of certain genes essential for the activation of T cells. Hence the production of IL-2 by T-helper cells, the maturation of cytotoxic T cells, and the production of some other lymphokines, such as interferon-γ, are all inhibited.

The overall action of ciclosporin is to suppress reversibly both cell-mediated and antibody-specific adaptive immune responses.

Indications: Ciclosporin is used for the prevention of graft and transplant rejection, and prevention of GVHD.

Route of administration: Oral, intravenous.

Adverse effects: Unlike most immunosuppressive agents, ciclosporin does not cause myelosuppression. It is markedly nephrotoxic to the proximal tubule of the kidney, and renal damage almost always occurs. This may be reversible or permanent. Hypertension occurs in 50% of people.

Less serious side-effects include mild hepatotoxicity, anorexia, lethargy, gastrointestinal upsets, hirsutism and gum hypertrophy.

Infectious diseases

Objectives

After reading this chapter, you will:

- Have basic understanding of bacterial, viral, fungal and parasitic infections
- Know how drugs act to defend against these infections
- Know the indications, contraindications and adverse drug effects associated with these drugs.

ANTIBACTERIAL DRUGS

Concepts of antibacterial chemotherapy

Bacteria belong to the kingdom of prokaryotic organisms. Some bacteria are pathogenic to humans and responsible for a number of medically important diseases.

The principal treatment of infections is chemotherapy, which in its simplest definition is the use of chemicals (drugs) to combat disease (Ch. 1). Chemotherapy of infections aims to selectively target the invading bacteria while having minimal effect on the host. This is achieved by exploiting differences that exist between the structure and physiology of the prokaryotic bacterial cells and the host eukaryotic cell (Figs. 11.1 and 11.2).

Antibacterial agents can be:

- bacteriostatic (i.e. they inhibit bacterial growth but do not kill the bacteria)

or

- bactericidal (i.e. they kill bacteria).

Fig. 11.1 Site of action of cytotoxic drugs that act on dividing cells		
Site	**Exploitable difference**	**Antibacterial drug**
Peptidoglycan cell wall	Peptidoglycan cell walls are a uniquely prokaryotic feature not shared by eukaryotic (mammalian) cells. Drugs that act here are therefore very selective	Penicillins Cephalosporins Glycopeptides
Cytoplasmic membrane	Bacteria possess a plasma membrane within the wall which is a phospholipid bilayer, as in eukaryotes. However in bacteria the plasma membrane does not contain any sterols and this results in differential chemical behaviour that can be exploited	Polymyxins
Protein synthesis	The bacterial ribosome (50S+30S subunits) is sufficiently different from the mammalian ribosome (60S+40S subunits) that sites on the bacterial ribosome are good targets for drug action	Aminoglycosides Tetracyclines Chloramphenicol Macrolides Fusidic acid
Nucleic acids	The bacterial genome is in the form of a single circular strand of DNA plus ancillary plasmids unenclosed by a nuclear envelope, in contrast to the eukaryotic chromosomal arrangement within the nucleus. Drugs may interfere directly or indirectly with microbial DNA and RNA metabolism, replication and transcription	Antifolates Quinolones Rifampicin

Fig. 11.6 Classification of selected medically important viruses and the diseases they cause

Family	ss/ds	Viruses	Diseases
DNA viruses			
Herpes viruses	ds	Herpes simplex (HSV)*	Cold sores, genital herpes
		Varicella zoster (VZV)*	Chickenpox, shingles
		Cytomegalovirus (CMV)*	Cytomegalic disease
		Epstein–Barr virus (EBV)*	Infectious mononucleosis
Poxviruses	ds	Variola	Smallpox
Adenoviruses	ds	Adenoviruses	Acute respiratory disease
Hepadnaviruses	ds	Hepatitis B	Hepatitis
Papovaviruses	ds	Papilloma	Warts
Parvoviruses	ss	B19	Erythema infectiosum
RNA viruses			
Orthomyxoviruses	ss	Influenza A* and B*	Influenza
Paramyxoviruses	ss	Measles virus	Measles
		Mumps virus	Mumps
		Parainfluenza	Respiratory infection
		Respiratory syncytial*	Respiratory infection
Coronaviruses	ss	Coronavirus	Respiratory infection
Rhabdoviruses	ss	Rabies virus	Rabies
Picornaviruses	ss	Enteroviruses	Meningitis
		Rhinoviruses	Colds
		Hepatitis A	Hepatitis
Calciviruses	ss	Norwalk virus	Gastroenteritis
Togaviruses	ss	Alphaviruses	Encephalitis, haemorrhagic fevers
		Rubivirus	Rubella
Reoviruses	ds	Rotavirus	Gastroenteritis
Arenavirus	ss	Lymphocytic choriomeningitis	Meningitis
		Lassavirus*	Lassa fever
Retroviruses	ss	HIV I, II*	AIDS

*viruses for which effective chemotherapy exists; ds, double stranded; ss, single stranded

Inhibition of attachment to or penetration of host cells

Amantadine

Mechanism of action: Amantadine blocks a primitive ion channel in the viral membrane (named M_2) preventing fusion of a virion to host cell membranes, and inhibits the release of newly synthesised viruses from the host cell (Fig. 11.7).

Route of administration: Oral.

Indications: Amantadine is used for the prophylaxis and treatment of acute influenza A in groups at risk. It is not effective against influenza B.

Adverse effects: Some patients (5–10%) report non-serious dizziness, slurred speech and insomnia. Neurological side-effects and renal failure can occur at high concentrations.

Therapeutic notes: Emergence of resistance to amantadine associated with clinical failure has been reported in 25–50% of patients. Amantadine is not used widely because of problems with resistance, its narrow spectrum of activity and because influenza vaccines are often preferred.

Neuraminidase inhibitors

Zanamivir belongs to the neuraminidase inhibitor class of drugs.

Mechanism of action: Zanamivir inhibits the release of newly synthesised viruses from the host cell by inhibiting the enzyme (neuraminidase) which is responsible for cleaving the peptide links between virus and host.

Route of administration: Zanamivir is delivered by inhalation, though its sister drug oseltamivir may be given orally.

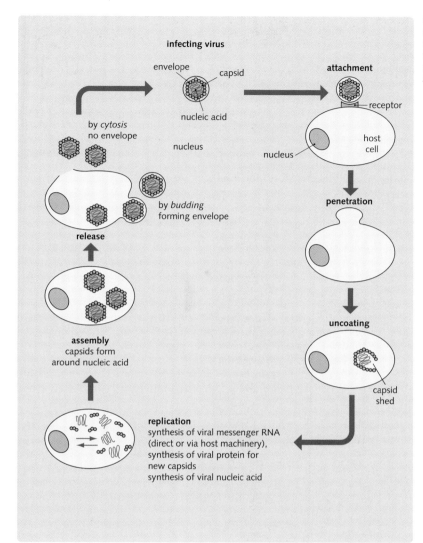

Fig. 11.7 Stages in the infection of a host's cell and replication of a virus. Several thousand virus particles may be formed from each cell. (Reproduced with permission from Mims et al. *Medical Microbiology*, 2nd edn. Mosby, 1998.)

Indications: Treatment of influenza A or B virus within 48 hours after onset of symptoms when influenza is endemic in the community.

Contraindications: Breastfeeding.

Adverse effects: Gastrointestinal disturbances.

Immunoglobulins

Examples of immunoglobulins include human normal immunoglobulin (HNIg/gamma globulin) and specific immunoglobulins, e.g. hepatitis B (HBIg), rabies (RIg), varicella zoster (VZIg) and cytomegalovirus (CMVIg) immunoglobulins.

Mechanism of action: Immunoglobulins bind specifically to antigenic determinants on the outside of virions. By specifically binding to a virus, the immunoglobulins may neutralize it by coating the virus and preventing its attachment and entry into host cells.

HNIg is prepared from pooled plasma of ~1000 donors and contains antibodies to measles, mumps, varicella and hepatitis A.

Specific immunoglobulins are prepared by pooling the plasma of selected donors with high levels of the antibody required.

Route of administration: Intramuscular, though immunoglobulins can be given intravenously.

Indications: HNIg is administered for the protection of susceptible contacts against hepatitis A, measles, mumps and rubella. Specific immunoglobulins may attenuate or prevent hepatitis and rabies following known exposure, and before the onset of signs and symptoms, e.g. following exposure to a rabid animal. VZIg and CMVIg are indicated for prophylactic use to prevent chickenpox, and cytomegalic disease in immunosuppressed patients at risk.

Contraindications: Immunoglobulins should not be given to people with known antibody against IgA.

Adverse effects: Malaise, chills, fever and (rarely) anaphylaxis.

Therapeutic notes: Protection with immunoglobulins is immediate and lasts several weeks. HNIg may interfere with vaccinations for 3 months.

Inhibition of nucleic acid replication

Aciclovir and related drugs
Aciclovir, famciclovir and valaciclovir are all closely related anti-viral drugs.

Mechanism of action: Aciclovir and related drugs are characterized by their selective phosphorylation in herpes-infected cells. This takes place by a viral thymidine kinase rather than host kinase, as a first step.

Phosphorylation yields a triphosphate nucleotide that inhibits viral DNA polymerase and viral DNA synthesis.

These drugs are selectively toxic to infected cells because, in the absence of viral thymidine kinase, the host kinase activates only a small amount of the drug. In addition, the DNA polymerase of herpes virus has a much higher affinity for the activated drug than has cellular DNA polymerase (Fig. 11.7).

Route of administration: Topical, oral, parenteral.

Indications: Aciclovir and related drugs are used for the prophylaxis and treatment of herpes simplex and varicella zoster virus infections, superficial and systemic, particularly in the immunocompromised.

Adverse effects: Side-effects are minimal. Rarely, renal impairment and encephalopathy occur.

Therapeutic notes: The herpes genome in latent (non-replicating) cells is not affected by aciclovir therapy and so recurrence of infection after cessation of treatment is to be expected.

CMV is resistant to aciclovir because its genome does not encode thymidine kinase.

Ganciclovir
Mechanism of action: Ganciclovir is a synthetic nucleoside analogue, structurally related to aciclovir. It also requires conversion to the triphosphate nucleotide form, though by a different kinase. Ganciclovir acts as a substrate for viral DNA polymerase and as a chain terminator aborting virus replication.

Route of administration: Oral, intravenous.

Indications: While as active as aciclovir against HSV and VZV, ganciclovir is reserved for the treatment of severe CMV infections in immunocompromised people, owing to its side-effects.

Adverse effects: Reversible neutropenia in 40% of patients. There is occasional rash, nausea and encephalopathy.

Therapeutic notes: Maintenance therapy with ganciclovir at a reduced dose may be necessary to prevent recurrence of CMV.

Ribavirin (tribavirin)
Mechanism of action: Ribavirin is a nucleoside analogue that selectively interferes with viral nucleic acid synthesis in a manner similar to aciclovir.

Route of administration: For respiratory syncytial virus (RSV) by inhalation; for Lassa virus intravenously.

Indications: Severe respiratory syncytial virus bronchiolitis in infants. Lassa fever.

Adverse effects: Reticulocytosis, respiratory depression.

Therapeutic notes: The necessity of aerosol administration for RSV limits the usefulness of this effective drug.

Nucleoside analogue reverse transcriptase inhibitors
Examples of nucleoside reverse transcriptase inhibitors include zidovudine (AZT), and the newer drugs, abacavir, didanosine (ddI), lamivudine (3TC), stavudine (d4T) and zalcitabine (ddC).

Mechanism of action: These nucleotide analogues all require intracellular conversion to the corresponding triphosphate nucleotide for activation. The active triphosphates competitively inhibit reverse transcriptase, and cause termination of DNA chain elongation once incorporated. Affinity for

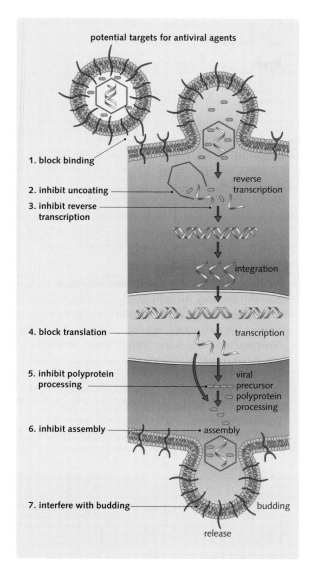

potential targets for antiviral agents

1. block binding

2. inhibit uncoating

3. inhibit reverse transcription

reverse transcription

integration

4. block translation

transcription

5. inhibit polyprotein processing

viral precursor polyprotein processing

6. inhibit assembly

assembly

7. interfere with budding

budding

release

Fig. 11.8 The HIV replicative cycle and potential sites of antiviral drug action.

viral reverse transcriptase is 100 times that for host DNA polymerase (Fig. 11.8, site 3).

Route of administration: Oral.

Indications: Nucleoside reverse transcriptase inhibitors are used for the management of asymptomatic and symptomatic HIV infections, and the prevention of maternal–fetal HIV transmission.

Adverse effects: Side-effects of AZT are uncommon at the recommended low dosage in patients with asymptomatic or mild HIV infections, but more

common in acquired immune deficiency syndrome (AIDS) patients on higher dosage regimens.

Toxicity to human myeloid and erythroid progenitor cells commonly causes anaemia and neutropenia, i.e. bone marrow suppression. Other common side-effects include nausea, insomnia, headaches and myalgia.

The major dose-limiting effects of ddI are pancreatitis and peripheral neuropathy, and of ddC and d4T, peripheral neuropathy.

Therapeutic notes: Drug resistance evolves to all the current nucleoside reverse transcriptase inhibitors by the development of mutations in reverse transcriptase, although the kinetics of resistance development varies for the different drugs (e.g. 6–18 months for AZT). Combined therapies may have a place in increasing efficacy synergistically and reducing emergence of resistant strains.

Non-nucleoside reverse transcriptase inhibitors

Efavirenz and nevirapine are examples of drugs within this class.

Mechanism of action: Efavirenz and nevirapine both bind to reverse transcriptase near the catalytic site, leading to a conformational change that inactivates this enzyme.

Route of administration: Oral.

Contraindications: Breastfeeding.

Adverse effects: Generally well tolerated. Rash, dizziness and headache may occur.

Therapeutic notes: Resistance can develop quickly when subtherapeutic doses are employed.

Inhibition of post-translational events

Protease inhibitors

Examples of protease inhibitors include saquinavir, and the newer drugs, ritonavir, indinavir, nelfinavir and amprenavir.

Mechanism of action: Protease inhibitors prevents the virus-specific protease of HIV cleaving the inert polyprotein product of translation into various structural and functional proteins (see Fig. 11.8, site 5).

Route of administration: Oral.

Indications: Protease inhibitors are used for the management of asymptomatic and symptomatic HIV infections, in combination with nucleoside reverse transcriptase inhibitors.

215

Fig. 11.12 Classification of medically important protozoan species causing disease in humans

Sub-phyla	Defining characteristics	Medically important species	Disease
Amoebae (sarcodina)	Amoeboid movement with pseudopods	*Entamoeba histolytica*	Amoebiasis (amoebic dysentery)
Flagellates (mastigophora)	Flagella that produces a whip-like movement	*Giardia lamblia* *Trichomonas vaginalis* *Leishmania* spp. *Trypanosoma* spp.	Giardiasis Trichomonal vaginitis Leishmaniasis Trypanosomiasis (sleeping sickness and Chagas' disease)
Cilates (ciliophora)	Cilia beat to produce movement	—	—
Sporozoans (sporozoa)	No locomotor organs in adult stage	Plasmodium spp.	Malaria

global importance. Parasitic protozoa replicate within the host's body and are usually divided into four subphyla according to their type of locomotion (Fig. 11.12).

Malaria

Malaria is the most important protozoal disease in tropical medicine. It is responsible for 2 million deaths per year and much morbidity in the 200 million people worldwide who are infected. Malaria is caused by four species of plasmodial parasites that are transmitted by female anopheline mosquitoes.

Antimalarial drugs target different phases of the life cycle of the malarial parasite (Fig. 11.13). This life cycle proceeds as follows:

- When an infected mosquito feeds on a human it injects sporozoites into the bloodstream from its salivary glands.
- The sporozoites rapidly penetrate the liver where they transform and grow into tissue schizonts containing large numbers of merozoites. In the case of *Plasmodium vivax* and *P. ovale*, some schizonts remain dormant in the liver for years (hypnozoites), before rupturing to cause a relapse.
- The large tissue schizonts rupture after 5–20 days, releasing thousands of merozoites that invade circulating red blood cells (RBCs), and multiply inside the cell.

- The host's RBCs rupture, leading to the release of more merozoites. These then invade and destroy more RBCs. This cycle of invasion/destruction causes the episodic chills and fever that characterize malaria.
- Some merozoites develop into gametocytes. If these are taken up by a feeding mosquito, the insect becomes infected, thus completing the cycle.

A decent knowledge of the plasmodial life cycle is a prerequisite to understanding the mechanism and site of action of antimalarial drugs.

The clinical features and severity of malaria depend upon the species of parasite and the immunological status of the person infected. Clinically significant malaria is less common in adults who have always lived in endemic areas, as partial immunity develops.

The four types of plasmodium causing malaria are:

- *P. falciparum* – widespread and causes malignant tertian (fever every third day) malaria. There is no exo-erythrocytic stage, so that, if the erythrocytic forms are eradicated, relapses do not occur.

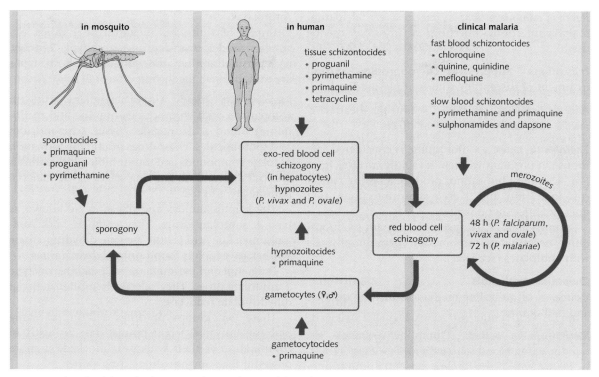

Fig. 11.13 Life cycle of the malarial parasite and point of action of chemotherapeutic agents.

- *P. vivax* – widespread and causes benign, tertian relapsing malaria. Exo-erythrocytic forms may persist in the liver for years and cause relapses.
- *P. malariae* – rare and causes benign quartan (fever every fourth day) malaria. There is no exo-erythrocytic stage, so that, if the erythrocytic forms are eradicated, relapses do not occur.
- *P. ovale* – mainly African and causes a rare form of benign relapsing malaria. Exo-erythrocytic forms may persist in the liver for years and cause relapses.

Approaches to antimalarial chemotherapy

Antimalarial drugs are usually classified in terms of their action against different stages of the parasite (see Fig. 11.13). They are used to protect against or cure malaria or to prevent transmission.

Prophylactic use
The aim of prophylactic use is to prevent the occurrence of infection in a previously healthy individual who is at potential exposure risk.

Suppressive prophylaxis involves the use of blood schizonticides to prevent acute attacks; causal prophylaxis involves the use of tissue schizonticides or drugs against the sporozoite to prevent the parasite becoming established in the liver.

Curative (therapeutic use)
Antimalarial drugs can be used curatively (therapeutically) against an established infection.

Suppressive treatment aims to control acute attacks, usually with blood schizonticides; radical treatment aims to kill dormant liver forms, usually with a hypnozonticide, to prevent relapsing malaria.

Antimalarial drugs

4-aminoquinolines
Chloroquine is an example of a 4-aminoquinoline.

Mechanism of action: Chloroquine is a rapidly acting blood schizonticide (see Fig. 11.13). It is concentrated 100-fold in erythrocytes that contain plasmodial parasites; this occurs because ferriprotoporphyrin IX, a degradation product of haemoglobin digestion by the parasites, acts as a chloroquine receptor. It is unclear how the high chloroquine concentrations kill the parasites; possibly, the digestion of haemoglobin is inhibited.

Adverse effects: Gastrointestinal disturbance, and neurotoxic effects (dizziness) may occur.

Therapeutic notes: A single dose of piperazine is usually effective for treating roundworm infection; threadworm infestation may require a longer course (7 days).

Benzimidazoles

Examples of benzimidazoles include mebendazole, thiabendazole and albendazole.

Mechanism of action: Benzimidazoles bind with high affinity to a site on tubulin dimers, thus preventing the polymerization of microtubules. Subsequent depolymerization leads to complete breakdown of the microtubule.

The selectivity of benzimidazoles arises because they are 250–400 times more potent in helminth than in mammalian tissue. The process takes time to have effect, and the worm may not be expelled for days.

Route of administration: Oral.

Indications: Benzimidazoles are used in the treatment of hydatid disease, and many nematode infestations (see Fig. 11.14).

Contraindications: Benzimidazoles should not be given to pregnant women as they are teratogenic and embryotoxic.

Adverse effects: Occasional gastrointestinal disturbance. Thiabendazole causes more frequent gastrointestinal disturbance, headache and dizziness. Serious hepatotoxicity rarely occurs.

Therapeutic notes: Dosage regimens of benzimidazoles range from a single dose for pinworm infestation to multiple doses for up to 5 days for trichinosis.

Diethylcarbamazine

Mechanism of action: It is not clear exactly how diethylcarbamazine exerts its filaricidal effect. It has been suggested that it damages or modifies the parasites in such a way as to make them more susceptible to host immune defences.

Diethylcarbamazine kills both microfilariae in the peripheral circulation and adult worms in the lymphatics.

Route of administration: Oral.

Indications: Diethylcarbamazine is the drug of choice for lymphatic filariasis caused by *Wucheria bancrofti*, *Loa loa* and *Brugia malayi* (see Fig. 11.14).

Adverse effects: Gastrointestinal disturbance, headache, lassitude.

Material from the damaged and dead worms causes allergic side-effects, including skin reactions, lymph gland enlargement, dizziness and tachycardia, lasting from 3 to 7 days.

Therapeutic notes: To minimize the dangerous sudden release of dead worm material, the initial dose of diethylcarbamazine is started low and then increased and maintained for 21 days.

Ivermectin

Mechanism of action: Ivermectin immobilizes the tapeworm *Onchocerca volvulus* by causing tonic paralysis of the peripheral muscle system. It does this by potentiating the effect of γ-aminobutyric acid at the worm's neuromuscular junction.

Route of administration: Oral.

Indications: Ivermectin is the drug of choice for *Onchocerca volvulus*, which causes river blindness and may be the most effective drug for chronic *Strongyloides* infection (see Fig. 11.14).

Adverse effects: Ocular irritation, transient electrocardiographic changes and somnolence. An immediate immune reaction to dead microfilariae (Mazzotti reaction) can be severe.

Levamisole

Mechanism of action: Levamisole stimulates nicotinic receptors at the neuromuscular junction and results in a spastic paralysis, which causes faecal worm expulsion.

Route of administration: Oral.

Indications: Treatment of choice for *Ascaris lumbricoides* round worm infection (se Fig. 11.14).

Adverse effects: Mild nausea and vomiting.

Objectives

After reading this chapter, you will:

- Have a good understanding of cancer and the cell cycle
- Know the different classes of drugs that are used to treat cancer and how their mechanisms of action result in beneficial and adverse effects.

CONCEPTS OF CANCER CHEMOTHERAPY

Cancer

Cancers are malignant neoplasms (new growths). Despite their variability, cancers share the characteristics of:

- Uncontrolled proliferation
- Local invasiveness
- Tendency to spread (metastasis)
- Changes in some aspects of original cell morphology/retention of other characteristics.

Cancers account for 20–25% of deaths in the Western world; attempts to cure or palliate cancer use three principal methods: surgery, radiotherapy and chemotherapy. These methods are not mutually exclusive, often being used in combination, e.g. adjuvant chemotherapy after surgical removal of a tumour.

> Adjuvant chemotherapy is given after successful treatment of a cancer, where no remaining disease is found, for prophylaxis against re-occurrence.

> Mr Collins is a 60-year-old delivery man, who presents with a 6-week history of passage of fresh blood from his anus and diarrhoea (he is normally slightly constipated). He also admits to low appetite, significant weight loss and feeling fatigued. He is referred for investigative colonoscopy, which reveals an abnormal growth in the descending colon. A biopsy reveals adenocarcinoma of the colon. Staging CT scans show no other areas of disease. He is managed by surgical resection of the tumour. Following this he undergoes adjuvant chemotherapy consisting of six cycles of 5-fluorouracil.

Chemotherapy

Cancer chemotherapy is the use of drugs to inhibit the rate of growth of, or to kill, cancerous cells while having minimal effects on non-neoplastic host cells.

In a fashion similar to antimicrobial chemotherapy, the ideal anti-cancer drugs target malignant cells in preference to non-malignant cells. This is achieved by exploiting the molecular differences between them.

The most striking difference between cancerous and non-cancerous cells is their accelerated rate of cell division. This remains the main target for therapeutic intervention at present, though newer drugs are being developed which recognize other molecular differences.

The chemotherapeutic techniques currently used include:

- Cytotoxic therapy – which is the main approach
- Endocrine therapy
- Immunotherapy.

Cancers differ in their sensitivity to chemotherapy, from the very sensitive (e.g. lymphomas, testicular carcinomas) where complete clinical cures can be achieved, to the resistant (generally solid tumours, e.g. colorectal, squamous cell bronchial carcinoma).

Multiple-choice questions (MCQs)

Indicate whether each answer is true or false.

Chapter 1 Introduction to pharmacology

1. **The following are intracellular messengers:**
   a. Cyclic adenosine monophosphate.
   b. Diacylglycerol.
   c. Inositol tetraphosphate.
   d. γ-aminobutyric acid (GABA).
   e. Cyclic guanosine monophosphate.

2. **A partial agonist:**
   a. Brings about the same maximal response as a full agonist.
   b. Can have the same affinity for the receptor as the full agonist.
   c. Can occupy all available receptors.
   d. Always irreversibly binds the receptor.
   e. Has the same efficacy as a full agonist.

3. **An antagonist:**
   a. Has similar receptor binding affinity to the agonist.
   b. Has similar efficacy to the agonist.
   c. Is always competitive.
   d. With a dose ratio of 10 is a weak antagonist.
   e. Will shift the agonists dose–response curve to the right.

4. **Compliance:**
   a. Is measured in mmol/L.
   b. Is often high in small children.
   c. Can be enhanced with good communication.
   d. Will be poor if the drug regimen is simple to follow.
   e. Is not important in many diseases.

5. **Drugs administered:**
   a. Intravenously are subjected to first-pass metabolism.
   b. Topically cannot have systemic side-effects.
   c. Rectally avoid first-pass metabolism.
   d. Orally have the highest possible bioavailability.
   e. Intravenously are more rapidly metabolized than via the oral route.

6. **The rate of renal excretion of a drug is usually related to:**
   a. The free (not protein-bound) plasma drug concentration.
   b. The total plasma drug concentration.
   c. Tubular reabsorption.
   d. Lipid solubility of the drug.
   e. The volume of distribution of the drug.

7. **The volume of distribution:**
   a. Cannot be greater than total body water.
   b. Is dependent on the pH of the blood.
   c. Is dependent on the degree of protein binding.
   d. Albumin tends to bind acidic drugs.
   e. Thiopental tends to accumulate in the blood.

8. **Drugs:**
   a. Are commonly excreted by the liver.
   b. That are lipid soluble cannot cross the blood–brain barrier.
   c. Such as paracetamol are directly toxic to the liver.
   d. Can interfere with cytochrome P-450 in the liver and alter the metabolism of other drugs.
   e. Are monitored for adverse effects even after being granted a licence for clinical use.

9. **Regarding adverse effects:**
   a. Thalidomide is contraindicated in pregnant women.
   b. Aspirin is safe in patients with glucose 6-phosphate dehydrogenase deficiency.
   c. Glucocorticoids can be used to treat hydralazine-induced autoimmune reactions.
   d. Family history of adverse effects is useful in anaesthesia.
   e. Most information on adverse drug reactions is obtained during phase 2 of drug development.

Chapter 2 Cardiovascular system

10. **Cardiac rate decreases:**
    a. As a result of β-blocker use.
    b. As a result of caffeine.
    c. As a result of adrenaline.
    d. In shock.
    e. In phaeochromocytoma.

11. **Cardiac rate increases:**
    a. As a result of parasympathetic stimulation.
    b. As a result of sympathetic stimulation.
    c. As a result of thyroxine.
    d. As a result of atropine.
    e. As a result of salbutamol.

61. Gastro-oesophageal reflux disease (GORD):

a. Can be exacerbated by smoking, alcohol and obesity.
b. Should always be referred to a specialist.
c. Can be treated simply with oral antihistamines.
d. Can cause metabolic acidosis.
e. Should not be treated with a PPI.

62. Proton pump inhibitors:

a. Include the drug fluconazole.
b. Include the drug lansoprazole.
c. Inhibit the H^+/K^+ ATPase irreversibly.
d. Seldom cause side-effects.
e. Are contraindicated in Zollinger–Ellison syndrome.

63. Antacids:

a. Act to reduce gastric acid secretion from parietal cells.
b. Include the alginate drugs.
c. Raise the pH of the stomach.
d. Are first-line drugs in eradicating *Helicobacter pylori*.
e. Include aluminium hydroxide.

64. Regarding *Helicobacter pylori*:

a. *H. pylori* is more common in humans and ferrets than other mammals.
b. Infection with *H. pylori* will undoubtedly result in peptic ulceration.
c. *H. pylori* secretes urease, which converts urea to carbon dioxide and water.
d. *H. pylori* eradication commonly relies on double therapy.
e. *H. pylori* is not involved in duodenal ulceration.

65. Regarding nausea and vomiting:

a. Emetic drugs should be used if corrosive agents have been ingested.
b. The vomiting centre is sensitive to dopamine.
c. The phenothiazines are useful antiemetics.
d. Ondansetron is a dopamine receptor antagonist.
e. Metoclopramide can cause extrapyramidal side-effects.

66. Antispasmodic drugs:

a. Include dicyclomine.
b. Include methylcellulose.
c. Should not be used in GORD.
d. Can inhibit parasympathetic innervation of the gut.
e. Are usually given rectally.

67. Regarding laxative drugs:

a. Lactulose encourages peristalsis.
b. Senna encourages peristalsis.
c. Laxatives are indicated in bowel obstruction.
d. Docusate sodium is a bulk-forming laxative.
e. Codeine is an analgesic and a laxative.

68. Regarding diarrhoea:

a. Diarrhoea commonly requires antibiotics in the Western world.
b. Fluid replacement should always be given intravenously.
c. Loperamide is given intramuscularly.
d. Morphine is often administered for diarrhoea.
e. *Clostridium difficile* is the commonest diarrhoea-causing pathogen in the Western world.

69. Inflammatory bowel disease (IBD):

a. Responds well to laxatives.
b. Is treated with long-term intravenous steroids.
c. Can be cured by surgical resection.
d. Is treated with aspirin derivatives.
e. Seldom results in nutritional deficiencies.

70. Regarding obesity:

a. Obesity is associated with diabetes mellitus and osteoarthritis.
b. Obesity should initially be treated with drugs.
c. Obesity is often treated with amphetamines.
d. Orlistat inhibits pancreatic lipase, and subsequent absorption of fat from the gut.
e. Leptin is used to induce satiety (fullness).

71. Which of the following are correctly paired:

a. Pancreatic supplementation is indicated in Crohn's disease.
b. Pancreatin replaces the endocrine function of the pancreas.
c. Colestyramine binds bile acids and prevents their reabsorption from the gut.
d. Ursodeoxycholic acid is used to treat gall stones.
e. Pancreatin must not be used after total pancreatectomy.

Chapter 9 Pain and anaesthesia

72. Pain:

a. Is sensed by nociceptors.
b. Can be objectively measured.
c. Usually has a well-defined cause.
d. Can be inhibited by antimalarial drugs.
e. Perception is simply the activation of nociceptors.

73. Opiate analgesic drugs:

a. Can be bought over the counter.
b. Often cause diarrhoea.
c. Should not be given intravenously.
d. Can cause respiratory depression in overdose.
e. Can cause smooth muscle contraction.

74. Regarding headache:

a. Headache is a common and non-sinister symptom.
b. NSAIDs are the first-line treatment for headache.

c. Nausea associated with headache requires hospital admission.
d. Serotonin (5-HT) agonists are indicated for acute migrainous attacks, constricting cerebral blood vessels.
e. Antihistamines are indicated for the acute migrainous attack.

75. **Regarding analgesia:**
   a. Analgesia for mild pain is best treated with paracetamol or aspirin.
   b. Co-proxamol should only be given for analgesia if morphine alone is not sufficient.
   c. The body produces its own endogenous opioids.
   d. Transdermal fentanyl is useful for patients susceptible to nausea.
   e. Weak opioids are used in myocardial infarction

76. **Which of the following are matched appropriately:**
   a. Neuralgic pain may respond to antiepileptics.
   b. Neuralgia commonly occurs due to demyelination.
   c. Amitriptyline is a selective serotonin reuptake inhibitor.
   d. Isoflurane is used to induce anaesthesia.
   e. Lidocaine is applied directly onto the cornea.

77. **Local anaesthetics:**
   a. Block potassium channels.
   b. Can be given intravenously.
   c. Include cocaine.
   d. Can be given with a vasoconstrictor.
   e. Can be used in heart failure.

78. **General anaesthetics:**
   a. Cause excitation of respiratory centres.
   b. Can be administered intravenously.
   c. Include thiopental.
   d. Are generally lipid insoluble.
   e. Can cause hypotension.

Chapter 10 Inflammation, allergic diseases and immunosuppression

79. **Inflammation/the inflammatory response:**
   a. Is an immunologically acquired process.
   b. Relies on endogenous agonist–receptor interactions.
   c. Can be inhibited by opiates.
   d. Relies on the mediators histamine and dopamine.
   e. Involves mast cells.

80. **Non-steroidal anti-inflammatory drugs:**
   a. Include paracetamol.
   b. Inhibit the lipoxygenase enzyme.
   c. Inhibit the cyclooxygenase enzyme.
   d. Inhibit the phospholipase A_2 enzyme.
   e. Include clopidogrel.

81. **Regarding cyclooxygenase (COX):**
   a. Aspirin inhibits cyclooxygenase reversibly.
   b. COX-1 is only expressed during the inflammatory response.
   c. Cyclooxygenase converts arachidonic acid to the prostanoids.
   d. COX-2 inhibitors are contraindicated in patients with cardiovascular disease.
   e. Inhibition of cyclooxygenase can worsen the symptoms of asthma.

82. **Steroidal anti-inflammatory drugs:**
   a. Are commonly used to treat aches and sprains.
   b. Are contraindicated in reversible airways disease.
   c. Have a delayed onset of action.
   d. Inhibit lipocortin synthesis.
   e. Can be administered intravenously.

83. **Considering rheumatoid arthritis (RA):**
   a. RA should not be treated with paracetamol.
   b. RA is an autoimmune disease.
   c. RA does not respond to non-steroidal anti-inflammatory drugs.
   d. Antimalarial drugs, such as chloroquine, are often used in the management of RA.
   e. Treatment with disease-modifying antirheumatic drugs (DMARDs) requires annual screening of the full blood count, and liver and renal function.

84. **Regarding gout:**
   a. Gout results from pyrophosphate crystals in joints.
   b. Gout is a slowly developing disease, and seldom presents acutely.
   c. Aspirin should be avoided in its management.
   d. Colchicine inhibits leucocyte migration, and it causes nausea and vomiting in about 80% of patients.
   e. Allopurinol is a methylxanthine.

85. **Regarding allergy:**
   a. IgA is the common mediator in allergic response.
   b. The new antihistamines are non-sedating.
   c. Histamine increases vascular permeability.
   d. Antihistamines are contraindicated in patients with diabetes mellitus.
   e. Histamine causes smooth muscle contraction.

86. **Regarding immunosuppression:**
   a. Ciclosporin is a prodrug.
   b. Azathioprine is cytotoxic to dividing cells.
   c. Ciclosporin exerts its actions by promoting certain genes essential for T-cell activation.
   d. Mycophenolate mofetil selectively inhibits T- and B-lymphocyte proliferation.
   e. Mineralocorticoids, not glucocorticoids, have immunosuppressant activity.

Short-answer questions (SAQs)

1. Discuss the use of premedication in anaesthesia.

2. Discuss the therapy of hay fever.

3. Describe the classes of drugs used in the treatment of peptic ulcers.

4. What are the main classes of drug used to treat fungal diseases, and what are their mechanisms of action?

5. Which drugs exert their action by modifying γ-aminobutyric acid (GABA) synaptic transmission, and when are they used clinically?

6. Explain the analgesic effect of opioids.

7. Outline the drugs used in the treatment of asthma.

8. Explain the concept of selective toxicity with reference to cytotoxic drugs used in the treatment of cancer.

9. Discuss the different classes of drug used as laxatives.

10. Describe the neurochemical imbalance found in the brains of people with Parkinson's disease, and list the classes of drug used to correct this imbalance.

11. Compare and contrast suxamethonium and atracurium.

12. Explain first-pass metabolism.

13. Describe the therapeutic uses of vasoconstrictors.

14. Explain the differences between lidocaine (lignocaine) and amiodarone in their use as anti-arrhythmics.

15. Compare and contrast competitive and non-competitive antagonists.

16. Explain the effects and clinical use of warfarin.

17. Explain how local anaesthetics inhibit nerve conduction.

18. Give an outline of the drug treatment of diabetes mellitus.

19. Explain the clinical use of anticholinesterases and how this is influenced by their duration of action.

20. Explain the role of cyclic adenosine monophosphate (cAMP) as an intracellular messenger in the cardiovascular system.

Extended-matching questions (EMQs)

For each scenario described below choose the *single* most likely option from the list of options. *Each option may be used once, more than once or not at all.*

1. G-protein linked receptors

A. Activation of phospholipase C
B. Activation of guanylyl cyclase on the membrane of endothelial cells
C. Fast synaptic neurotransmission
D. Phosphorylation of tyrosine residues
E. Activation of protein kinase C
F. Inactivation of protein kinase C
G. Malignancy
H. Inactivation of adenylyl cyclase
I. Activation of adenylyl cyclase
J. None of the above

Instruction: Match one of the options listed above to the lead-in given below.

1. DAG and IP_3 cause ☐

2. Bradykinin causes ☐

3. Cholera causes ☐

4. Pertussis causes ☐

5. DAG and IP_3 production follows ☐

2. Pharmacokinetics

A. Redistribution
B. Reduction
C. Absorption
D. Oxidation
E. Phase 2 metabolism
F. Phase 1 metabolism
G. First-pass metabolism
H. Hydrolysis
I. Creatinine clearance
J. Dithranol

Instruction: Match one of the options listed above to the descriptions given below.

1. The drug is often one taken orally, absorbed through the intestinal wall, goes directly to the liver through the portal venous system and gets metabolized there before reaching the target organ. ☐

2. The drug is oxidised, reduced or hydrolysed resulting in an increase in polarity of the drug and provision of a site for further reactions. ☐

3. The drug is conjugated, resulting in it becoming more hydrophilic and thus more readily excretable. ☐

4. Warfarin, the anticoagulant, is inactivated in this way to result in the transformation of a ketone group into a hydroxyl group. ☐

5. Drugs leave the circulation and enter tissues perfused by blood. ☐

3. Emergency and nervous system drugs

A. Propofol
B. Levodopa only
C. Levodopa plus carbidopa
D. Carbidopa
E. Flumazenil
F. *N*-Acetylcysteine
G. Lidocaine
H. Intravenous morphine
I. Ibuprofen
J. Nitrous oxide

Instruction: Match one of the options listed above to the statements given below.

1. To treat Parkinson's disease it is best to give ☐

2. A patient is in serious respiratory depression following an excessive alcohol consumption while on a benzodiazepine. The most appropriate treatment would be ☐

3. A young victim of assault makes an impulsive decision to take a paracetamol overdose but regrets it immediately and calls for help. On arrival at hospital she should be given ☐

4. A local anaesthetic is required to allow excision of a small mole. ☐

5. A road traffic accident victim, who was forced into the central reservation, is assessed by paramedics and found to have a patent airway and circulation but is in extreme pain. ☐

4. Antibiotics and antivirals

A. Aciclovir
B. Penicillin
C. Fluconazole
D. Bleomycin

E. Chloroquine

F. Praziquantel

G. Ganciclovir

H. Rifampicin

I. Chloramphenicol

J. Trimethoprim

Instruction: Match one of the options listed above to the descriptions given below.

1. A bactericidal drug that prevents peptide cross-linking within the microbial cell wall is given to a 26-year-old woman presenting with an uncomplicated urinary tract infection to take for a course of 7 days.

2. A bacteriostatic drug was used to treat a respiratory tract infection in a 30-year-old man, who subsequently developed a hypersensitivity complex affecting the eyes, skin and mucous membranes. Treatment was immediately stopped.

3. A patient was put on a regimen of drugs to treat his tuberculosis. After his commencement he noted that his urine and tears had turned orange-red.

4. A 17-year-old student develops a red and tingling area of skin just above his lips. He is diagnosed as having a cold sore.

5. A patient who was on treatment for non-Hodgkin's lymphoma for many years developed shortness of breath resulting in reduced exercise capacity. Chest X-ray revealed lung fibrosis. It was thought to be caused by one of the cytotoxic antibiotic drugs he was taking, which worked by fragmenting DNA.

5. Cardiovascular system drugs

A. Quinidine

B. Lidocaine

C. Heparin

D. Glyceryl trinitrate

E. Erythropoietin

F. Amiodarone

G. Atorvastatin

H. Digoxin

I. Verapamil

J. Aspirin

Instruction: Match one of the options listed above to the descriptions given below.

1. An antianginal drug that involves the formation of nitric oxide, thereby dilating systemic veins.

2. An antiarrhythmic drug that blocks voltage-gated sodium channels, which slows phase 0 of the cardiac action potential and therefore increases the effective refractory period.

3. An antiarrhythmic drug that slows phases 0 and 3 of the cardiac action potential, prolonging the cardiac action potential duration and the effective refractory period

4. An antiarrhythmic drug that shortens phase 2 of the cardiac action potential by calcium antagonism.

5. A cardiac glycoside with positive inotropic action that shifts the Frank–Starling ventricular function curve upwards.

6. Drug interactions

A. Moclobemide

B. Clozapine

C. Insulin

D. Diazepam

E. Ethanol

F. Phenytoin

G. Phenelzine

H. Aspirin

I. Vigabatrin

J. Hydrochlorothiazide

Instruction: Match one of the options listed above to the descriptions given below.

1. A French man who eats cheese and drinks wine daily is given medication for depression and becomes acutely ill with severely raised blood pressure. He is prescribed an irreversibly acting drug.

2. A young woman who has been taking epilepsy medication and has just started taking an oral contraceptive pill. Two months later, she finds that she is pregnant.

3. This drug was given to a student experiencing hallucinations, although it can cause potentially fatal neutropenia in 1% of the population. She drinks lots of high energy drinks, containing caffeine to study late. This is thought to inhibit metabolism of this drug (normally by cytochrome P450), resulting in an increase in serum levels and side-effects.

4. A patient taking anxiolytic medication recently drank to excess while out one night. He was found on the street by paramedics who noted that he was not breathing.

5. A middle-aged man with bipolar affective disorder is found to have high serum levels of lithium. His general practitioner has recently started him on a diuretic to treat his hypertension.

7. Endocrine system drugs

A. Increase oral contraceptive
B. Isophane insulin
C. Glibenclamide
D. Insulin aspart and insulin zinc suspension
E. Take her off oral contraceptive
F. Prednisolone
G. Carbimazole
H. Levothyroxine
I. Beclometasone
J. Metformin

Instruction: Match one of the options listed above to the descriptions given below.

1. A 30-year-old woman presents to her general practitioner with increasing sweating, anxiety and weight loss despite an ever-increasing appetite. She is diagnosed with an endocrine condition and given medication. ☐

2. A woman who is on the oral contraceptive pill and has asthma develops deep vein thrombosis. Appropriate management is required. ☐

3. A young man requires modification to his insulin regimen for type 1 diabetes. His doctor thinks he needs to change only his intermediate-acting insulin from the protamine zinc insulin to a different one. ☐

4. A 50-year-old man with heart failure has recently developed type 2 diabetes. He needs to take an oral antidiabetic drug. ☐

5. A middle-aged man has been taking treatment for his rheumatoid arthritis. He now has increased central abdominal fat, a moon-shaped face, purple striae, thin arms and legs, and hypertension. A drug he is taking was thought to be responsible. ☐

8. The kidney and urinary tract drugs

A. Mannitol
B. Amiloride
C. Aldosterone
D. Oxybutynin
E. Adrenaline
F. Methazolamide
G. Bumetanide
H. Doxazosin
I. Sildenafil
J. Bendroflumethiazide

Instruction: Match one of the options listed above to the descriptions given below.

1. A drug that inhibits the $Na^+/K^+/2Cl^-$ co-transporters in the luminal membrane of the loop of Henle. ☐

2. A drug that acts by relaxing the detrusor smooth muscle of the bladder and is, therefore, used as a treatment for urge incontinence. This drug should not be given to patients with glaucoma. ☐

3. A drug that blocks the sodium channels in the luminal membrane of the late distal convoluted tubule and collecting duct, thereby reducing potassium secretion into the lumen. ☐

4. A drug to help maintain an erection through relaxation of penile smooth muscle that can be given to patients with multiple sclerosis. Relaxation of the smooth muscle happens through inhibition of phosphodiesterase-mediated degradation of cGMP. ☐

5. A drug that inhibits the Na^+/Cl^- symporters in the luminal membrane of the early distal convoluted tubule. ☐

9. Gastrointestinal system drugs

A. Domperidone
B. Aluminium hydroxide
C. Omeprazole
D. Prednisolone
E. Loperamide
F. Hyoscine
G. Senna
H. Lactulose
I. Mesalazine
J. Ursodeoxycholic acid

Instruction: Match one of the options listed above to the descriptions given below.

1. A 33-year-old banker visits her general practitioner with burning pain behind her sternum. A diagnosis of oesophageal reflux is made. ☐

2. A 25-year-old patient with history of peptic ulcer disease is placed on aspirin following development of angina. Prophylactic treatment is indicated against ulcer reoccurrence and a drug which causes irreversible inhibition of H^+/K^+ ATPase is selected. ☐

3. A 50-year-old patient who develops pain due to metastases is placed on opiate pain relief and subsequently develops constipation. She is put on a stimulant laxative to increase intestinal motility. ☐

4. A 30-year-old woman, who suffers from motion sickness, needs to go on a business cruise. She is given an antiemetic which act by competitive antagonism of muscarinic receptors. ☐

5. A patient recently diagnosed with inflammatory bowel disease is placed on a maintenance drug. ☐

10. Respiratory system drugs

A. Salbutamol
B. Salmeterol
C. Aminophylline
D. Naloxone
E. Dry mouth
F. Immunosuppression
G. Ephedrine
H. Coughing
I. Morphine
J. Oxygen

Instruction: Match one of the options listed above to the descriptions given below.

1. An example of physical defence mechanism.

2. An adverse effect associated with a drug used to treat chronic obstructive pulmonary disease (COPD).

3. A long-acting agonist used by asthmatic people for immediate relief of symptoms.

4. An intravenous xanthine given to treat a young adult, following admission to hospital with a life-threatening asthma attack.

5. A drug used to as a respiratory stimulant in those with drug-induced respiratory depression.

Chapter 1 Introduction to pharmacology

1. a. True   generated by the activation of a G-protein, and adenylyl cyclase.
    b. True   generated along with inositol phosphate $(IP)_3$ by activated phospholipase C.
    c. False IP_3 is inositol triphosphate.
    d. False   GABA is a neurotransmitter, not an intracellular messenger.
    e. True   generated by the activation of the guanylyl cyclase enzyme.

2. a. False   despite the affinity being the same, the partial agonist can never bring about the same response as the full agonist.
    b. True   see 2a.
    c. True   though it can still not bring about the same response as the full agonist.
    d. False   binding is usually reversible, though can be irreversible.
    e. False   see 2a. Efficacy is the ability of the agonist to bring about a response once bound to the receptor.

3. a. True   the binding capacity of agonists and antagonists is usually similar.
    b. False   the antagonist will have very little, if any, ability to activate the receptor and bring about a response.
    c. False   non-competitive antagonists, also known as irreversible antagonists, have a similar effect irrespective of the agonist concentration.
    d. False   a dose ratio of 10 implies the antagonist is very potent.
    e. True   higher doses of agonists will be required to bring about the same physiological effect.

4. a. False   compliance is how well the patient adheres to the drug regimen prescribed by the doctor.
    b. False   compliance in children depends on both the child and the parent to cooperate with the drug regimen.
    c. True   a good doctor–patient relationship improves compliance.
    d. False   the simpler the regimen, the higher the degree of compliance.

e. False   compliance is essential in most diseases, especially infectious diseases such as tuberculosis.

5. a. False   intravenous drugs bypass first-pass metabolism.
    b. False   high doses of potent steroids can result in systemic effects.
    c. False   blood draining the rectum is filtered through the liver before entering the systemic circulation.
    d. False   unpredictable absorption from the gut, and first-pass metabolism makes oral drugs less bioavailable.
    e. True   intravenous drugs will have more rapid speed on onset, and subsequent metabolism than oral drugs.

6. a. True   the rate of excretion increases with increasing drug concentration.
    b. False   the free concentration is the determinant.
    c. True   tubular secretion and tubular reabsorption are important for many drugs.
    d. False   lipid-soluble drugs are predominantly metabolized in the liver.
    e. False   the volume of distribution of the drug will influence the plasma half-life but not the rate of renal excretion.

7. a. False   some drugs distribute extensively into tissues, and they can have values in excess of total body water.
    b. True   in theory, as the degree of ionization of the drug will determine its solubility in the various components of a body.
    c. True   in the blood or tissues.
    d. True   basic drugs tend to be bound by globulins.
    e. False   very lipid soluble drugs build up in fat.

8. a. False   drugs are metabolized by the liver, but excreted by the kidneys and in the gastrointestinal tract.
    b. False   lipid insoluble drugs cannot cross the blood–brain barrier.
    c. False   the metabolites of paracetamol are hepatotoxic.
    d. True   many drugs can either induce or inhibit liver enzymes, altering the metabolism of other drug classes.
    e. True   the yellow card scheme in the UK allows drug reactions to be monitored.

9. a. True   it is teratogenic.
   b. False   aspirin is an oxidant drug so haemolysis would occur.
   c. True   glucocorticoids are immunosuppressive.
   d. True   it is important when choosing the muscle relaxant.
   e. False   it is during phase 4.

Chapter 2 Cardiovascular system

10. a. True   β-adrenoceptors are located in the heart, they increase heart rate via G-proteins. Therefore, their blockade results in a decrease in heart rate.
   b. False   Nicotine causes nicotinic acetylcholine receptor excitation, affecting both sympathetic and parasympathetic systems and effects include tachycardia and glandular secretions, respectively.
   c. False   adrenaline is a sympathetic system neurotransmitter.
   d. False   one of signs of shock is a weak yet rapid pulse.
   e. False   this is a tumour of the sympathetic nervous system.

11. a. False   parasympathetic innervation of the heart via the vagus nerve slows cardiac rate.
   b. True   sympathetic innervation of the heart increases heart rate and contractility.
   c. True   excessive thyroxine increases the basal metabolic rate and heart rate, and can predispose to arrhythmias (atrial fibrillation).
   d. False   atropine is an anticholinergic, inhibiting parasympathetic inhibition on the heart.
   e. False   salbutamol is a β-adrenoceptor agonist, and as such can increase heart rate.

12. a. True   all class I agents block sodium channels.
   b. True   adenosine causes transient delay in conduction.
   c. False   propranolol is a class II agent, while sotalol is a class III agent.
   d. True   all class III agents block potassium channels.
   e. False   nicorandil is used to prevent angina.

13. a. False   opiate analgesia is often required in acute angina attacks.
   b. False   patients require a nitrate free period, as they can become insensitive to their effects.
   c. True   verapamil and diltiazem act predominately on the heart to slow the rate and force of contraction; nifedipine acts on the vasculature to cause vasodilatation.

   d. False   anticoagulation in unstable angina is achieved with heparin.
   e. True   β-adrenoceptor antagonists reduce myocardial oxygen demand, and lengthen diastole when myocardial perfusion occurs.

14. a. True   α- and β-adrenoceptor activation regulate vascular tone.
   b. False   nitric oxide relaxes vascular smooth muscle, reducing vascular tone.
   c. True   angiotensin II is a potent vasoconstrictor.
   d. False   essential hypertension has an unknown cause, renal artery stenosis is a cause of secondary hypertension.
   e. True   ACE inhibitors can themselves cause hyperkalaemia by their inhibitory action on aldosterone.

15. a. False   septic shock results in nitric oxide release and vasodilatation.
   b. False   the role of steroids in shock remains unclear, though their action will be delayed as they alter gene expression.
   c. False   adrenaline's main action in shock is to increase vascular tone, and it relaxes smooth muscles of the airways.
   d. True   shock results in hyperfusion and hypoxia of peripheral tissues.
   e. True   sympathetic activation as a result of hypotension drives the symptoms of anxiety.

16. a. True   HMG CoA reductase inhibitors are also known as statins, and inhibit HMG CoA reductase, which is in the pathway of cholesterol biosynthesis.
   b. False   xanthine oxidase converts purines to uric acid, and xanthine oxidase inhibitors are used in the treatment of gout.
   c. True   bezafibrate is more effective in reducing serum triglycerides than cholesterol.
   d. False   alfacalcidol is a vitamin D derivative used in renal failure.
   e. True   colestyramine binds bile acids in the gut, preventing their reabsorption, and promoting the breakdown of cholesterol to replace this loss.

17. a. True   low-molecular-weight heparins are being used more often now since dosing is less frequent and effects are more predictable.
   b. False   rTPa is not commonly antigenic, while streptokinase is derived from bacteria, and is antigenic.
   c. True   fibrinolysis is contraindicated in most active bleeding disorders, and after trauma or surgery.

d. False   fibrinolytics are given by intravenous infusion only.

e. True   warfarin is indicated for prophylactic use following massive pulmonary embolism or deep vein thrombosis.

18. a. False   ibuprofen reversibly inhibits cyclooxygenase, and it has no antiplatelet effects.

b. True   aspirin irreversibly inhibits cyclooxygenase, preventing the formation of thromboxane A_2, which is responsible for platelet aggregation.

c. True   clopidogrel inhibits the activation of the glycoprotein IIb/IIIa receptor, and is a useful alternative in aspirin-sensitive patients.

d. True   dipyridamole inhibits cAMP degradation, and results in poor platelet aggregation.

e. False   heparin potentiates the action of anti-thrombin III, and has no effect on platelet aggregation.

19. a. True   pernicious anaemia is an autoimmune disease resulting in inadequate intrinsic factor, which is responsible for vitamin B_{12} absorption from the gut.

b. True   iron in the large bowel is oxidized to dark coloured iron oxides.

c. False   erythropoietin is ineffective in treating anaemia unless adequate iron stores are present, see 19e.

d. True   primary and secondary haemochromatosis result in cirrhosis secondary to iron deposition in the liver.

e. False   erythropoietin is naturally synthesized in the kidney, but acts in the bone marrow. Erythropoietin is used to treat anaemia in renal failure.

Chapter 3 Respiratory system

20. a. False   β-adrenoceptor antagonists (β-blockers) may make asthma worse, by inhibiting endogenous β-adrenoceptor activation, which causes smooth muscle relaxation.

b. True   β-adrenoceptor agonists act to relax smooth muscle, causing bronchodilatation.

c. True   ibuprofen and the other NSAIDs inhibit cyclooxygenase, and divert arachidonic acid synthesis down the lipoxygenase pathway, which generates leukotrienes (bronchoconstrictors).

d. False   asthma is marked by reversible airways narrowing.

e. False   oxygen should be administered at 100%. Oxygen restriction is sometimes indicated in chronic obstructive pulmonary

21. a. False   beclometasone is a steroid drug, and is used in asthma prophylaxis, and it has no bronchodilating properties.

b. True   theophylline is a methylxanthine, and inhibits cAMP breakdown. Increased cAMP results in smooth muscle relaxation.

c. False   sodium cromoglicate is a mast-cell stabilizer, and used in asthma prophylaxis, having no bronchodilating properties.

d. True   salmeterol is a long-acting $β_2$-adrenoceptor agonist.

e. True   ipratropium bromide is an antimuscarinic, and inhibits parasympathetic bronchoconstriction.

22. a. True   this is a commonly reported side-effect, and results from skeletal muscle activity.

b. False   see 22d.

c. False   ankle oedema is not reported although peripheral vasodilatation may occur.

d. True   activation of β-adrenoceptors in the heart results in tachycardia.

e. False   this is, however, a common side-effect of inhaled corticosteroids.

23. a. False   COPD is an irreversible airways disease, asthma is reversible.

b. False   smoking is the leading cause of COPD, although pollution can be a risk factor.

c. True $α_1$-antitrypsin reduces protease damage, without it emphysema can occur.

d. True   Examples of such combination drugs include Combivent® and Duovent®.

e. True   it reduces the viscosity of bronchial secretions.

24. a. False   pulmonary surfactant is used to reduce the surface tension of the alveolus in respiratory distress syndrome (RDS) of neonates.

b. False   naloxone is used to reverse opiate overdose. Flumazenil is used to reverse benzodiazepine overdose.

c. True   opiates act in the cough centre to inhibit the cough reflex.

d. True   ephedrine causes vasoconstriction, and reduction in oedema and secretions of the nasal mucosa.

e. False   naloxone has a much shorter half-life than most of the opiates it is used to counteract, and often given repeatedly until the opiate overdosed on is metabolized.

Index

Note: Page numbers in *italics* refer to figures and tables.

A

abacavir, 214
abciximab, 51–2
abnormal impulse conduction & generation, 30
absence seizures, 100, 101, *103*
absorption, drug, 12–13
acarbose, 127
accommodation, 114
acetazolamide, 105, 116
acetic acids, *185*, 187
acetylcholine (ACh), 5, 67, 71, 154, *155*
  drugs inhibiting release of, 69
  drugs inhibiting synthesis of, 68–9
  drugs inhibiting vesicular packaging of, 69
  parasympathetic nervous system, 77
  release of, 69, 70
acetylcholinesterase (AChE), 67, 68, *68*
acetylsalicylic acid *see* aspirin
aciclovir, 214
acid, 112
acid-related disease, 155–7
  see also specific disease
acid secretion, 154, *155*, 155–6
acne, 191, *191*, *194*
acquired immune deficiency syndrome (AIDS), 215, 216, 224
acquired resistance, 202–3
acrolein, 231
actin, 69
actinomycin D, 232
action potential
  cardiac, 26, *26*, *27*
  nerve, 65, *65*, *66*
acute secretory diarrhoea, 162
adalimumab, 189
adenoma, 121
adenosine, 34
adenosine diphosphate (ADP), 47, 123
adenosine triphosphate (ATP), 123, *148*, 224
adenoviruses, *212*
adenylase cyclase, 169
adenylyl cyclase, 7–8, 27, 37, 154
adjuvant chemotherapy, 227
adrenal medulla, 73
adrenaline, 34, 43, *75*
  anaphylactic shock, 195, *196*
  effect on blood vessels, 73

adrenaline *(continued)*
  inactivation, 76
  open-angle glaucoma, 116
adrenocortical steroids, 233
adrenocorticotrophic hormone (ACTH), 129, *129*, 130
adsorbents, *160*, 162–3
affect, flattening of, 95
affective disorders, 90–5
  bipolar, 91
    treatment of, 94–5
  unipolar, 90–1
    site of action of drugs for, *93*
    treatment of, 91–4
afferent arterioles, 144, 145
affinity, 9, 10
African Caribbeans, hypertension in, 39
African trypanosomiasis, 223–4
agonist drugs, 4, *9*, 9–10
AIDS *see* acquired immune deficiency syndrome (AIDS)
albendazole, *225*, 226
albumin, 13
alcohol, *15*, 16
  misuse of, *108*, 110
alcuronium, 69
aldosterone, 29, 38, 128, 146, *148*
  antagonists, 149
aldosterone-induced proteins (AIP), *148*
alemtuzumab, 234
alendronate, 141
alginates, 157
alkaline salts, 157
alkylating agents, 228, *229*, 230–1
allergens, 56, *57*, 194
allergic disorders, 194–6, *195*
  drug therapy of, 195–6, *196*
allergic reactions to drugs, 20
allergic rhinitis, 61–2, *195*, *196*
allopurinol, *15*
  gout, 190, *190*
allylamines, 219
α-adrenoceptor, 32, 42
  activation, 37, *37*
  agonists, 116, 117
  antagonists, 149
    for hypertension, *40*
    for reversing mydriasis, 117
  blockade, 99
  effects mediated by, 73
α_1-adrenoceptor, 73
  antagonists, 40